Health *in* Rural Canada

Health *in* Rural Canada

Edited by Judith C. Kulig and Allison M. Williams

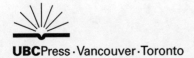

UBCPress · Vancouver · Toronto

20 19 18 17   5 4

Printed in Canada on FSC-certified ancient-forest-free paper
(100% post-consumer recycled) that is processed chlorine- and acid-free.

___

Library and Archives Canada Cataloguing in Publication

Health in rural Canada / edited by Judith C. Kulig and Allison M. Williams.

Includes bibliographical references and index.
Also issued in electronic format.
ISBN 978-0-7748-2172-8 (bound); ISBN 978-0-7748- 2173-5 (pbk.)

1. Rural health – Canada. 2. Health status indicators – Canada. 3. Rural
health services – Canada. I. Kulig, Judith Celene. II. Williams, Allison M.

RA771.7.C3H42 2012   362.1′042570971   C2011-907066-9

___

Canadä

UBC Press gratefully acknowledges the financial support for our publishing
program of the Government of Canada (through the Canada Book Fund), the
Canada Council for the Arts, and the British Columbia Arts Council.

This book has been published with the help of a grant from the Canadian
Federation for the Humanities and Social Sciences, through the Aid to
Scholarly Publications Program, using funds provided by the Social Sciences
and Humanities Research Council of Canada.

UBC Press
The University of British Columbia
2029 West Mall
Vancouver, BC V6T 1Z2
www.ubcpress.ca

We would like to dedicate this book to

rural Canadians who work to sustain health in their families and communities each day;

rural health researchers from across Canada who, through their passion, interest, and expertise, have worked tirelessly to increase the understanding of rural health; and

our undergraduate and graduate students and research colleagues who have inspired us to create this volume.

Contents

Part 2: Rural Health Human Resources

Part 3: Rural Health Services Delivery

Part 4: Rural Health Policy and Research

      Communities / 409
          B. Krieg

Part 7: Aging in Rural Contexts

23   Diversity among Older Adults in Rural Canada: Health in
      Context / 427
          N. Keating and J. Eales

24   Looming Dementia Care Crisis: Are Canadian Rural and
      Remote Settings Ready? / 447
          D.A. Forbes and P. Hawranik

25   Health- and Social-Care Issues in Aging Resource
      Communities / 462
          M. Skinner, N. Hanlon, and G. Halseth

26   Rural Women's Health Promotion Needs and Resources:
      A Photovoice Perspective / 481
          B. Leipert, T. Landry, C. McWilliam, M.L. Kelley, D. Forbes,
          P. Wakewich, and J. George

27   The Future of Rural Health Research: Concluding
      Thoughts / 503
          J.C. Kulig and A.M. Williams

      Contributors / 512

      Index / 515

Figures and Tables

Tables

Foreword

When I was growing up in the 1940s in a small town, now a ghost town, we were fortunate to have a first-aid clinic staffed by a worker whose knowledge was gleaned through osmosis, we were told, by association with his older physician brothers. When an elective tonsillectomy was deemed appropriate for whatever ailed us, I and five other children from the community were driven early one morning to his physician brother who practised seven miles away. After the surgery, we returned home late in the evening to be cared for by our family members in what must have been a pioneering but historically unrecognized day surgery program. Five of us survived, but the sixth was less fortunate, bleeding to death in the night with no professional supervision or instructions, coordinated follow-up, or homecare that might have altered the outcome. The heartbroken mother of the child shouldered the entire guilt of electing surgery on behalf of her son, who might have lived without the procedure. The shrieking and crying of the inconsolable mother at the funeral pierce my thoughts even to this day, permanently etched in my memory. The entire community shared her grief and struggled to accept their fate, believing that there was no other choice under the circumstances.

That was my first encounter with rural health care – my first encounter with health care, for that matter. I hope that through the intervening years rural health care has improved and that better outcomes are now realistic expectations for most, if not all, Canadians who inhabit rural and remote parts of this country. If we have yet to reach that utopian vision, let's hope that all possible efforts are being directed toward achieving that worthwhile goal.

What will it take to get us there? We have to recognize that rural, remote, northern, and Aboriginal communities are unique and must be viewed and defined in their own right, not by their non-urbanicity. We must recognize the heterogeneity of such communities and not assume that they are homogeneous in their characteristics. We must acknowledge that there are health gradients and health inequities affecting the populations of these communities. We must commit to refocusing our attention and energy on rural issues. We need to explore and understand the factors that determine the health of these communities and the health of those individuals who live in them, and we must be willing to believe that they might be different from the population at large. Some have argued that rurality itself is a major determinant of health. Finally, we need a strong and sustainable rural health research effort in this country that provides evidence of rural health inequities and differences, identifies healthy rural communities and pockets of healthy individuals, and showcases best practices, concepts, and solutions that work. We need support for knowledge translation relevant to rural communities. We need to ensure opportunities and support for innovative ideas and future research that promises to change how we view the totality of rural health.

If we have made progress in rural health issues, credit should go to the many individuals, organizations, and governments that have made rural health issues clearly visible on the radar screen. Health Canada for many years, even preceding the creation of its Office of Rural Health, which unfortunately is no longer in operation, sponsored research competitions to encourage rural health research. The short-lived Office of Rural Health, the report of the Conference on Rural Health (which the office sponsored), and the subsequent Ministerial Advisory Council on Rural Health articulated the need to focus on rural health as its own entity. The Canadian Society of Rural Physicians has always been a strong advocate for the special needs of rural health care. The Canadian Society for Rural Health Research has created a Canadian network of researchers.

Strong advocates for rural research have also emerged from academia. The rural health research group at Laurentian University sponsored a conference in 1993 on the theme of "Redressing the Imbalance." The

University of Northern British Columbia sponsored several conferences in 2001 involving participants from rural and Aboriginal communities, giving them a voice that had not been heard before. The Canadian Institutes for Health Research produced a report on rural health research and made rural health a cross-cutting theme across its thirteen institutes.

Committed academic researchers across Canada continue to explore rural health issues, and many of them are contributors to this volume. Topics range from population health status, health services, health human resources, cultural aspects, and special needs of rural, remote, and northern communities. It is important to document the findings of these researchers in a way that is accessible to future students and researchers so that lessons learned do not disappear. We need to build a library of reports, research evidence, stories, and experiences that record the life of rural Canada, to create and build a discipline called rural health and life. This volume will contribute enormously to that endeavour, and the editors and authors deserve our appreciation and gratitude for moving us toward that goal.

Mamoru Watanabe, Professor Emeritus
Faculty of Medicine, University of Calgary

Acknowledgments

Dr. Judith C. Kulig and Dr. Allison M. Williams both acknowledge the financial and material support from their respective faculties (Faculty of Health Sciences, University of Lethbridge, and School of Geography and Earth Sciences, Faculty of Science, McMaster University).

Dr. Kulig also acknowledges the financial support of the Vice-President Academic's Office (University of Lethbridge); the time required to complete this edited volume was due in part to the receipt of a University Scholar Award (2009-11) from the University of Lethbridge.

Dr. Williams also acknowledges the support of the Ontario Women's Health Council (OWHC) and the Canadian Institutes for Health Research (CIHR), Institute for Gender and Health, for her OWHC/CIHR Mid-Career Award in Women's Health. This award allowed her to devote time to this volume.

Health *in* Rural Canada

Chapter 1   Health and Place in Rural Canada

Allison M. Williams and Judith C. Kulig

Rural Canada accounts for about 90 percent of the country's land mass and is home to almost a third of Canada's population. Many Canadians define themselves through an idea of Canada as largely rural; our national identity is rooted historically in the immigration of our ancestors to the rural areas of this country when it was being developed. Our ongoing links to the rural landscape are based on our dependence on resources, including foods and minerals, as well as our need for recreation and renewal. Still persistent in the country's collective imagination is a sense of Canada's rural and remote places as defining spaces of Canadian national identity, from the varied rural landscapes of the Group of Seven artists, whose work has become an icon of Canadian nationhood, to Canadian musicians such as Gordon Lightfoot and Anne Murray, who sing about life and livelihood in rural Canada. Our rural landscapes are what draw world travellers to visit us, with fifteen UNESCO biosphere reserve sites in Canada, many of which either encompass rural areas or are surrounded by them (e.g., Niagara Escarpment, Ontario, or Clayoquot Sound, British Columbia). Canada's First Nations mastered survival in rural and remote corners of the country, teaching Europeans how to live in the wilderness. Early European settlers set the foundation for Canada's economic success, which is still based on primary industries, the vast majority of which are located in rural and remote areas. In the past couple of decades, there has been a recognized shift toward a new national identity reflective of urban multicultural centres. A preoccupation with cities has impacted our cultural identity, making less visible the crucial need for studies of dynamic Canadian rural spaces.

Depending on the definition of the word *rural* used, between 19 percent and 30 percent of Canadians are formally defined as living in rural Canada (Bollman and Clemenson 2008); rural people are also known for their diverse and distinct cultural and demographic characteristics compared with their urban counterparts. For example, rural areas have fewer immigrant and visible minority populations, higher proportions of First Nations, and unique religious groups such as the Anabaptists (i.e., Amish, Hutterites, and Mennonites). Furthermore, rural areas have higher proportions of dependants, both children and older adults (Dandy and Bollman 2008); this is contrasted with low proportions of those of working age (Canadian Institute for Health Information [CIHI] 2006; Ministerial Advisory Council on Rural Health 2002).

These demographic characteristics play a large role in the comparative vulnerability that rural Canadians experience across a number of population health determinants. Rural Canadians experience a greater number of population health risks compared with urban Canadians. They generally have lower socio-economic status due to higher unemployment rates and lower education levels than do urban Canadians (Kirby and LeBreton 2002). This contributes to comparatively poorer health status; to illustrate, rural residents have a shorter life expectancy and higher mortality and infant mortality rates than the Canadian average (CIHI 2006; Kirby and LeBreton 2002). In contrast to urban residents, rural residents show higher levels of high blood pressure and obesity, higher levels of arthritis/rheumatism and depression, and lower levels of self-reported functional health, self-assessed health status, and health-promoting behaviours (CIHI 2006; Mitura and Bollman 2003). Furthermore, higher rates of accident, suicide, and disability are experienced in rural populations, partly explained by the prevalence of primary sector employment in rural areas. Strasser (2003) has specified that these noted health disparities between rural and urban geographies are found around the world, further substantiating the Canadian Health Commission's assertion that "geography is a determinant of health" (Romanow 2002). If we can identify a clear health gap between urban and rural populations, how can we work to reduce it? It is imperative that we gain a better understanding of these disparities through research that provides enhanced comprehension of how and why they occur.

Because much of the discussion on rural health in Canada focuses on a deficit model, there is a distorted perception of the risks and benefits of rural living. For example, overshadowed are results such as those in the CIHI (2006) report on the health of rural Canadians, which found that there are statistically significant differences among rural residents reporting a "sense of belonging"[1] compared with their urban counterparts. Many rural residents choose to live in such an environment, emphasizing the connection with physical geography and its positive impact in their lives.

One of the fastest-growing populations in Canada is among Aboriginal peoples. From 1996 to 2006, the Aboriginal population grew at a rate of 45 percent, compared with only 8 percent for the non-Aboriginal population. It is expected that by 2017 there will be 1.4 million Aboriginal people in Canada, an increase of 4 percent. The increase is related not only to a higher fertility rate but also to a sense of identity, as individual Aboriginals evidence an interest and comfort in identifying themselves as such (Statistics Canada 2010). As a group, Aboriginal peoples are the fastest-growing segment in Canadian society (Indian and Northern Affairs Canada 2009). On average, Aboriginal peoples are younger than other Canadians and therefore have higher fertility rates and are more often young families.

Aboriginal peoples illustrate both their strength and their vulnerability as a group. Their vulnerability is easily discernible when considering their health status; this group experiences HIV infections 2.8 times higher than the average Canadian. The life expectancy for First Nations is approximately 7 years less than the average Canadian; infant mortality is 1.5 times higher among First Nations groups and 4 times higher among the Inuit (Health Canada 2009). Suicide rates are also much higher among this population: among the average Canadian population, suicide rates are 13/100,000, whereas among the Inuit they are 79/100,000 and among the on-reserve First Nations 28/100,000 (CIHI 2004). The vulnerability of this group suggests that their needs must be prioritized if any change in rural health status is to occur. This book contains a section (Part 6) dedicated to addressing questions and issues pertaining to the specific health needs/status/care of Aboriginals in Canada.

As the first comprehensive volume addressing rural health research in Canada, this collection provides breadth while sharing a theme: *health and place*. It adds to the growing international literature available from Australia (Liaw and Kilpatrick 2008; Smith 2007) and the United

Figure 1.1   All provinces, districts/areas, and towns mentioned in this book

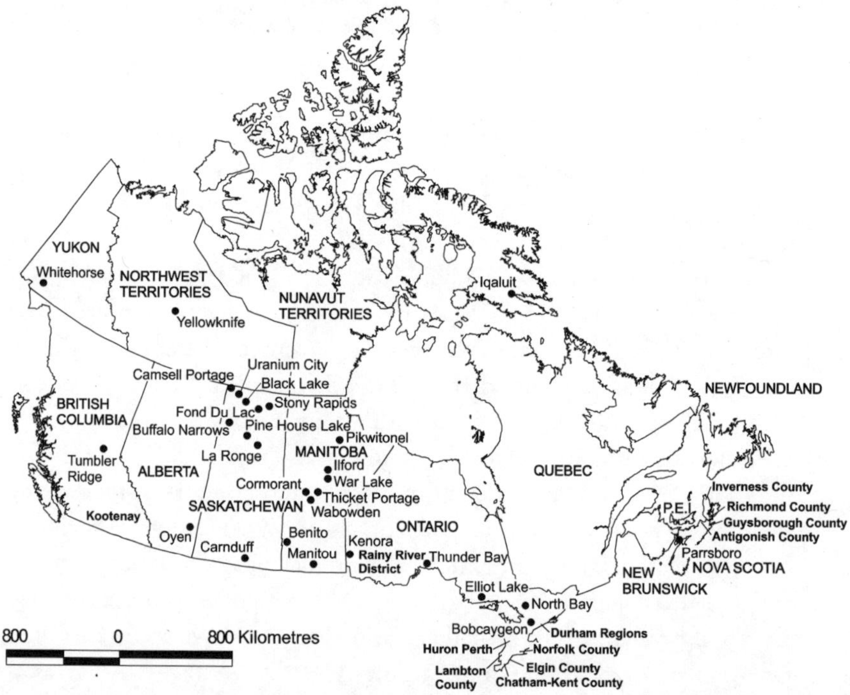

States (Glasgow et al. 2004; Loue and Quill 2001) that focuses exclusively on the meaning of rural and its impact on both health status and health outcome. Through its examination of the richness and diversity of rural health issues in Canada, the book best meets the needs of both established and emerging health researchers while providing useful information for policy makers involved in decision making for all groups across the population health spectrum.

As noted in Figure 1.1, most Canadian provinces and territories are represented in the research contained in this collection, albeit to differing degrees; Atlantic Canada, the northern territories, and Nunavut will no doubt strengthen their research voices in the future. Similarly, work pertaining to minority groups, such as newly arrived immigrants and refugees and various rural-based religious communities, is still sparse and, as a result, has correspondingly less representation in this collection; this gap will likely be filled by the next generation of rural researchers.

The contributing authors use a variety of theoretical frameworks, reflected in the employment of a wide range of research designs and analytical methods. The richness of this collection is in the multitude of disciplinary perspectives represented, often working in collaborative teams. Certainly, within Canada, the majority of rural health research is driven by an interdisciplinary focus, allowing for a more complex analysis and a deeper understanding of specific health issues. Thus, contributing research groups have included a variety of professional and academic disciplines, such as nursing, social work, geography, epidemiology, and sociology.

At the core of this volume is the theme of health and place. Within it, three broad and significant sub-themes are highlighted: *rural places matter to health, rural places are unique,* and *rural places are dynamic.* Using the chapters as illustrations, we attempt to establish the importance of the need to understand the unique qualities of rurality across a number of geographical scales. We begin by providing an overview of the Canadian health system, detailing how rural services are structured and funded. Next we define what rural means and how a common definition was decided on for this collection. A comprehensive understanding of rural health issues in Canada is an important step in understanding the health of our nation in general. Given the connections that we all hold to the rural landscape and its inhabitants, a volume such as this is necessary in broadening our knowledge base while also helping to ensure sustainability of our rural areas.

Canadian Rural Health Services

To understand how health services are delivered in rural Canada, one must first review how Canadian health care is governed, funded, and delivered. To address *governance,* we turn to the Canada Health Act, enacted in 1984; it represents five principles of health care in Canada: accessibility, universality, portability, comprehensiveness, and public administration. This legislation conceptualized health in terms of social justice and aspired to ensure equitable access to health care for all. Medicare guaranteed citizens access to medically necessary services regardless of their geographical locations, but in reality it guarantees only that people be assessed for services; it does not guarantee that they will receive them (Health Canada 2007). Consequently, great disparities in service access exist, such as those between urban and rural populations.

To address the issue of *funding,* the Constitution divided federal and provincial powers such that the former would acquire the resources to finance health care but the latter would govern the actual *delivery* of health-care products and services. Provincial governments receive annual transfer payments from the federal government to finance health-care delivery. Each Canadian province and territory thereby has a unique health-care system since the delivery design is province specific. As the federal government has struggled with deficits, transfer payments to the provinces have been reduced, leaving provincial/territorial jurisdictions less inclined to honour the principles of the Canada Health Act.

The exception to provincial/territorial delivery of health services is First Nations and Inuit communities (i.e., registered under the Indian Act) that receive care in partnership with the federal government. First Nations and Inuit Health Branch (FNIHB) either directly provides a variety of services on reserve to individuals and families or transfers funds to the local communities to provide the services that they need.

An example of the jurisdictional specificity of health-care delivery can be found in the recent changes instituted in Ontario. Fourteen Local Health Integration Networks (LHINs) were formed in the past few years (announced in 2004 and in place by 2006); each has geographical boundaries that encompass what was formerly approximately three times the number of health districts. Two of the fourteen LHINs (i.e., the Northeast and Northwest LHINs) cover substantial rural hinterland, representing the medically under-serviced area of northern Ontario, defined as all the area north of Manitoulin Island. Each LHIN is responsible for planning, funding, and coordinating health services such as hospitals, community care access centres (CCACs), community health centres (CHCs), mental health and addiction agencies, community support services, and long-term care for the communities in its region/under its jurisdiction.

As mentioned, the development and delivery of rural health services inevitably differ across provinces and territories and ultimately have impacts on the quantity and quality of rural health services. Let us compare, to illustrate the point, recent developments in health-care delivery in two provinces, New Brunswick and Alberta. The provincial government in New Brunswick has chosen to focus on resource allocation, indicating that its health mandate will focus on rural issues by developing a rural health institute and working on recruitment and retention of health-care professionals (Province of New Brunswick 2008). In contrast, Alberta has been reforming the structure of its system, working to create a "superboard" to deliver its health services: in 2009, all nine regions and three provincial entities (Alberta Cancer Board, Alberta Mental Health Board, and Alberta Alcohol and Drug Abuse Commission) were amalgamated into one large regional health service system governed by a president and a chief executive officer with vice-presidents in set geographical zones throughout the province. Thus, in this configuration, individuals focus on specific issues such as women's health and palliative care from a provincial level. There is also a single chief operating officer for the rural health delivery system within the province. Furthermore, evidence-based decisions regarding rural health-care services in Alberta ensure consistency from one rural community to another despite their inherent recognized differences (Duckett 2009). This goal of consistency or standardization stands in stark contrast to the aims and arguments advanced in this book, which call for greater recognition of the specific and unique characteristics of rural places and the many contextual nuances that make them individual and dynamic.

Defining Rural

What exactly do we mean by rural Canada? Defining what is rural has become the subject of lively debates at conferences and other such forums. One report concluded that, despite a review of over 150 publications related to rural nursing, there was no universal definition of the term "rural" or "remote" (Kulig et al. 2003). Pitblado (2005) has noted that using technical (geographical distance) and social (indices) approaches can help to define these elusive terms. *The National Study on Rural and Remote Nursing Practice,* based on survey data from registered nurses (RNs), concluded that it is more appropriate to focus on the meaning of rurality shared by rural residents rather than a single specific definition (Kulig et al. 2008). Similarly, Williams and Cutchin (2002) suggest a multi-faceted definition of rural based upon socio-cultural characteristics (i.e., cultural aspects of place), measurable descriptive features (i.e., land use, demographic structure), and local understandings of rural. Such a definition naturally encourages holistic, interdisciplinary research to address research topics within and across rural settings.

Adding to the debate regarding the definition of rural are the attempts to differentiate among rural, remote, and northern. Perhaps, like rurality, it might be more appropriate to focus on the more complex meanings of remote and northern rather than general and limiting definitions. Just as it is challenging to generalize about the definition or meaning of rural given that rural geographies often encompass remote and northern areas of Canada, so too it is difficult to generalize about the rural health experiences lived across these geographies. For example, there are significant differences among delivering a child, receiving diagnostic tests, and having surgery depending on whether one lives in the isolated North, on the edge of an urban area, or within a farming district. Documentation of these differences has been lacking in Canada, and thus far our understanding of health differences and similarities among rural geographies in our country, as well as between rural and urban geographies, is limited. Despite this, many researchers inevitably need to use one of a number of specific definitions, based on either objective or subjective approaches, pending the question being asked. Recognizing that rurality is complex and multi-dimensional, we use the shorthand "rural" when generally referring to the composite of rural, remote, and northern.

Generally speaking, there are three main definitions of rural: (1) census rural; (2) Rural and Small Town (RST), which has since been extended to Metropolitan Influenced Zones (MIZ), and (3) predominantly rural region (see Box 1.1). The definition used is often based on the purpose of the specific research question or analysis. For example, the predominantly rural region definition is best employed when conducting rural policy analysis with a regional focus, such as a comparison of transportation for health-care access. In contrast, the RST or MIZ definition can be useful when examining community-level issues such as comparing retention of health professionals across rural communities.

For many rural health researchers, the RST definition is an appropriate choice because it designates whole towns or communities as rural and allows for analysis of specific issues that impact these geographical areas. Unless otherwise noted, this is the chosen definition for this book. The RST definition refers to residents who are "outside the main commuting zone of 10,000 or more" (Bollman and Clemenson 2008, 9). Using this definition, approximately 19 percent of Canadians would be considered rural.

BOX 1.1   Definitions of Rural

1   *Census rural* typically refers to the population living outside settlements of 1,000 or more inhabitants and with a population density of 400 or more inhabitants per square kilometre (Statistics Canada 2007).

2   *Rural and Small Town (RST)* refers to individuals in towns or municipalities outside the commuting zones of larger urban centres (with 10,000 or more population) (duPlessis et al. 2001, 6). Larger urban centres refer to both Census Metropolitan Areas (CMAs) and Census Agglomerations (CAs). The RST population is also discussed in light of the degree of influence of larger urban centres. There are three categories: Strong Metropolitan Influenced Zone (MIZ) (30 percent or more of residents commute to a larger urban centre), Moderate MIZ (5-29 percent of residents commute to any urban core), and Weak MIZ (0 percent of residents commute to an urban core).

3   *Predominantly rural regions* refer to having more than 50 percent of the population living in a rural community with a population density of fewer than 150 persons per square kilometre (OECD 1994). Such regions are further classified as rural metro-adjacent (predominantly rural census divisions adjacent to metropolitan centres), rural non-metro-adjacent (rural census divisions not adjacent to metropolitan centres), and rural northern (predominantly rural census divisions found either entirely or mostly above specific lines of parallel in provinces [e.g., fiftieth line of parallel in Newfoundland] as well as all of Yukon, Northwest Territories, and Nunavut) (Ehrensaft and Beeman 1992).

Health and Place

Spaces are primarily physical, such as geographies based on physical or administrative boundaries. Space is organized into social *places* or bounded settings that hold meaning and identity and where social relations are constituted. Harrison and Dourish (1996, 69) provide a simple way to understand this distinction using an analogy of house and home: "We are located in space, but we act in place. Furthermore places are spaces that are valued. The distinction is rather like that between a house and a home; a house might keep out the wind and the rain, but a home is where we live."

Disease and health (care) exist in both space and place, across a wide range of scales. Small geographical scales include the spaces and places of health-care settings (e.g., hospital wards or nursing home rooms), whereas larger scales encompass rural regions that are shaped by even larger state- or global-level processes, such as globalization.

The research exploring and documenting place and its relationship to health has grown exponentially over the past decade, with contributions from a wide range of disciplines, from medical health sciences and community epidemiology through to the social sciences, where numerous disciplines have been involved. Arguably, health geographers have been at the cutting edge of this scholarship, having a firm disciplinary base in space and place and more recently in place and its relationship to health. A number of good reviews of health and place research by geographers outline the numerous scales at which place can be operationalized in examining substantive issues: health inequalities (Curtis 2004; Hayes 1999; Smyth 2007), care and caring (Parr 2003), health-care work (Andrews and Evans 2008), and telemedicine (Cutchin 2002). In this work, health is defined broadly, encompassing both ill health (i.e., disease) as well as positive health (i.e., well-being and quality of life). One key area of inquiry has been the place-sensitive attention to a number of non-geometric constructions of space, such as culture, gender, and sexuality (Kearns 1995; Kearns and Moon 2002). This often theoretically driven work embraces the world of difference with respect to how we as humans perceive ourselves and experience health (care) in place.

Much of this work has used qualitative methods, such as a case study approach, in arguing how place or locality impacts health. In this genre of health and place research, specific localities operate as field sites, and the effect of place on health is examined across a number of different indices, from the availability of health services to the degree of social capital experienced. One such work examined the changes experienced in community care services as a result of health system restructuring across two locales in Ontario – one in a medically under-serviced area (Sault Ste. Marie) in northern Ontario, the other in a well-serviced area in southern Ontario (Guelph) – highlighting the impacts on the health of the populations in question (Williams 2006). Other such work has examined settings of care, such as home, long-term care facility, or hospital, making a case for how the immediate settings of care and the social relations within such settings impact health (McLean 2007). A similar case study approach is used in much of the environment and health research, where hazards and risks are examined often at the local level. Certainly, much of the work on farming accidents and risks to health, such as bovine spongiform encephalopathy (BSE), can be placed in this category of research.

Another genre of health and place research uses sophisticated quantitative methods, such as multi-level modelling, to search for area effects or between-area variations in (ill) health. The statistical models used take account of spatial differences in numerous socio-demographic characteristics of populations, such as differences in age, sex, education, and income (individual or compositional characteristics), but cannot explain, at most scales of analysis, the small but significant amount of between-area variation in (ill) health. This significant variation is understood to be the result of contextual or place characteristics, also known as area effects. These contextual characteristics are often derived from aggregate statistics, describing features such as housing (age and size), economic structure (industrial base, economy), green space (parkland), social capital, sense of place, community identity, or availability of services, such as those used for recreation (pools, gyms). Considerable research has examined these issues at smaller scales – the neighbourhood and the region – but comparatively less has been conducted targeting larger scales. In this volume, a number of chapters illustrate such area effects at larger scales, including between urban and rural areas and across a continuum of rural areas. Increasingly, mixed methods are appearing in health and place research, providing both breadth and depth. All of rural research needs to acknowledge, consider, and incorporate the unique contexts of rural communities. As Chapter 15 demonstrates, the implications extend into the ethics of health research in rural communities. What do confidentiality and anonymity mean, for instance, and how are they achieved in cohesive rural communities? How are the boundaries and roles of the research participants defined in these communities? Related to this is the appropriate dissemination of research results that can ensure the voices of rural people are heard within policy and service contexts.

Figure 1.2 shows a number of health and place themes apparent throughout the chapters. The first sub-theme is *place matters to health,* evident in health inequalities across the urban-rural continuum. The second is that *there is great diversity in rural places,* with each locality or place providing a unique, nuanced health experience. The third and

Figure 1.2   Health and place themes with corresponding book sections

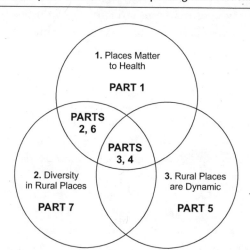

last sub-theme is that *rural places are dynamic,* and thus so are their impacts on health.

We will now discuss each of these sub-themes with reference to the chapters. These discussions on the health and place sub-themes do not comply with the order of the chapters in the Contents, where the sectional grouping of chapters reflects the similarity in the substantive material presented. Rather, the following thematic discussions tie chapters together by their shared representation of each of the three respective sub-themes. We have done this in an effort to promote critical dialogue among chapters as well as encourage critical comparison across each section of the book. Importantly, there is overlap across the chapters and themes, with the research findings illustrating the interconnections among and the complexities of rural health issues. For example, the link between sense of belonging and positive mental health is important to the sub-themes of rural place matters to health and rural places are dynamic, as discussed below. We will return to the sub-themes in the concluding chapter when we discuss policy implications and research recommendations.

Rural Places Matter to Health

The first and most common theme in the collection is that place does matter to health. Place is not only key to identity but also operates as a social resource, often defining our life chances, the degree of risk that we experience, and, ultimately, our health (care) and well-being. Living and working in rural areas have impacts on health status, partly due to the results of shortcomings in health-care services. The findings presented here illustrate and confirm that in rural areas health status and care services delivery are different compared with urban places. For example, compared with urban areas, life expectancy is lower in rural and remote areas, and mortality rates are higher in more rural and remote areas. In presenting a broad picture of the health of rural populations by comparing differences between rural and urban Canada with respect to life expectancy, health behaviour, and quality-of-life indicators, we learn that rural residents are more likely to exhibit less healthy behaviours than urban residents. Furthermore, health status has stagnated among rural dwellers, and among rural residents less than forty-five years of age there are higher death rates mostly due to injury, suicide, and accident. The enduring health status disparities suggest that care is not available or not accessed in rural places.

A central realization in the theme place matters to health is that the discussion has to take into account difference, whether defined by culture, gender, or sexuality. The links between culture and the socio-political context of health status help to clarify the health status variation experienced by First Nations, Inuit, and Métis. This variation includes the experience and frequency of specific diseases but also the social support embedded in their culture that has positive impacts on health and ill health. In contrast, mental health status is actually better in rural and non-metropolitan areas compared with other disorders, in part because of the availability of social support in rural communities. Finally, the findings clarify that rural health status is linked to socio-economic status, illustrating that health-care services need to be embedded in economic and community development.

Ongoing challenges with recruiting and retaining health professionals in rural geographies mean that rural residents experience many obstacles in obtaining care due to lack of available services and personnel as well as geographical and transportation limitations. Our current understanding is that rural Canadians use a different range of services (e.g., there is more reliance on family physicians and less use of dental services) and that the contextual barriers to accessing certain kinds of services (e.g., mental health providers) are known but not always acknowledged through the current "one size fits all" health-care delivery system. We learn from the research presented here that health-care

providers are unavoidably mobile individuals, increasing the likelihood of migration from rural areas. In general, rural health providers
are older and are not being replaced at sufficient levels to match the
provider-to-population proportions in urban areas. Within the context
of an aging population and the evident inequality in health human
resources across the urban-rural continuum, there remains the need
for careful recruitment and retention planning for health-care providers. Beyond planning, actual preparation for working in the rural environment also needs to be carefully considered so that, for example,
the needs of those with mental health concerns are appropriately
addressed.

All of these variations and specific examples regarding rural health
status and the supply of health providers point to the need for a paradigm shift in how we operationalize health-care services in rural areas.
The research findings across the rural communities studied, together
with the divergent groups that were their focus, clearly indicate that
enhancing health status is linked to improving the economic and educational status of rural residents. Furthermore, community development efforts are tied to improving health status. These findings point to
creating policies with a rural lens to address the uniqueness of rural
communities through developing and implementing health services
that include the perspectives of rural peoples. In other words, genuine
endorsement from rural residents is essential and will further foster
their sense of belonging and acknowledge that rural life is important to
their urban counterparts. Finally, the research also clearly notes that
focusing on capacity building and the social determinants of health is
necessary to develop and implement appropriate health services that
will positively impact rural residents' health status.

Rural Places Have Great Diversity

The second theme in this book is that there is a great amount of diversity among rural geographies. Intuitively, we know that there are differences among rural communities from one geographical area of the
country to another. Numerous case studies are presented in many of
the chapters, noting differences in individual and community responses
to adversity and illness as well as how health-care services are developed
and provided to attend to these specific circumstances. Rural Canadians
believe that to paint all rural communities with one brush is inappropriate when developing and delivering health services. However, given

the number of rural towns across Canada, the impacts on health (care) are poorly understood. This confirms the importance of conducting future research that differentiates rural communities, their health status, and the types of services that are effective in addressing identified concerns. Many of the chapters have employed place-specific case studies as an approach, acknowledging nuances in the characteristics of each place of concern.

Rural communities are diverse, differentially affecting residents' experiences of (ill) health. How older residents experience aging or dementia varies across their respective rural settings. Former resource communities, commonly referred to as "instant towns," have a unique set of challenges with respect to caring for the aged (see Chapter 25). Recognizing that rural communities are generally under-served, some have concluded that cases of dementia are worse in certain communities precisely because of the insufficient health-care services and stark shortage of health-care providers (see Chapter 24). Much work is needed in developing the place-specific services and providing education for the range of health-care providers who care for the aged, especially those with dementia. These illustrations reinforce a common thread across the three sub-themes: rural health-care delivery needs to consider the unique nature of the individual within his or her specific rural community.

The examples of place-specific links provided here also make clear how the characteristics of place influence the availability of health care and, indirectly, health. One example of how place influences health-care availability is the multi-disciplinary, multi-sector, and multi-dimensional training centre discussed in Chapter 7. Through the provision of curriculum, field placements, continuing education, and professional development, this centre is enhancing the capacity of local health services. It is clear that capacity building is a key component of successful rural health-care service and delivery.

Other key features identified in the research for the successful delivery of health services to rural and remote locations are the establishment of trust and the creation of relationships with community members. Collaborative processes to develop these features while concomitantly addressing other challenges associated with the delivery of health services in such locations are therefore not a luxury but a necessity. Bridging health policy, health services, and research in the application of a conceptual model to guide and evaluate service development for palliative care is yet another example of how the diversity of rural

Canada needs to be considered when developing and implementing health-care service.

Rural Places Are Dynamic

The third sub-theme developed in this volume is that rural places are dynamic. Numerous changes are being experienced by rural places: population shifts, economic changes resulting from globalization (including the current recession), and climatic changes due to global warming. Some specific examples include the loss of employment within the oil and gas industry related to the recession, the increased number of wildfires, and the constant threats to the agricultural sector due to the increased incidence of viruses (e.g., avian flu) and other disorders, such as BSE, as discussed in Chapter 19. These examples highlight the fact that the future of rural Canada is uncertain. This makes it all the more important to undertake research that can contribute to resolving issues by developing and implementing unique programs and initiatives by and for the individuals and families who choose to maintain a rural lifestyle.

Furthering our understanding of dynamism in rural communities, the research findings connect place (rural and community) with condition (health and well-being). In addition, rural community well-being and resilience are linked to the availability of rural health-care services. We highlighted the diversity of rural communities above and the differences in the specific health conditions; of course, there are also common concerns experienced across the spectrum of rural populations. For example, in rural and remote Canada, individuals with mental health disorders and specific diseases such as HIV/AIDS experience stigma. In addition, they confront barriers in accessing and receiving care. Similarly, in rural and remote locations across Canada, caregivers looking after the aged and those who are palliative experience limited support in their demanding role(s).

Despite the local social support that rural Canadians experience, there is agreement that professional supports to communities are declining in availability and quality, as seen in the lack of health professionals and health programs addressing particular conditions and disorders. Rural Canadians are increasingly concerned that, although their relatives are aging in place, albeit with significant personal supports and costs, they themselves will not be able to do so. Thus, the dynamism of rural Canada, together with variation in the experience of (ill) health, calls for innovation.

Innovation in some cases has taken the form of adopting new technologies in providing health-care services (and even in continuing education). Technological innovation greatly influences the dynamism of rural places, bridging both distance and time. Given the extreme shortfall of health professionals (e.g., registered nurses, physicians, physiotherapists) in rural areas, creativity in providing care and supporting those who provide it is needed to ensure that health care remains accessible and available for rural residents. To illustrate, computer technology can be used to address diabetes and other chronic conditions among rural people, as discussed in Chapter 10. Our hope is that this volume will provide evidence that health-care services in rural areas need to remain in place and need to address the uniqueness of the rural context across the full spectrum, from health promotion to treatment, chronic care, and end-of-life support.

Conclusion

Focusing on the rural context as place and its interrelationship with the myriad of health issues discussed in this book will strengthen our knowledge and understanding of the complexity of rural health, especially across three thematic areas. The first theme, place matters to health, provided evidence of health variations across the urban-rural continuum. The second theme, diversity in rural places, confirmed that each place provides a unique, nuanced health experience. And the third theme, rural places are dynamic, suggests that the ever-changing nature of place will inevitably have irregular impacts on health. Debates about the definition and meaning of rural add to our understanding of place while challenging researchers to ask questions that will generate relevant information. Many other topics still need to be addressed to understand fully the range of health issues within rural communities, as will be further discussed in the concluding chapter.

Note

1 Sense of belonging is a concept related to levels of social attachment among individuals and is indicative of social engagement and participation within communities.

References

Andrews, G.J., and J. Evans. 2008. "Understanding the Reproduction of Health Care: Towards Geographies in Health Care Work." *Progress in Human Geography* 32, 6: 759-80.

Bollman, R., and H. Clemenson. 2008. "Structure and Change in Canada's Rural Demography: An Update to 2006." *Rural and Small Town Canada Analysis Bulletin* 7, 7: 1-29.

Canadian Institute for Health Information (CIHI), 2004. *Improving the Health of Canadians.* Ottawa: CIHI.

—. 2006. "How Healthy Are Rural Canadians? An Assessment of Their Health Status and Health Determinants." Ottawa: CIHI. http://secure.cihi.ca/.

Curtis, S. 2004. *Health and Inequality: Geographical Perspectives.* London: Sage.

Cutchin, M.P. 2002. "Virtual Medical Geographies: Conceptualizing Telemedicine and Regionalization." *Progress in Human Geography* 26, 1: 19-39.

Dandy, K., and R.D. Bollman. 2008. "Seniors in Rural Canada." *Rural and Small Town Canada Analysis Bulletin* 7, 8: 1-56. Catalogue No. 21-006X. Ottawa: Statistics Canada, http://www.statcan.ca/.

Duckett, S. 2009. *The Future of Health Care in Rural Communities.* Okotoks, AB: Sheep River Health Trust.

du Plessis, V., R. Beshiri, R. Bollman, and H. Clemenson. 2001. "Definitions of Rural." *Rural and Small Town Canada Analysis Bulletin* 3, 3: 1-43. Catalogue No. 21-006-XIE. Ottawa: Statistics Canada, http://www.statcan.ca/.

Ehrensaft, P., and J. Beeman. 1992. "Distance and Diversity in Nonmetropolitan Economies." In *Rural and Small Town Canada,* edited by R.D. Bollman, 193-224. Toronto: Thompson Educational Publishing.

Glasgow, N., M. Wright, L. Johnson, and N. Johnson. 2004. *Critical Issues in Rural Health.* Oxford: Blackwell Publishing.

Harrison, S., and P. Dourish. 1996. "Re-place-ing Space: The Roles of Place and Space in Collaborative Systems." In *Proceedings of the 1996 ACM Conference on Computer Supported Cooperative Work,* 67-76. New York: ACM Press.

Hayes, M. 1999. "'Man, Disease, and Environmental Associations': From Medical Geography to Health Inequalities." *Progress in Human Geography* 23, 2: 289-96.

Health Canada. 2007. *Health Care System: Health Care Act: Federal Transfers and Deductions.* Ottawa: Health Canada, http://www.hc-sc.gc.ca/.

—. 2009. *A Statistical Profile on the Health of First Nations in Canada: Self-Rated Health and Selected Conditions, 2002 to 2005.* Ottawa: Health Canada, http://www.hc-sc.gc.ca/.

Indian and Northern Affairs Canada (INAC). 2009. *Urban Aboriginal Population in Canada.* Ottawa: INAC, http://www.ainc-inac.gc.ca/.

Kearns, R.A. 1995. "Medical Geography: Making Space for Difference." *Progress in Human Geography* 19, 2: 251-59.

Kearns, R., and G. Moon. 2002. "From Medical to Health Geography: Novelty, Place, and Theory after a Decade of Change." *Progress in Human Geography* 26, 5: 605-25.

Kirby, M., and M. LeBreton. 2002. *The Health of Canadians: The Federal Role Volume 2: Recommendations for Reform.* Ottawa: Standing Senate Committee on Social Affairs, Science, and Technology.

Kulig, J., M.E. Andrews, N. Stewart, R. Pitblado, M. MacLeod, D. Bentham, C. D'Arcy, D. Morgan, D. Forbes, G. Remus, and B. Smith. 2008. "How Do Registered Nurses Define Rurality?" *Australian Journal of Rural Health* 16, 1: 28-32.

Kulig, J., E. Thomlinson, F. Curran, D. Nahachewsky, M. Macleod, N. Stewart, and R. Pitblado. 2003. "Rural and Remote Nursing Practice: An Analysis of Policy Documents." Report R03-2003 for the Nature of Nursing Practice in Rural and Remote Canada, University of Lethbridge.

Liaw, S-T., and S. Kilpatrick. 2008. *A Textbook of Australian Rural Health.* Canberra: Australian Rural Health Education Network.

Loue, S., and B. Quill, eds. 2001. *Handbook of Rural Health.* Cambridge, UK: Springer.

McLean, A. 2007. "The Therapeutic Landscapes of Dementia Care: Contours of Inter-subjective Spaces for Sustaining the Person." In *Therapeutic Landscapes,* edited by A. Williams, 315-22. Hampshire, UK: Ashgate.

Ministerial Advisory Council on Rural Health. 2002. *Rural Health in Rural Hands: Strategic Directions for Rural, Remote, Northern, and Aboriginal Communities.* Ottawa: Office of Rural Health, Health Canada.

Mitura, V., and R. Bollman. 2003. "The Health of Rural Canadians: A Rural-Urban Comparison of Health Indicators." *Rural and Small Town Canada Analysis Bulletin* 4, 6: 1-23.

Organization for Economic Cooperation and Development (OECD). 1994. *Creating Rural Indicators for Shaping Territorial Policies.* Paris: OECD.

Parr, H. 2003. "Medical Geography: Care and Caring." *Progress in Human Geography* 27, 2: 212-21.

Pitblado, J.R. 2005. "So, What Do We Mean by 'Rural,' 'Remote,' and 'Northern'?" *Canadian Journal of Nursing Research* 31, 1: 163-68.

Province of New Brunswick. 2008. *Transforming New Brunswick's Health Care System: The Provincial Health Plan 2003-2012. Major Initiatives.* Fredericton: Government of New Brunswick, http://www.gnb.ca/.

Romanow, R.J. 2002. *Building on Values: The Future of Health Care in Canada.* Ottawa: Commission on the Future of Health Care in Canada, http://dsp-psd.pwgsc. gc.ca/.

Smith, D.J. 2007. *Australia's Rural and Remote Health: A Social Justice Perspective.* 2nd ed. Victoria, Australia: Tertiary Press.

Smyth, F. 2007. "Medical Geography: Understanding Health Inequalities." *Progress in Human Geography* 32, 1: 119-27.

Statistics Canada. 2007. *2006 Census Dictionary.* Catalogue No. 92-566. Ottawa: Statistics Canada.

—. 2010. *Aboriginal Statistics at a Glance.* Ottawa: Statistics Canada, http://www.statcan. gc.ca/.

Strasser, R. 2003. "Rural Health around the World: Challenges and Solutions." *Family Practice* 20, 4: 457-63.

Williams, A. 2006. "Restructuring Home Care in the 1990s: Geographical Differentiation in Ontario, Canada." *Health and Place* 12, 2: 222-38.

Williams, A., and M. Cutchin. 2002. "The Rural Context of Health Care Provision." *Journal of Interprofessional Care* 16, 2: 107-15.

Part 1: Rural Health Status

Chapter 2 Rural Health Status and Determinants in Canada

M. DesMeules, R.W. Pong, J. Read Guernsey,
F. Wang, W. Luo, and M.P. Dressler

Key Points

- Compared with urban areas, rural areas reported higher proportions of people with low income and less formal education. On the other hand, rural residents reported a stronger sense of community belonging than did their urban counterparts.
- Health-related factors such as the prevalence of smoking and obesity were elevated in rural Canada, while analyses of other health influences, such as dietary practices and leisure time physical activities, indicated lower levels of practice in rural areas.
- Higher overall mortality rates among rural communities were related to causes such as circulatory disease, injury, and suicide. Residents of the most rural areas are often at the highest risk. In contrast, residents of rural communities that have the most commuting flow between large centres were at lower risk of dying than those in urban areas or other rural areas for certain health conditions.
- Generally, rural residents of Canada are more likely to be in poorer socio-economic conditions, to have lower educational attainments, to exhibit less healthy behaviours, and to have higher overall mortality rates than urban residents.

Rural communities differ from urban communities in many ways that can determine health status differences between rural and urban

Canada. This chapter is based on a report entitled *How Healthy Are Rural Canadians? An Assessment of Their Health Status and Health Determinants* (Canadian Institute for Health Information [CIHI] 2006). It is the first pan-Canadian study that presents a broad picture of the health of rural populations with regard to aspects such as life expectancy, health behaviour, quality-of-life indicators, chronic conditions, and injuries. It focuses on the analysis of national data from several sources to examine whether there are differences in health status between rural and urban Canadians. It explores disadvantages and disparities facing rural communities in Canada, with the intention of reaching a better understanding of rural health needs to better inform rural health programs and policies. A more detailed version of the report can be found at http://www.phac-aspc.gc.ca.

In the past, much of rural health research in Canada focused on accessibility of health services, and less attention was given to the other determinants of health. While the need for adequate health services is recognized (see Chapter 4, this volume), there might be more fundamental reasons behind the disparities identified in the literature than simply access to services. An adequate understanding of rural health requires the adoption of a much broader perspective. Rural communities face a number of socio-demographic and -economic challenges. In general, rural communities have different socio-economic and -demographic profiles than urban communities. Aging of the population, economic difficulties, and geographical isolation are among the factors that can contribute to health vulnerabilities in rural areas and small towns in developed countries.

Most rural communities have high dependency ratios, with larger proportions of children and youth (0-19 years of age) and seniors (older than 60 years of age) and a smaller proportion of working-age individuals (20-50 years of age). Many factors contribute to rural areas having an older population distribution, including the tendency of retirees to move to rural areas and the migration of rural youth to urban centres for further education and employment opportunities (Ministerial Advisory Council on Rural Health 2002).

Employment and education opportunities are critical to the well-being of people. Unfortunately, some rural areas are lacking in these opportunities and in social, cultural, and recreational facilities that support a growing population. In general, rural residents are less educated, have higher unemployment rates, and have lower incomes than urban residents. In 2001, the proportion of people aged twenty to thirty-four with less than a high school diploma was higher in rural (23 percent) than urban (14 percent) communities. Finally, rural/urban income disparities are still apparent, with families in rural communities having a median income of $49,449 compared with $56,817 for their urban counterparts (Statistics Canada 2004).

The ethnic composition of rural Canada also differs from that of urban areas. In 1996, rural Canada had the lowest proportion of immigrants, including recent immigrants and visible minorities, 88 percent of whom lived in urban regions. Another important characteristic of rural communities is their relatively high proportions of Aboriginal people. Canada has the second highest proportion (3.3 percent) of Aboriginal people in the total population; New Zealand ranks first with 14 percent of its total population being Aboriginal. Aboriginal people accounted for 2.2 percent of the population of Australia and 1.5 percent of the population of the United States (Statistics Canada 2003). In 2001, a little over half (51 percent) of the population who identified themselves as Aboriginal – First Nations, Inuit, and Métis – lived in rural Canada (Statistics Canada 2003); this 51 percent comprised 31 percent living on Indian reserves and settlements and 19.5 percent living in rural non-reserve areas (Curtis and Jones 1998, 645-72). These proportions have declined slightly since 1996 since the Aboriginal population is experiencing the same patterns of youth out-migration to urban areas.

"Place" embodies a lot of things and is often treated as a residual category. It is a shorthand way of describing a host of factors that might have health consequences for communities and populations. It is now argued that place should have a special status in the population-health discourse, particularly as an important explanatory variable (Curtis and Jones 1998, 645-72; Duncan, Jones, and Moon 1993, 725-33; Forbes and Wainright 2001, 801-16; Goins and Mitchell 1999, 147-56; Kearns and Gesler 1998; MacIntyre, MacIver, and Soomans 1993, 213-34; Stafford et al. 2001, 117-29). For this reason, the conceptualization and measurement of place have received more attention. A simplified framework has been developed as part of this research to portray the hypothesized relationships between major categories of health determinants, including place, and the health status of populations (see Figure 2.1). This framework is informed by a variety of studies on social support networks (Johnson 1996, 61-66; Krout 1989, 141-56), cultural values (Hoyt et al. 1997, 449-70; Rode and Shephard 1984, 1472-77), economic conditions (Amato and Jiping 1992, 229-40), educational attainment (Durlbery 1992, 191-98), occupation and work (Denis 1998,

Figure 2.1   A population-health framework for rural health

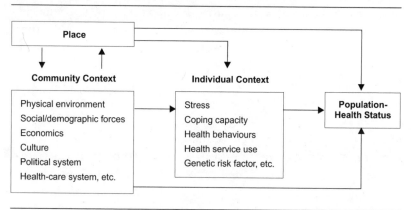

419-36; Jennissen 1992; Pratt 1990, 399-417; Wing and Wolf 2000, 786-93), and lifestyle (Young and Sevenhuysen 1989). It recognizes the compositional, contextual, and collective impacts of place and shows that the relationships between place and health status can be direct, indirect, or reciprocal.

Building on this framework, the overall research question driving this chapter is this: are people living in rural areas and small towns less healthy than those living in cities? The main objective is to describe the health status and identify key determinants of health that would permit us to explain why some rural communities are healthy and others less healthy. This study focuses on rural areas given that the body of knowledge on the health of rural communities in Canada is quite limited and that a better understanding of rural health issues is needed.

Methodology

Definition of Rural

Urban areas were used as the reference group against which different types of rural areas in Canada were compared. Critical to any type of rural research is how the term "rural" is defined or operationalized. For this study, the Rural and Small Town (RST) definition developed by Statistics Canada is adopted. It refers to the population living outside the commuting zones of larger urban centres – specifically, outside Census Metropolitan Areas (CMAs) and Census Agglomerations

(CAs). CMAs (containing populations of 100,000 or more) and CAs (with populations of 10,000 or more) contain large urban areas or urban cores, together with neighbouring census subdivisions (CSDs) or municipalities, that have a high degree of social and economic integration with the urban core.

The Metropolitan Influenced Zones (MIZ) classification of rural, also developed by Statistics Canada, is a refinement or an extension of the RST concept "to better show the effects of metropolitan accessibility on non-metropolitan areas" (du Plessis et al. 2002; McNiven, Puderer, and Janes 2000). CSDs[1] that lie outside a CMA or CA are classified into one of four zones of influence ranging from "strong" to "no" influence, according to the degree of influence that CMAs or CAs have on them.

- Strong MIZ: 30 percent or more of the employed labour force living in the CSD work in *any* CMA/CA.
- Moderate MIZ: at least 5 percent but less than 30 percent of the employed labour force living in the CSD work in *any* CMA/CA.
- Weak MIZ: more than 0 percent but less than 5 percent of the employed labour force living in the CSD work in *any* CMA/CA.
- No MIZ: includes all CSDs that have a small employed labour force (fewer than forty people) or no commuters to a CMA/CA.

MIZ commuting flows from a rural area or small town to all larger urban centres (with a population of 10,000 or more) for work were combined to determine the degree of influence of CMAs/CAs (Rambeau and Todd 2000). The classification and its methodology have been extensively validated by Statistics Canada (McNiven, Puderer, and Janes 2000). Commuter flow is used as a proxy for "access" to services such as health care, education, banking, shopping, and cultural and sports activities.

Strengths and Limitations

The four-category MIZ classification is based on administrative boundaries and takes into account the heterogeneity of rural communities. It also allows comparisons between urban communities (CMAs/CAs) and four categories of rural communities. On the other hand, this classification is not related to the social representations of rural and urban and does not examine the heterogeneity within the CMA/CA category.

Data Sources and Analytical Methods

The following data sources were used: Canadian annual mortality data, Canadian Cancer Registry, and Canadian Community Health Survey (CCHS) 2000-1. A file containing each CSD of Canada and its respective MIZ category was merged with each of these datasets.

Canadian Annual Mortality Data

Analytical Approach
Records from the Canadian annual mortality database were aggregated to the CSD level and then to the national and provincial levels for the period 1986-96. The CSD boundaries were those of the 1996 census. The Canadian annual mortality database uses the CSD of the patient's residence. In other words, it refers to where people lived as opposed to where they died (which could, in some cases, be the CSD of a hospital or long-term-care facility). The CSD data were subsequently assigned to a MIZ category to compare mortality rates for rural and urban areas, by age group and sex. The comparisons were made using age-standardized mortality rates (ASMRs) and standardized mortality ratios (SMRs). (For the methods used to determine the statistical significance of the SMRs and ASMRs, please see the full report at http://www.phac-aspc. gc.ca.) The standard population was that of the 1991 census. Causes of death, according to the ninth revision of the *International Classification of Disease* (ICD-9), were examined by ICD-9 chapters on the basis of their frequency in each age group. The selected causes of death (e.g., circulatory diseases, respiratory diseases, cancers, injuries, motor vehicle accidents [MVAs],[2] suicides, etc.) represent over 80 percent of all deaths.

Multivariate Analysis
The potential association between all-cause, suicide, and MVA mortality and area of residence, based on the MIZ classification, was examined in multivariate regression analyses (Poisson regression using CMA/CA as the reference category) to account for the effect of socio-demographic and -economic determinants of health, such as north/south location,[3] education, occupation, income, mobility, ethnic background, marital status, and average number of persons per household. Sex-combined information on these characteristics was derived from the 1996 census. Age-, sex-, and CSD-specific mortality counts for the three causes of death were computed for the period 1986-96.

Data Quality and Limitations

Complete census data were available for 78.6 percent of the 5,984 CSDs defined in 1996 because of the small populations in the remaining CSDs, but the share of the CSDs included in our study varied by MIZ: 75.3 percent CMA/CA, 99.1 percent Strong MIZ, 93.9 percent Moderate MIZ, 82.3 percent Weak MIZ, and 50.1 percent No MIZ. Area suppression (i.e., the suppression of data for CSDs with small populations) explains the unavailability of some census data at the CSD level. Area suppression results in the suppression of all information for geographical areas with populations below 40 persons. Also, data on income variables in areas with populations below 250 persons or fewer than 40 private households are suppressed. Note that the socio-economic variables are enumerated on the long census of population questionnaire, which is completed by a 20 percent sample of households. Thus, information for CSDs with a population of 250 inhabitants would be based on a sample of 50 census respondents.

Canadian Cancer Registry

Analytical Approach

A similar methodology was used for the analysis of cancer incidence data. Records were aggregated to the CSD level and then to the national and provincial levels for the period 1986–96. The CSD boundaries were those of the 1996 census. Age-standardized incidence rates (ASIRs) and ratios were calculated using the 1991 census population as a standard. All-cause and cause-specific incidence rates and ratios for forty cancer sites were calculated, by age group and sex. See the full report for methods of testing the significance of the SIRs and ASIRs.

Canadian Community Health Survey 2000-1

Analytical Approach

The analysis of the Canadian Community Health Survey was done in two stages. Bivariate analyses were first performed to examine the differences in health status between urban and rural communities. Age-standardized prevalence rates for over forty indicators were calculated by sex and urban/rural category using the 2001 census population as the standard. Data were weighted to take into account the complex sample design, to adjust for non-response, and to adjust for post-stratification. The bootstrap procedure was used to calculate 95 percent confidence intervals.

Multivariate Analysis

Following the bivariate analysis, multivariate logistic regression analyses were performed to ascertain the relationships between selected health determinants and place of residence. The goal of this analysis was to assess whether place of residence had an independent effect on specific health outcomes after several determinants of health had been controlled for. Key health status outcomes were chosen: self-rated health, stress levels, chronic conditions, body mass index, and smoking.

Data Quality and Limitations

The CCHS is a sample of all CSDs in Canada, which does not include all the CSDs used in this analysis. As well, persons living on Indian reserves or crown lands, the clientele of institutions, full-time members of the Canadian Armed Forces, and residents of certain remote regions are excluded; therefore, the associations or the proportions reported for some of the most rural/remote areas might be underestimated.

Deriving Life and Health Expectancy Measures

Life tables are a valuable tool for health evaluation. Although their primary use is to model life expectancy at birth, life tables can be used to derive health expectancy, years of life lost, and many other models depicting the burden of disease or poor health for a population.

Life Expectancy

The Canadian annual mortality data for the most recent years available (1999-2001) were used to calculate age- and sex-specific mortality rates by MIZ categories. Life expectancy by sex and MIZ were then obtained and compared by rural category according to previous methods (Chiang 1984; Manuel, Goel, and Williams 1998, 52-56).

Health-Adjusted Life Expectancy

Health expectancy describes a family of indices that combine mortality (i.e., life expectancy) with different measures of health-related quality of life, of which health-adjusted life expectancy (HALE) is one particular measure (Manuel et al. 2000, 73-80). HALE is a measure that incorporates both the quantity and the quality of life by representing the number of expected years of life equivalent to years lived in full health, based on the average experience in a population. For a more detailed discussion of the methods for calculating HALE, see the full report at http://www.phac-aspc.gc.ca.

General Statistical Notes and Limitations

Throughout this report, the estimates are provided with 95 percent confidence intervals. Reported statistics are taken to be significantly different if the 95 percent confidence intervals do not overlap. In the text, rates described as "significantly different" can be taken to be statistically significantly different at the 95 percent level. The small population in Weak or No MIZ sometimes restricts the amount of data available to calculate the rates. The level of uncertainty associated with rates calculated for these areas is certainly greater than for areas with larger populations (e.g., CMAs/CAs). Consequently, confidence intervals have been calculated and accompany the presented rates or ratios so that the level of uncertainty associated with them is clearly stated. These confidence intervals do not describe the uncertainty associated with potential bias, such as the uncertainty in proper CSD identification.

Results

Although some health measures did not show pronounced rural/urban differences, and some outcomes were actually found to be worse in urban areas, rural areas generally showed a health disadvantage for many of the measures examined in this study. Despite rural Canadians reporting a stronger sense of community and less stress, health status worsened with increased rurality; the exception was most cancer rates, which were found to be higher in urban areas. Generally speaking, rural residents were more likely to be living in poorer socio-economic conditions, to have lower educational attainments, to exhibit behaviours that were less healthy, and to have higher overall mortality rates than their urban counterparts.

Health Status

Life expectancy at birth was generally higher in urban compared with rural areas, and the differences were greater among men. Life expectancy in men ranged from 76.7 years in CMAs/CAs to 73.9 years in No MIZ areas. Among women, life expectancy was at its highest in CMAs/CAs, at 81.4 years, and at its lowest in Weak MIZ areas, at 81.3 years.

Higher overall mortality risks among rural residents seemed to be driven by higher death rates from causes such as circulatory disease, injury, and suicide (see Chapter 3, this volume, for more detailed analysis of deaths due to injury and suicide). Residents of the most rural areas were often at the highest risk of death. In contrast, for certain health conditions, residents in Strong MIZ communities were at lower risk of dying than those in urban or other rural areas. Using a detailed breakdown of age group, it becomes apparent that greater overall mortality risk in rural areas is driven mainly by those under the age of forty-five (see Chapter 3).

Circulatory disease mortality risk was significantly higher in all MIZ categories among both men and women aged zero to sixty-five years or older (for both sexes combined, Moderate MIZ: SMR = 1.07; Weak MIZ: SMR = 1.06; No MIZ: SMR = 1.10), with the exception of Strong MIZ areas (both sexes combined, SMR = 1.00). The highest proportions of death due to circulatory disease occurred among men aged forty-five to sixty-four years.

The incidence rates of most cause-specific cancers were lower in rural areas than in urban areas. Two exceptions were lip cancer in men and cervical cancer (see Chapter 3, this volume, for possible reasons for this latter finding). Overall, cancer mortality rates were slightly lower in rural than urban areas (among men, CMA/CA: 247.0 per 100,000; Weak MIZ: 238.7 per 100,000; among women, CMA/CA: 155.1 per 100,000; Weak MIZ: 149.9 per 100,000).

For the most part, respiratory disease mortality risks were significantly higher among rural residents (both sexes combined, Moderate MIZ: SMR = 1.08; Weak MIZ: SMR = 1.10; No MIZ: SMR = 1.10). Residents of Strong MIZ areas, however, had a reduced risk of dying from respiratory conditions compared with those living in cities (both sexes combined, SMR = 0.94).

A reduced risk of dying from diabetes was observed among men living in Strong MIZ areas compared with their urban counterparts (Strong MIZ: SMR = 0.81). Women living in the most rural areas had higher risks of dying from diabetes than those living in cities and Strong MIZ areas (Strong MIZ: SMR = 0.98; Moderate MIZ: SMR = 1.17; Weak MIZ: SMR = 1.16; No MIZ: SMR = 1.32).

Canadians living in Strong, Weak, and No MIZ areas reported a higher prevalence of arthritis/rheumatism compared with their urban counterparts (both sexes combined, CMA/CA: 15.4 percent; No MIZ: 17.5 percent).

Multivariate analyses were used to examine the association between mortality and place of residence while adjusting for various socio-economic and -demographic factors. This association remained statistically significant after a number of health determinants had been controlled for. The results show that higher mortality risks in rural areas remained for all-cause mortality (relative risks [RRs] ranging from 1.10 to 1.32 for men aged 0-44 years and from 1.08 to 1.27 for women in the same age group) (see Table 2.1), MVA-related deaths (RRs ranging from 1.61 to 1.90 for men aged 45-64 years and from 1.69 to 2.98 for women), and suicide-related deaths (RRs ranging from 1.28 to 1.67 for men aged 65 years or older and from 0.66 to 0.81 for women). In other words, place of residence still had an independent and statistically significant effect on all-cause mortality as well as mortality due to MVAs and suicides, in specific age groups, after some health determinants had been accounted for.

Not having completed secondary school and having a low median household income were strong predictors of increased mortality risk in both men and women. Ethnic composition also had a strong effect on mortality risk: a proportion of less than 10 percent (versus more than 10 percent) of Aboriginal people within the census subdivision was associated with a 53 percent to 61 percent reduction in mortality risk, and a proportion of immigrants of less than 5 percent was associated with a 5 percent reduction of the mortality risk. Slightly higher mortality risks were also associated with small household size (i.e., fewer than three individuals per household). People living in CSDs located in the north had a 26 percent increased risk of dying from any cause compared with people living in CSDs located in the south.

Health Determinants

Rural areas reported higher proportions of people with low income (CMA/CA: 32.4 percent; No MIZ: 49.9 percent) and low levels of formal education (CMA/CA: 27.8 percent; No MIZ: 43.0 percent). On the other hand, more rural residents than urban residents reported a strong sense of community belonging (CMA/CA: 56.2 percent; No MIZ: 76.8 percent), a measure of social capital.

Table 2.1   Adjusted relative risk (RR) estimates for the association between place of residence and all-cause mortality, people aged zero to forty-four years, Canada, 1986-96

	Relative risk		
Variable	Men (95% CI)	Women (95% CI)	Total population (95% CI)
Place of residence			
CMA/CA	Reference	Reference	Reference
Strong MIZ	1.10 (1.07, 1.14)*	1.08 (1.03, 1.12)*	1.11 (1.08, 1.15)*
Moderate MIZ	1.17 (1.14, 1.21)*	1.19 (1.15, 1.24)*	1.20 (1.17, 1.23)*
Weak MIZ	1.20 (1.16, 1.23)*	1.18 (1.12, 1.22)*	1.20 (1.18, 1.24)*
No MIZ	1.32 (1.23, 1.41)*	1.27 (1.15, 1.40)*	1.33 (1.25, 1.42)*
Completed secondary school			
75-100%	Reference	Reference	Reference
50-74%	1.20 (1.17, 1.24)*	1.13 (1.09, 1.18)*	1.20 (1.17, 1.23)*
25-49%	1.27 (1.21, 1.33)*	1.17 (1.10, 1.24)*	1.26 (1.21, 1.31)*
0-24%	1.74 (1.45, 2.07)*	1.31 (1.01, 1.71)*	1.63 (1.39, 1.91)*
Married			
≥50%	Reference	Reference	Reference
<50%	1.20 (1.18, 1.22)*	1.14 (1.11, 1.16)*	1.18 (1.16, 1.20)*
Median household income			
≥$40,000	Reference	Reference	Reference
$20,000 - <$40,000	1.20 (1.18, 1.22)*	1.16 (1.13, 1.19)*	1.20 (1.17, 1.22)*
<$20,000	1.36 (1.23, 1.51)*	1.52 (1.33, 1.75)*	1.43 (1.31, 1.57)*
Unemployment			
≥15%	Reference	Reference	Reference
10% - <15%	0.96 (0.94, 0.98)*	0.98 (0.95, 1.03)	0.92 (0.90, 0.94)*
<10%	0.87 (0.85, 0.89)*	0.95 (0.92, 1.00)	0.91 (0.89, 0.93)*
Medical occupations			
≥5%	Reference	Reference	Reference
<5%	1.06 (1.04, 1.08)*	1.04 (1.02, 1.07)*	1.06 (1.04, 1.08)*
Aboriginals			
≥10%	Reference	Reference	Reference
<10%	0.71 (0.68, 0.74)*	0.66 (0.62, 0.70)*	0.71 (0.68, 0.73)*
Immigrants			
≥5%	Reference	Reference	Reference
<5%	0.95 (0.93, 0.97)*	0.95 (0.93, 0.98)*	0.96 (0.95, 0.98)*
Movers (inter CSD)			
≥20%	Reference	Reference	Reference
<20%	0.90 (0.88, 0.92)*	0.93 (0.91, 0.95)*	0.90 (0.88, 0.91)*
Average number of persons per family			
≥3%	Reference	Reference	Reference
<3%	1.19 (1.16, 1.22)*	1.15 (1.12, 1.18)*	1.18 (1.16, 1.20)*
North vs. south			
North	1.25 (1.19, 1.32)*	1.24 (1.15, 1.33)*	1.26 (1.21, 1.32)*
South	Reference	Reference	Reference

Note: * RR estimate statistically different from reference (1.00) at $p < .05$.
Sources: Statistics Canada, Canadian Annual Mortality Data, 1986-96; Statistics Canada, 1996 Census.

Health Behaviours

The age-standardized proportions of smoking and second-hand smoke exposure were elevated in rural Canada (respectively, CMA/CA: 24.9 percent; No MIZ: 32.4 percent; CMA/CA: 27.0 percent; No MIZ: 34.2 percent), and the proportion of those eating more than five fruits and vegetables per day was lower in rural areas (CMA/CA: 38.2 percent; No MIZ: 31.1 percent). Three health outcomes selected for investigation were significantly associated with place of residence: for two, self-rated fair or poor health and overweight/obesity (body mass index > 25.0), risk was higher in a rural setting. Self-report of fair/poor health was greater in the Weak MIZ and No MIZ areas (13.6 percent and 14.4 percent respectively) than in urban areas (CMA/CA: 12.0 percent), and levels of obesity were higher in a rural setting (CMA/CA: 46.9 percent; No MIZ: 57.2 percent). For the outcome of a quite stressful to extremely stressful life, however, CMA/CA residents were more at risk (26.1 percent versus 22.8 percent in No MIZ).

In the multivariate regression analysis of smoking and place of residence, the association was no longer statistically significant after a number of determinants of health had been controlled for (see Table 2.2). Socio-demographic, -economic, and health predictors of smoking included in the analysis indicated that the risk of being either an occasional or a daily smoker was significantly greater for those of Aboriginal descent, aged less than forty-five years, regular consumers of alcohol, physically inactive, and reporting poor or fair health. Lower income, lower educational attainment, and higher levels of stress were also significantly associated with the risk of smoking.

For both Canadian men and women, the risk of being obese was still significantly associated with place of residence even after covariates had been accounted for in multivariate regression analysis (see Table 2.3). Factors associated with a higher risk of being obese or overweight included Aboriginal origin, having one or more chronic diseases, not having worked in the previous twelve months, being only moderately active (compared with active) or inactive in leisure time activities, not eating the recommended five or more servings of fruits or vegetables each day, and reporting activity limitations in daily activities. Predictors of a decreased risk of obesity were being a current smoker, getting older, regularly consuming alcohol (women only), and having a low income (men only).

Table 2.2   Adjusted odds ratios (OR) estimates for the association between place and smoking, by sex, Canada, 2000-1

Variable (Referent group = 1.0)	Men smoking	Women smoking
Place of residence[1]		
Strong MIZ	1.01 (0.91-1.12)	0.98 (0.89-1.09)
Moderate MIZ	1.04 (0.95-1.13)	0.99 (0.91-1.08)
Weak MIZ	0.96 (0.89-1.03)	0.95 (0.88-1.03)
No MIZ	1.03 (0.85-1.26)	1.11 (0.92-1.33)
Age[2]		
<45 years of age	1.87 (1.75-2.00)*	2.06 (1.93-2.20)*
Aboriginal status: yes	2.59 (2.08-3.21)*	3.78 (3.18-4.51)*
Race: non-Caucasian (excluding Aboriginal populations)[3]	0.63 (0.56-0.71)*	0.29 (0.25-0.33)*
Income[4]		
Middle high	1.30 (1.20-1.40)*	1.35 (1.24-1.47)*
Middle low	1.49 (1.36-1.63)*	1.50 (1.37-1.64)*
Low	2.27 (2.03-2.54)*	2.08 (1.88-2.31)*
Education[5]		
Secondary degree/no post degree	1.48 (1.37-1.59)*	1.56 (1.46-1.67)*
Less than secondary degree	1.91 (1.77-2.06)*	1.67 (1.55-1.80)*
Worked past 12 months: no	0.66 (0.58-0.75)*	—
Alcohol consumption: regular	1.56 (1.46-1.67)*	1.47 (1.38-1.56)*
Self-rated health: poor/fair	1.24 (1.13-1.36)*	1.28 (1.18-1.38)*
Stress level[6]		
A bit stressful	1.15 (1.07-1.24)*	1.13 (1.05-1.21)*
Quite a bit/extremely stressful	1.37 (1.27-1.48)*	1.51 (1.39-1.64)*
Physical activity[7]		
Moderate	—	—
Inactive	1.46 (1.37-1.55)*	1.26 (1.19-1.33)*

Notes:
Confidence intervals were determined using 500 bootstrap weights to account for the complex survey design.
— Excluded during modelling.
* Statistically significant at $p < .05$.
1 Referent group is CMA/CA.
2 Referent group is ≥45 years of age.
3 Referent group is Caucasian.
4 Referent group is high income.
5 Referent group is postsecondary degree.
6 Referent group is not very/not at all stressful.
7 Referent group is active.
Source: Statistics Canada, Canadian Community Health Survey, 2000-1.

Compared with living in a CMA/CA, living in a rural area did not negatively affect all three selected health outcomes. For self-rated health, the association between reporting fair/poor health and place of residence was no longer significant after a number of health determinants had been taken into account (see Table 2.3). Some of the predictors of poor or fair health for both men and women were having one or more chronic diseases, being overweight, being depressed, not having worked in the previous twelve months, not being married, smoking, and not having a strong sense of belonging to the community.

With regard to a stressful life, residents (both male and female) of Moderate and Weak MIZ were still at significantly less risk than CMA/CA residents after regression analysis. The factors associated with reporting higher levels of stress were being a current smoker, having one or more chronic diseases, having a weak sense of belonging to the community, and being divorced, separated, or widowed.

Discussion

In general, rural residents are less healthy than urban Canadians. Although they experience some health advantages, typically they have higher mortality rates and shorter life expectancies, with injuries, motor vehicle accidents, and suicides being major contributors to deaths. Those living in the most rural areas experience the highest disadvantages in relation to deaths due to injuries, cardiovascular diseases, and diabetes.

Previous descriptions of mortality have shown conflicting results: some studies have reported poorer outcomes in rural and remote areas, whereas others have conferred an advantage on rural populations. Our report shows that, for all age groups up to sixty-four years, the all-cause mortality risks were higher in rural than urban areas, with the highest risks of premature death (prior to the age of sixty-five years) being identified among children and adolescents (see Chapter 3, this volume).

The association between all-cause mortality and place of residence was not explained by the selected determinants of health included in our regression analysis for men and women aged 0 to 44 years. Place of residence still had an independent and statistically significant effect on the all-cause risk of mortality in this age group. Compared with people living in a CMA/CA, the total population aged 0 to 44 living in a rural and remote area had an 11 percent to 33 percent increase in mortality risk. Socio-economic factors such as low income and level of education

Table 2.3 Adjusted odds ratios (OR) estimates for the association between place and selected health indicators of Canadian men and women, 2000-1

Variable (Referent group = 1.0)	Men			Women		
	Self-rated health	BMI ≥25	Stress level	Self-rated health	BMI ≥25	Stress level
Place of residence[1]						
Strong MIZ	0.97 (0.83-1.13)	1.20 (1.08-1.32)*	0.95 (0.85-1.06)	0.98 (0.85-1.14)	1.21 (1.10-1.33)*	0.95 (0.86-1.04)
Moderate MIZ	1.05 (0.93-1.18)	1.21 (1.12-1.30)*	0.85 (0.78-0.93)*	0.86 (0.76-0.98)*	1.19 (1.10-1.27)*	0.85 (0.78-0.92)*
Weak MIZ	1.12 (1.00-1.27)	1.26 (1.17-1.35)*	0.86 (0.79-0.94)*	1.05 (0.94-1.17)	1.30 (1.21-1.40)*	0.84 (0.79-0.91)*
No MIZ	0.97 (0.78-1.22)	1.41 (1.18-1.69)*	0.94 (0.70-1.23)	1.24 (0.96-1.59)	1.33 (1.11-1.60)*	0.86 (0.73-1.02)
Age: different for each category[2]	1.04 (1.03-1.04)*	0.75 (0.69-0.82)*	0.79 (0.73-0.85)*	1.03 (1.02-1.03)*	0.78 (0.73-0.84)*	0.71 (0.66-0.76)*
Body mass index[3]						
25-30 (overweight)	2.07 (1.43-3.00)*	n/a	n/a	1.33 (1.12-1.58)*	n/a	n/a
>30 (obese)	1.42 (1.24-1.62)*			1.40 (1.26-1.57)*		
Marital status[4]						
Divorced/separated/widowed	1.15 (1.01-1.29)*	n/a	1.13 (1.03-1.24)*	—	n/a	1.18 (1.10-1.26)*
Single	1.54 (1.34-1.76)*		0.72 (0.66-0.78)*	1.27 (1.12-1.44)*		—
Aboriginal status: yes	n/a	1.68 (1.38-2.04)*	n/a	n/a	1.73 (1.45-2.05)*	n/a
Race: non-white	—	0.50 (0.45-0.55)*	0.81 (0.72-0.91)*	1.37 (1.16-1.63)*	0.58 (0.52-0.65)*	0.81 (0.73-0.90)*
Income[5]						
Middle high	1.24 (1.08-1.43)*	0.87 (0.81-0.93)*	0.85 (0.79-0.91)*	1.30 (1.12-1.50)*	1.10 (1.03-1.17)*	0.83 (0.78-0.89)*
Middle low	1.63 (1.41-1.87)*	0.77 (0.70-0.83)*	—	1.66 (1.42-1.95)*	1.06 (0.99-1.14)	0.88 (0.82-0.95)*
Low	2.08 (1.75-2.46)*	0.65 (0.59-0.73)*	1.33 (1.19-1.50)*	2.18 (1.84-2.59)*	—	—

Education [6]

Secondary degree/no post degree	1.27 (1.12-1.43)*	0.93 (0.87-0.99)*	0.81 (0.75-0.88)*	1.19 (1.07-1.33)*	1.08 (1.01-1.15)*	0.79 (0.75-0.84)*
Less than secondary degree	1.79 (1.60-2.00)*	1.06 (0.98-1.14)	0.74 (0.69-0.80)*	1.72 (1.54-1.91)*	1.32 (1.23-1.41)*	0.73 (0.68-0.79)*
Worked past 12 months: no	1.64 (1.35-2.00)*	1.43 (1.24-1.64)*	0.77 (0.65-0.90)*	1.40 (1.13-1.72)*	1.33 (1.19-1.50)*	0.87 (0.77-0.99)*
Smoking: yes	1.28 (1.16-1.42)*	0.64 (0.60-0.68)*	1.29 (1.21-1.38)*	1.29 (1.17-1.41)*	0.74 (0.70-0.78)*	1.43 (1.34-1.52)*
Alcohol consumption: regular	n/a	—	n/a	n/a	0.71 (0.67-0.75)*	n/a

Notes:

Confidence intervals were determined using 500 bootstrap weights to account for the complex survey design.

— Excluded during modelling; n/a: not applicable.

* Statistically significant at p < .05.

1 Referent group is CMA/CA.

2 Referent group for stress level is ≥45 years of age; referent group for "BMI ≥25" is ≥60 years of age; age variable is continuous for modelling of self-rated health.

3 Referent group is BMI 18.5-24.9.

4 Referent group is married/common-law.

5 Referent group is high income.

6 Referent group is postsecondary degree.

Source: Statistics Canada, Canadian Community Health Survey, 2000-1.

achieved contribute to this increased mortality risk, as do ethnic background and geographical location (north versus south). Age has a bearing on how strong the association is between place of residence and
all-cause mortality (those aged 45-64 and 65+ showing increasingly
lower risk), but other features of living in a remote area, not considered
in this analysis, clearly contribute to rural residents' disadvantage in this
regard. Chapter 4 in this volume discusses some of the aspects of rural
life that affect residents' willingness or ability to access health-care services and thus potentially reduce their risk of serious illness, disability,
or death. There is some evidence that rural residents perceive health as
merely the absence of disease, and in a culture of self-reliance and independence they might not deem health promotion and preventive
medicine to be important or see the need to seek help until they are
seriously ill. As well, family physicians are greatly under-represented in
rural areas, specialists even more so.

One benefit of living in a rural area was found to be a lower incidence of cancer. The overall incidence rates were lower in rural than
CMA/CA areas, with the exception of lip cancer in men and cervical
cancer. Overall mortality rates too were slightly lower in the rural
population, although this varied by age and sex. These findings seem to
be somewhat anomalous given the poorer access to health-care services
and the higher prevalence of "unhealthy" behaviours noted in rural
populations, and they raise the question of whether a lower exposure to
environmental pollutants/toxins might be conferring an advantage.

Smoking, exposure to smoke, and a less than healthy diet were more
prevalent among rural residents, although the association of smoking
and place of residence was no longer significant in multivariate regression analysis. The poorer diet and greater risk of obesity found outside
the CMAs/CAs might be consistent with a population that does not
value preventive measures or has not been reached or influenced by
health education messages. Self-reported fair or poor health was also
significantly associated with rural residence, although the relation was
again found to be no longer significant when covariates were included
in the regression analysis. Some of the predictors of a poor or fair health
report were having one or more chronic diseases, being overweight,
being depressed, not having worked in the previous twelve months, not
being married, smoking, and not having a strong sense of belonging to
the community. Rural residents were less likely to report having a quite
stressful to extremely stressful life, and this association still held for
Moderate and Weak MIZ in multivariate regression analysis.

A strong sense of belonging to the community is more common among rural residents and might be one of their more important social capital tools. Social capital has been defined in many ways (van Kemenade 2003) and generally refers to links between an individual and his or her immediate social environment; it includes concepts such as social networks, mutual trust, civic participation, community engagement, and other institutional relations that can affect the health of individuals. It is generally accepted that a healthy social climate, which results in residents having a sense of belonging and pride in their community, contributes to the health of communities and populations (Albrecht, Clarke, and Miller 1998; Baum 1999; Brown and Kulig 1997). Indeed, some authors have suggested that community characteristics have a greater impact on health status than the availability of medical care (Mansfield et al. 1999; Molinari, Ahern, and Hendryx 1998). Ross (2002) has found that community belonging is associated with self-perceived health, even taking into account socio-economic status, the presence of chronic disease, health behaviours, stress, and other factors (see Chapter 8, this volume, for a discussion of issues related to mental health and well-being). On the other hand, suicide mortality risks among men were significantly higher in rural areas for all age groups compared with urban men. There is a need to study the mechanisms of how concepts such as social capital and community capacity contribute directly and indirectly to the health of a community.

Although some determinants of health are more difficult to modify than others, possible avenues for addressing urban/rural health disparities might include regional economic development programs; occupational health and safety measures to address deaths due to injury and poisoning; improved rural road conditions and road safety awareness; rural-friendly approaches to disease prevention and health promotion; and early detection programs aimed at secondary prevention of chronic diseases such as cardiovascular diseases. Successful strategies need to be identified to address rural/urban disparities in health status. Although we can learn from existing best practices, real breakthroughs require rural-specific health policies and interventions that are relevant to rural settings.

Notes

1 "Census subdivision" is the general term applying to municipalities as determined by provincial equivalent (e.g., Indian reserves, Indian settlements, and unorganized territories).
2 MVA (rather than motor vehicle collision [MVC]) is the variable used as part of a "mortality due to injury" analysis using ICD-9 codes E810 to E825.
3 The north/south category is also CSD based. CSDs were assigned to the north if their representative points fell north of the north-south line. Each MIZ is assigned one of the following categories: north, north transition, south transition, or south (McNiven and Puderer 2000).

References

Albrecht, S.L., L.L. Clarke, and M.K. Miller. 1998. "Community, Family, and Race/Ethnic Differences in Health Status in Rural Areas." *Rural Sociology* 63: 235-52.
Amato, P.R., and Z. Jiping. 1992. "Rural Poverty, Urban Poverty, and Psychological Well-Being." *Sociological Quarterly* 33, 2: 229-40.
Baum, F. 1999. *Social Capital and Health: Implications for Health in Rural Australia.* Adelaide: National Rural Health Alliance.
Brown, D., and J. Kulig. 1997. "The Concept of Resiliency: Theoretical Lessons from Community Research." *Health and Canadian Society* 4, 1: 29-50.
Canadian Institute for Health Information (CIHI). 2006. *How Healthy Are Rural Canadians? An Assessment of Their Health Status and Health Determinants.* Ottawa: CIHI.
Chiang, C.L. 1984. *The Life Table and Its Applications.* Malabar, FL: Robert E. Krieger.
Curtis, S., and I. Jones. 1998. "Is There a Place for Geography in the Analysis of Health Inequality?" *Sociology of Health and Illness* 20: 645-72.
Denis, W.B. 1998. "Causes of Health and Safety Hazards in Canadian Agriculture." *International Journal of Health Services* 18, 3: 419-36.
Duncan, C., K. Jones, and G. Moon. 1993. "Do Places Matter? A Multi-Level Analysis of Regional Variation in Health Related Behaviour in Britain." *Social Science and Medicine* 37: 725-33.
du Plessis, V., R. Beshiri, R.D. Bollman, and H. Clemenson. 2002. *Definitions of "Rural."* Ottawa: Statistics Canada, Agricultural Division.
Durlbery, S. 1992. "Preventive Health Behavior among Black and White Women in Urban and Rural Areas." *Social Science and Medicine* 34: 191-98.
Forbes, A., and S.P. Wainwright. 2001. "On the Methodological, Theoretical, and Philosophical Context of Health Inequalities Research: A Critique." *Social Science and Medicine* 53: 801-16.
Goins, R.T., and J. Mitchell. 1999. "Health-Related Quality of Life: Does Rurality Matter?" *Journal of Rural Health* 15, 2: 147-56.
Hoyt, D.R., R.D. Conger, J.G. Valde, and K. Weihs. 1997. "Psychological Distress and Help Seeking in Rural America." *American Journal of Community Psychology* 25: 449-70.
Jennissen, T. 1992. *Health Issues in Rural Canada.* Ottawa: Library of Parliament, Research Branch.
Johnson, J.E. 1996. "Social Support and Physical Health in the Rural Elderly." *Applied Nursing Research* 9: 61-66.
Kearns, R.A., and W.M. Gesler. 1998. *Putting Health into Place: Landscape, Identity, and Well-Being.* Syracuse: Syracuse University Press.

Krout, J.A. 1989. "Rural versus Urban Differences in Health Dependence among the Elderly Population." *International Journal of Aging and Human Development* 28, 2: 141-56.

MacIntyre, S., S. MacIver, and A. Soomans. 1993. "Area, Class, and Health: Should We Be Focusing on Places or People?" *International Social Policy* 22: 213-34.

Mansfield, C.J., J.L. Wilson, E.J. Kobrinkski, and J. Mitchell. 1999. "Premature Mortality in the United States: The Roles of Geographic Area, Socioeconomic Status, Household Type, and Availability of Medical Care." *American Journal of Public Health* 89, 6: 893-98.

Manuel, D., V. Goel, and J. Williams. 1998. "The Derivation of Life Expectancy for Local Areas." *Chronic Diseases in Canada* 19, 2: 52-56.

Manuel, D.G., V. Goel, J.I. Williams, and P. Corey. 2000. "Health-Adjusted Life Expectancy at the Local Level in Ontario." *Chronic Diseases in Canada* 21, 2: 73-80.

McNiven, C., and H. Puderer. 2000. "Delineation of Canada's North: An Examination of the North-South Relationship in Canada." Geography Working Paper Series No. 2000-3. Ottawa: Statistics Canada, http://www.statcan.gc.ca/.

McNiven, C., H. Puderer, and D. Janes. 2000. *Census Metropolitan Area and Census Agglomeration Influenced Zones (MIZ): A Description of the Methodology*. Ottawa: Statistics Canada.

Ministerial Advisory Council on Rural Health. 2002. *Rural Health in Rural Hands: Strategic Directions for Rural, Remote, Northern, and Aboriginal Communities*. Ottawa: Health Canada.

Molinari, C., M. Ahern, and M. Hendryx. 1998. "The Relationship of Community Quality to the Health of Women and Men." *Social Science and Medicine* 47, 8: 1113-20.

Pratt, D.S. 1990. "Occupational Health and the Rural Worker: Agriculture, Mining, and Logging." *Journal of Rural Health* 6, 4: 399-417.

Rambeau, S., and K. Todd. 2000. *Census Metropolitan Area and Census Agglomeration Influenced Zones (MIZ) with Census Data*. Ottawa: Statistics Canada.

Rode, A., and R.J. Shephard. 1984. "Ten Years of 'Civilization': Fitness of Canadian Inuit." *Journal of Applied Physiology* 56, 6: 1472-77.

Ross, N. 2002. "Community Belonging and Health." *Health Reports* 13, 3: 33-39. Statistics Canada Catalogue No. 82-003.

Stafford, M., M. Bartley, R. Mitchell, and M. Marmot. 2001. "Characteristics of Individuals and Characteristics of Areas: Investigating Their Influence on Health in the Whitehall II Study." *Health and Place* 7: 117-29.

Statistics Canada. 2003. *Aboriginal Peoples of Canada: A Demographic Profile*. Ottawa: Statistics Canada.

–. 2004. *Statistical Area Classification: Highlight Tables for Canada, Provinces, Territories, 2001 Census*. Ottawa: Statistics Canada.

van Kemenade, S. 2003. "Social Capital as a Health Determinant: How Is It Defined?" Working Paper 02-07. Ottawa: Health Canada Policy Research Communications Unit, http://www.hc-sc.gc.ca/.

Wing, S., and S. Wolf. 2000. "Intensive Livestock Operation, Health, and Quality of Life among Eastern North Carolina Residents." *Environmental Health Perspective* 108, 3: 233-38.

Young, T.K., and G. Sevenhuysen. 1989. "Obesity in Northern Canada Indians: Patterns, Determinants, and Consequences." *American Journal of Clinical Nutrition* 49, 5: 786-93.

Chapter 3   **Children, Youth, and Young Adults and the Gap in Health Status between Urban and Rural Canadians**

A. Ostry

Key Points

- Socio-economic conditions vary in a fairly steady gradient moving from urban to remote regions in Canada, and these differences across regions are large. Mortality rates move in a similar gradient for most causes (i.e., they tend to be worse moving from urban to remote regions) except in the case of Strong Metropolitan Influenced Zones (MIZ), where overall rates tend to be lower than they are in urban places and other rural MIZ.
- Even after controlling for the variation in demographic and socio-demographic conditions across MIZ, mortality rates for most causes of death remain higher in rural and remote regions.
- The differences in mortality across the urban-rural continuum are mainly driven by people under age 45 and particularly due to deaths caused by injury, accident, and suicide. In particular, males 15 to 19 years old contribute disproportionately to this variation in mortality.
- Finally, compared with urban Canada, rural Canada has poor socio-economic conditions and is vulnerable to economic downturns. Given the major role that socio-economic differences appear to play in the health status of rural Canadians, it is important to link strategies to improve health with strong economic and community development programs targeted at the needs of rural and remote Canadians.

A number of studies conducted over the past decade have shown consistent deficits in health status among rural compared with urban Canadians (Mitura and Bollman 2003, 2004; Statistics Canada 2000). These studies tended to be on a fairly small scale or were crude, particularly in terms of how the term "rural" was defined for study purposes. This changed in 2006 with the publication, by the Canadian Institute for Health Information (CIHI), of the report *How Healthy Are Rural Canadians? An Assessment of Their Health Status and Health Determinants*. This report utilized hard mortality outcomes obtained from the Canadian Mortality Database (CMD); a new Statistics Canada system for more finely coding rural regions (MIZ); and the Canadian Community Health Survey (CCHS) in 2002, which, because of its huge sample size (130,000), captured responses from approximately 30,000 rural Canadians, making it, at one stroke, the largest-ever survey of the living situation and health status of rural residents of this country.

The overall purpose of this chapter is to illustrate the size, scope, and nature of current differences in health status between urban and rural Canadians in order to develop recommendations for a targeted rural health research and policy agenda utilizing results of this CIHI report. The specific purpose is to articulate more clearly the extent to which differences in health status among rural children, youth, and young adults are the main drivers of the "gap" in health status between urban and rural Canadians. In the methods section, I briefly outline how the terms "rural" and "urban" are used in the CIHI report and in my resynthesis of the report's results. In the second section, I synthesize and present salient findings from the report. I then outline the rationale for a policy and research agenda to reduce the health deficit in rural Canada based mainly on the results of this investigation.

Methods and Analyses Used in the CIHI Report

The reader is referred to the previous chapter for a detailed outline of the methods used in the CIHI report. As noted in Chapter 2, each census subdivision (CSD) in Canada was coded into one of the MIZ categeories (McNiven, Puderer, and Janes 2000). In this chapter, I present some results for each of the seven MIZ categories. However, for most results, I have proceeded as in the previous chapter, by amalgamating four MIZ zones (Strong, Moderate, Weak, and No MIZ) into a "rural" category and compared it to the three remaining "urban" MIZ categories.

There is little consensus on how to define rurality (du Plessis, Beshiri, and Bollman 2001; Pitblado 2005; Pong and Pitblado 2001). However, several empirical methods developed for different purposes by various groups of researchers can be applied to Canadian communities. These definitions have been developed by organizations such as Statistics Canada, the OECD (Organization for Economic Cooperation and Development), and Canada Post. The Standard Area Classification (SAC) Codes (developed by Statistics Canada) were chosen mainly because the definition considers multiple levels of information, such as metropolitan adjacency, population size, and the influence that metropolitan zones have on a community as reflected in the commuting characteristics of the labour force. It is therefore more nuanced than most other definitions that rely solely on population counts or density. As in Chapter 2, the MIZ classifications are used here to present the results.

Results

Variation in the Social Determinants of Health between Urban and Rural Areas in Canada

As outlined in Chapter 2, and based on results from the 2000-1 CCHS, strong gradients across the rural-urban continuum were observed for socio-economic determinants of health. Given these results, together with the knowledge that negative health behaviours and negative health outcomes are almost always strongly associated with adverse socio-economic circumstances, it is likely that people living in rural areas will be less healthy than those in urban locations (Evans, Barer, and Marmor 1994; Frank 1995; Heymann et al. 2005). It is also likely, given the fairly steady gradient of increasingly adverse socio-economic conditions moving from urban to remote places, that the pattern of health behaviours and health outcomes will similarly (at least to the extent that they are wholly or largely driven by socio-economic determinants) show strong gradients across each of these rural zones.

Variation in Health Outcomes between Urban and Rural Residents of Canada

Table 3.1 is a descriptive summary of the main urban versus rural differences extracted from the CIHI rural health report (2006) across a number of health behaviours, illnesses, and mortality outcomes. As already discussed, the presentation of results has been simplified by collapsing the seven MIZ codes into two: urban and rural.

It is clear, when viewing the first column in the table, that the prevalence of most adverse health behaviours and health outcomes is higher in rural compared with urban Canada. There are some exceptions where outcomes are better in rural compared with urban areas. For example, the prevalence of stress, mental disorders, almost all cancer

Table 3.1 Summary of results from CIHI report on the health of rural Canadians

Health behaviours	Prevalence	After control for socio-economic status
Smoking	higher rural	no difference
Exposure to second-hand smoke	higher rural	not tested
Five servings of fruit	lower rural	not tested
Leisure time and physical activity	little difference	not tested
Self-reported health indicators		
Poor self-reported health status	higher rural	no difference
Obesity	higher rural	higher rural
Stressful life	lower rural	lower rural
Low self-esteem	lower rural	
Mental disorders	lower rural	
Arthritis and rheumatism	higher rural	
Diabetes	higher rural for women	higher rural for women
Mortality		
All causes 0-64 years of age	higher rural	higher rural
All causes >64 years of age	little difference	slightly higher
Circulatory disease	higher rural	not tested
High blood pressure	no difference	
All cancers	lower rural	lower rural
Lung cancer	lower rural	no difference
Colorectal cancer	lower rural	no difference
Breast cancer	lower rural	lower rural
Cervical cancer	higher rural	higher rural
Prostate cancer	lower rural	lower rural
Respiratory disease	higher rural	higher rural
Asthma	lower rural	
Injury and poisoning	higher rural	higher rural
Other injury and poisoning (drownings, falls, burns, accidental poisonings)	higher rural	higher rural
Motor vehicle accidents	higher rural	higher rural
Suicide	higher for rural men unclear for women	higher rural

Source: CIHI (2006).

deaths, and asthma is lower in rural places. In contrast, the prevalence of smoking, eating fewer than five servings of fruit, poor self-reported health, obesity, arthritis and rheumatism, all-cause mortality for those less than age 65, and age-standardized mortality due to respiratory and circulatory diseases, diabetes, injuries and poisonings, motor vehicle accidents (MVAs), and suicides is higher in rural compared with urban places.

Given that, in general, rural Canadians experience more adverse socio-economic circumstances, the results in Table 3.1 are not surprising. It is expected and found in most sub-populations that smoking and mortality from MVAs and circulatory diseases are higher among poorer and less-educated populations, such as those encountered in greater proportion in rural Canada. However, there are interesting anomalies (e.g., except for cervical cancer, cancer rates are lower in rural places) in looking at differences in health outcomes in rural versus urban regions of Canada. And, although these associations between adverse socio-economic circumstances and poorer health in rural places are clearly present, deeper investigation is required to understand whether or not the associations are entirely due to the large regional differences in socio-economic circumstances or whether there are other factors that explain these differences.

Table 3.1, in rough fashion, illustrates the descriptive differences (i.e., whether prevalence was lower or higher in rural or urban regions) for several important health behaviours and outcomes between rural and urban regions. In the next section, illustrated in Table 3.2, complexity is added to this descriptive understanding of urban/rural differences in three ways: (1) by presenting mortality rates to illustrate the absolute sizes of urban/rural differences; (2) by breaking these rates down for several major causes of death; and (3) by comparing the results found in urban regions in relation to each of the four rural MIZ, to explore more deeply differences in the prevalence of health outcomes across several different types of rural regions.

A Quantitative Overview of the Variation in Health Outcomes between Urban and Rural Residents of Canada

Table 3.2 shows that, in all cases (except all-cancer mortality in women), age-standardized mortality rates are higher in most (but not all) rural MIZ compared with urban MIZ in Canada. The last column (which calculates the percent difference in mortality rates in remote compared with urban regions) indicates that death from injury, poisoning,

Table 3.2 Annual mortality rates (per 100,000) in urban and rural Canada

Population	Urban	Strong MIZ	Moderate MIZ	Weak MIZ	Remote	Difference remote/ urban (%)
All-cause mortality						
All	694.6	667.8*	739.7*	735.9*	792.4*	14.1
Men	908.0	838.9*	946.3*	940.7*	1010.4*	11.3
Women	542.4	515.2*	563.5*	557.7*	585.1*	7.9
Circulatory diseases						
All	273.4	274.8	292.2*	289.7*	301.7*	10.4
Men	354.5	339.8*	368.6*	366.9*	377.7*	6.5
Women	214.1	215.1	226.5*	221.9*	229.2*	7.1
Respiratory diseases						
All	59.2	55.8*	64.0*	65.1*	65.5*	10.6
Men	88.8	79.8*	93.2*	92.1*	91.8	3.4
Women	42.1	37.8*	42.6	44.8*	43.2	2.6
All-cancer mortality						
All	191.3	177.4*	193.4	189.4	197.0*	3.0
Men	247.0	221.3*	245.4	238.7*	250.1	1.3
Women	155.1	140.8*	152.2*	149.9*	150.1	-3.2
Diabetes						
All	15.7	14.3*	16.9*	16.8*	18.8*	19.7
Men	18.8	15.4*	18.1	18.0	19.2	2.1
Women	13.6	13.3	15.9*	15.8*	18.5*	36.0
Injuries and poisonings						
All	43.0	54.5*	65.7*	68.1*	97.1*	125.8
Men	61.9	79.2*	97.3*	101.2*	142.5*	130.2
Women	25.6	29.0*	33.3*	34.0*	48.5*	89.5
Suicides						
All	.12.3	12.8	16.3*	16.2*	23.7*	92.7
Men	19.3	21.4*	27.3*	27.1*	38.4*	99.0
Women	5.7	4.0*	5.1	4.9*	7.9*	38.6

* Differences were statistically significant at $p < .05$.
Source: Statistics Canada, Canadian annual mortality data, 1986-96.

and suicide shows the greatest difference between urban and remote locations.

These mortality data indicate, first, the paradox that, while the prevalence of adverse mental health outcomes is lower in rural compared with urban areas (although not statistically significantly lower), suicide rates are higher (see Table 3.1). At first glance, this is a rather counterintuitive result. Second, the tables indicate that mortality due to suicide, injury, and poisoning increases in a fairly steady gradient moving from urban to rural places. Third, results for Strong MIZ regions almost always indicate the lowest rates of any region. Fourth, the differences for injury and poisoning mortality among men are the most dramatic between urban and remote places (61.9 compared with 142.5 per 100,000 – a difference of 130.2 percent).

Variation in Health Outcomes between Urban and Rural Residents of Canada by Age and Gender

To explore these issues further, it is necessary first to determine whether these mortality patterns vary across the rural-urban continuum depending on age and/or gender. The CIHI authors conducted sub-analyses separately for males and females with age groups 0-4, 5-19, 20-44, 45-64, and 65+. Analyzed in this fashion, the picture of differences that emerges in health across the rural-urban continuum is much more complex. Differences in age-standardized all-cause mortality across the rural-urban continuum are most pronounced for girls (and young women) and hardly evident for older women. The pattern observed for women is similar for males in the five different age groups, although the absolute mortality rates across all age groups are much higher among males. To summarize, observed general variations in health outcomes across the rural-urban continuum are driven mainly by differences across this continuum among people under age 45.

In Figure 3.1, males and females under age 45 are divided into three age groups (0-4, 5-19, 20-44), and percent differences in all-cause mortality between those living in urban compared with remote regions (i.e., residents of No MIZ only) are presented. Figure 3.1 demonstrates that the difference in all-cause mortality between urban and remote residents is slightly greater for boys and young men compared with girls and young women and that these differences are most pronounced for girls and boys 5 to 19 years old. In fact, all-cause mortality rates for boys 5 to 19 years old and girls living in remote areas of Canada were approximately 160 percent greater than those for their counterparts living in urban locations.

These data indicate that differences in health outcomes across the rural-urban continuum are primarily driven by older children and teens and to a lesser extent young to middle-aged adults and very young children and infants. In the next section, I explore the particular causes of death that are most responsible for the large differences observed across the rural-urban continuum for young Canadians.

Figure 3.1   Percentage difference in all-cause mortality rates for girls, boys, young women, and young men in urban compared with remote areas in Canada, 1986-96

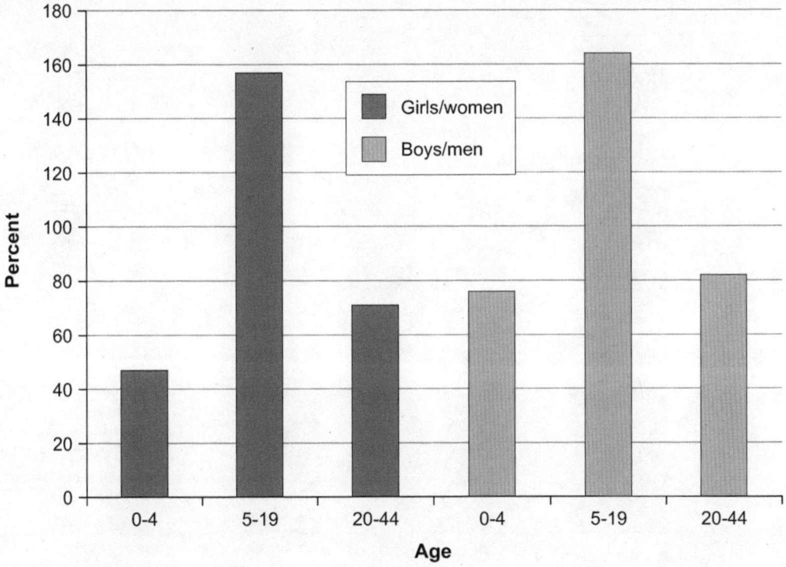

Source: CIHI (2006).

Variation in Health Outcomes between Urban and Rural Residents of Canada by Age, Gender, and Cause of Death

For boys and young men, deaths from injuries and poisonings, MVAs, and suicides account for the largest proportion of overall deaths in these age groups. They also account for much of the large variation in mortality rates across the rural-urban continuum observed for these age groups. Figure 3.2 shows these data for boys 5 to 19 years old only.

Mortality from MVAs in remote regions is 32.5 and in urban regions 11.1 per 100,000; this is a difference of 170 percent. In the case of suicides, rates are 27.1 in remote regions compared with 6.9 per 100,000 in urban regions, a difference of over 250 percent. Figure 3.2 presents results only for boys 5 to 19 years old. Replication of these calculations for young men (20-44) and older men (45-65) reveals a similar pattern but with a shallower gradient across the rural-urban continuum with increasing age. Thus, for example, among men aged 44 to 65, the excess in suicide mortality for those residing in remote places is "only" approximately 50 percent compared with about 250 percent among 5 to 19 year olds.

Figure 3.2   Age-standardized mortality rates due to injuries and poisonings, other injuries, motor vehicle accidents, and suicides (per 100,000) among males five to nineteen years old by urban and remote place of residence, Canada, 1986-96

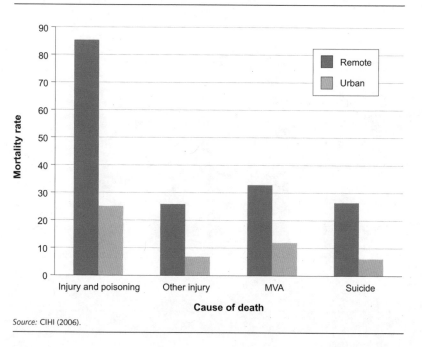

Source: CIHI (2006).

Injury, poisoning, accident, and suicide play a major role in rural/ urban mortality variations among boys and young men. But is this true for girls and young women? Figure 3.3 compares injury and poisoning mortality rates for boys and girls and young men and women across the rural-urban continuum. Males in the three age categories and in each region across the rural-urban continuum have much higher mortality rates from injuries and poisonings than females. And, while there is a gradient for injury/poisoning deaths among females across the rural-urban continuum, it is steeper for boys and young men, indicating that the risk of death moving from urban to remote locations from this cause is particularly severe for boys and young men compared with girls and young women.

Injuries, accidents, and suicides are very important factors among those under age 45 (particularly males) in explaining the gap in health outcomes between rural and urban Canada. It is well known that suicide rates in British Columbia's rural places are generally much higher for Aboriginal compared with non-Aboriginal British Columbians

Figure 3.3   Age-standardized mortality rates due to injuries and poisonings (per 100,000) among girls, boys, young women, and young men by place of residence, Canada, 1986-96

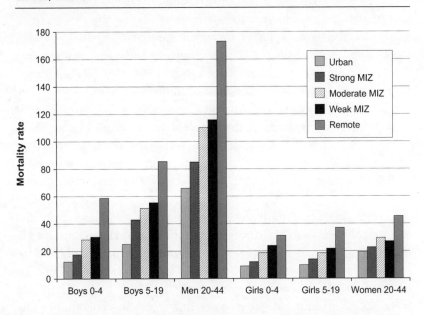

Source: CIHI (2006).

(Chandler and Lalonde 2008). At least some of the excess suicide mortality seen in rural British Columbia is likely driven by these higher rates among Aboriginals. Unfortunately, it is impossible given the dataset used in this investigation to determine suicide rates for Aboriginals separately from non-Aboriginals.

The "Health Gap" after Controlling for Socio-Economic Conditions

As demonstrated in Chapter 2 and earlier in this chapter, even *after controlling for socio-economic circumstances,* all-cause mortality for those under age 65 is higher in rural regions, as is mortality specifically from cervical cancer, respiratory disease, diabetes (for women only), injury and poisoning, MVA, suicide, and the prevalence of arthritis and rheumatism. Thus, other factors, perhaps different for different outcomes and age groups, beyond those due to the more adverse socio-economic circumstances facing most rural Canadians might at least partly explain the differences observed across the rural-urban continuum, for these outcomes.

Multivariate analyses of all-cause mortality, after fully controlling for demographic and socio-economic differences, indicate that, for all three age groups (0-44, 45-64, 65+), residing in rural places exerted an independent effect. However, the strength of association of place of residence with these analyses increased moving from analyses with those over age 65 to the 44-64 age group, with the strongest associations found among the youngest age group (0-44). For this age group, after controlling for socio-economic conditions, men and women living in rural and remote regions had all-cause mortality rates ranging from 11 to 33 percent higher than those living in urban places. These differences were statistically significant. Unfortunately, because of data limitations, CIHI was unable to conduct multivariate analyses for injuries, poisonings, and MVAs. However, they were conducted for suicides using age groups 15-24, 25-44, 45-64, and 65+. For males of all age groups, after controlling for demographic and socio-economic differences, there was still an independent and statistically significant effect due to place of residence characterized by an increasing rate of suicide mortality moving from urban to remote places. The risk for males 15 to 24 years old was particularly high. For rural and remote males 15 to 24 years old, after controlling for socio-economic conditions, the risk of death from suicide was from 20 to 58 percent higher than for urban males of this age. Among rural and remote females 15 to 24 years old, after control, the risk of death from suicide was from 27 to 225 percent higher than for urban females of this age. This pattern of greater risk for rural and remote females was not observed for all other female age groups.

Discussion

Five main conclusions can be drawn from these analyses. First, socio-economic conditions vary in a fairly steady gradient moving from urban to remote regions in Canada, and the sizes of these differences across regions are large. Second, mortality rates move in a similar gradient for most causes (i.e., they tend to be worse moving from urban to remote regions), except in the case of Strong MIZ, where rates overall tend to be lower than they are in urban places and other rural MIZ. Third, even after controlling for the variation in demographic and socio-demographic conditions across MIZ, mortality rates for most causes of death remain higher in rural and remote regions. Fourth, these differences in mortality across the urban-rural continuum are mainly driven by people under age 45 and particularly due to deaths caused by injury, accident, and suicide. And fifth, mortality from these outcomes among males, particularly in the 15-19 age range, contributes disproportionately to the variation in mortality across MIZ.

These observations should be useful in terms of broadly developing research and policy to improve the health of rural Canadians over the medium and long terms. At a basic level, these results provide evidence that more prevention and treatment resources should be made available for Canada's rural population since the health needs of rural Canadians are greater, on average, than those of urban Canadians. Also, thinking about these results from the perspective of social determinants of health, it is clear that a significant proportion (varying depending on the outcome under consideration) of the gradient in health outcomes across the rural-urban continuum can be explained by the systematic socio-economic disadvantages experienced by rural Canadians. Considered from a social determinants framework, this finding clearly implies that rural economic development must be prioritized, not only for the sake of economic growth, but also as an explicit strategy to improve the health of rural Canadians.

The results from this report build a case for not just increasing funding to develop better treatment and prevention in rural versus urban places or to promote greater economic development in these parts of Canada but also, in the process, specifically targeting young people, particularly teens and young adults. The CIHI results show definitively that the differences in health status across the rural-urban continuum are small for those over age 45; clearly, the rural health disadvantage is largely a problem among children, youth, and young adults. Given that poverty among children and youth in Canada (in all regions) is very high relative to other industrial nations, this means that child and youth health must be a specifically articulated priority for health policy makers in this country.

As noted above, for certain outcomes, such as MVAs, a significant proportion of the difference in rates across the rural-urban continuum is not well explained by the socio-economic differences across these regions. For these kinds of outcomes, more research is needed to determine which unique aspects of rural living, beyond socio-economic determinants, are salient. Again, in terms of MVAs, the findings of higher collision rates in rural places are not new (Dryden et al. 2003; Kmet and MacArthur 2006). It is well known that motor vehicle accidents are a larger problem in rural compared with urban regions.

More research is needed to better understand links between risk-taking behaviours and MVAs in rural places in terms of "hotspots" and seasonal variations. The latter might be a particular problem compounded by Canada's severe winters. As well, in terms of policy responses, the availability of rapid air and road ambulance services and well-equipped trauma facilities in rural hospitals is likely to have a large payoff in reduced mortality from road collisions.

In terms of other injuries, they can occur while rural people are engaged in outdoor recreational pursuits. The higher-risk recreational environments in many rural and remote regions, along with higher male risk-taking behaviours, can be a relatively lethal combination (Boland et al. 2005; Miles-Doan and Kelly 1995).

The results for suicide are alarming, particularly for young women and men. Research from Australia, Norway, and the United Kingdom found that the largest increases in suicide rates for young adults since the 1970s occurred among residents in rural regions (Dudley et al. 1998; Kelly, Charlton, and Jenkins 1995; Mehlum, Hytten, and Gjertsen 1999). The high rates in rural Canada seen in this study might also reflect recent increases.

It is well known that in Canada suicide rates among Aboriginal youth are higher than among non-Aboriginal youth (Chandler and Lalonde 2008; Lalonde 2006). Given the often high proportion of Aboriginals living in remote regions of Canada, this could explain, to some extent, the extremely high rates observed in these regions. However, in multivariate analyses in this CIHI study, ethnic background, including Aboriginal ancestry, was controlled for, yet the differences in suicide mortality in rural versus urban places remained high.

As in the case for MVAs, results for suicide appear to indicate that, even after controlling for ethnic and socio-economic factors, rates are higher in rural regions. It might be, as demonstrated by Chandler and Lalonde (2008), that the situation for Aboriginals living in rural areas is much different than it is for non-Aboriginals. Building on Durkheim (1987), they have shown clearly that Aboriginal communities that have negotiated strong land claims and tended to retain strong Aboriginal cultural practices have dramatically lower suicide rates than communities with less strength along these dimensions. These results indicate that strong communities are important in prevention of suicide in rural Aboriginal communities and point to the possibility that, for non-Aboriginals, rural community integrity might be key in lowering suicide rates. This implies that research on community development, change, and its impacts on health in the rural context will be key to developing a better understanding of higher suicide rates in rural communities and, consequently, policies to counter them.

The CIHI study raises some interesting paradoxes. First, it is unclear why cancer mortality appears lower in rural compared with urban places (except for cervical cancer among women). This is particularly interesting for lung cancer and needs more exploration given that mortality from other respiratory illness tends to be higher in rural Canada and that smoking rates are much higher in rural regions. This observation requires further research since the risk for cervical cancer is much higher in rural compared with urban places. Multivariate analyses indicate that the socio-economic differences across the rural-urban continuum explain much of the difference in rates. There is strong evidence that young women in rural places are at particular risk of contracting sexually transmitted infections. For example, in British Columbia, infection rates for chlamydia among rural women are much higher than they are among urban women (Division of STI/HIV Prevention and Control 2006). These data, from British Columbia at least, indicate that young rural women might be engaging in more risky sexual behaviours than their urban counterparts. Given the strong association of adverse socio-economic conditions with cervical cancer and other STDs, the particularly bleak economic outlook for young women in many rural places might require research and policy attention in a bid to understand better this important issue for rural health (Goldenberger et al. 2008).

Several empirical studies conducted in Canada indicate that in fact the prevalence of mental health outcomes such as depression is lower in rural places. In a large case control study of suicide among sawmill workers in British Columbia, Ostry et al. (2006) demonstrated that rates were lower among workers who lived and worked in rural areas and who moved from urban to rural areas compared to urban workers. Yet, according to the CIHI study, suicide rates for men are higher in rural compared with urban places. These findings are hard to explain given the results obtained by Ostry et al. (at least in British Columbia and for sawmill workers) and the lower levels of self-reported stress and self-reported mental health among residents of rural places. These anomalous findings indicate that much more research is required, probably across different sub-populations living in different types of rural places, to better understand the high rates observed in the CIHI study.

Also, in all the mortality analyses, Strong MIZ appear to be the healthiest places to live in Canada. These places are close to large CMAs and have at least 30 percent of their population commuting to the local urban centres. Why these somewhat distant suburbs of urban places are fairly healthy places relative to both their urban neighbours and more rural and remote places needs to be explored further.

References

Boland, M., A. Staines, P. Fitzpatrick, and E. Scallan. 2005. "Urban-Rural Variation in Mortality and Hospital Admission Rates for Unintentional Injury in Ireland." *Injury Prevention* 11, 1: 38-42.

Canadian Institute for Health Information (CIHI). 2006. *How Healthy Are Rural Canadians? An Assessment of Their Health Status and Health Determinants.* Ottawa: CIHI, http://www.phac-aspc.gc.ca/.

Chandler, M.J., and C.E. Lalonde. 2008. "Cultural Continuity as a Protective Factor against Suicide in First Nations Youth." *Horizons* 10, 1: 68-72.

Division of STI/HIV Prevention and Control. 2006. *STI/HIV in Northeastern BC.* Vancouver: British Columbia Centre for Disease Control.

Dryden, D.M., L.D. Saunders, B.H. Rowe, L.A. May, N. Yiannakoulias, L.W. Svenson, D.P. Schopflocher, and D.C. Voaklander. 2003. "The Epidemiology of Traumatic Spinal Cord Injury in Alberta, Canada." *Canadian Journal of Neurological Sciences* 30, 2: 113-21.

Dudley, M., N. Kelk, T. Florio, B. Waters, J. Howard, and D. Taylor. 1998. "Coroners' Records of Rural and Non-Rural Cases of Youth Suicide in New South Wales." *Australian and New Zealand Journal of Psychiatry* 32, 2: 242-51.

du Plessis, V., R. Beshiri, and R. Bollman. 2001. "Definitions of Rural." *Rural and Small Town Canada Analysis Bulletin* 3, 3: 1-17.

Durkheim, E. 1987. *Suicide.* New York: Free Press.

Evans, R., M. Barer, and T. Marmor. 1994. *Why Are Some People Healthy and Others Not?* New York: Aldine de Gruyter.

Frank, J. 1995. "The Determinants of Health: A New Synthesis." *Current Issues in Public Health* 1: 233-40.

Goldenberger, S., J. Shoveller, M. Koehoorm, and A. Ostry. 2008. "Barriers to STI Testing among Youth in a Canadian Oil and Gas Community." *Health and Place* 14, 4: 718-29.

Heymann, J., C. Hertzman, M. Barer, and R.G. Evans. 2005. *Healthier Societies: From Analysis to Action.* Oxford: Oxford University Press.

Kelly, S., J. Charlton, and R. Jenkins. 1995. "Suicide Deaths in England and Wales, 1982-1992: The Contribution of Occupation and Geography." *Population Trends* 80: 16-25.

Kmet, L., and C. MacArthur. 2006. "Urban-Rural Differences in Motor Vehicle Crash Fatality and Hospitalization Rates among Children and Youth." *Accident Analysis and Prevention* 38, 1: 122-27.

Lalonde, C.E. 2006. "Identity Formation and Cultural Resilience in Aboriginal Communities." In *Promoting Resilience in Child Welfare,* edited by R.J. Flynn, P. Dudding, and J. Barber, 52-71. Ottawa: University of Ottawa Press.

McNiven, C., H. Puderer, and D. Janes. 2000. *Census Metropolitan Area and Census Agglomeration Influenced Zones (MIZ): A Description of the Methodology.* Catalogue No. 92F0138MIE2000002. Ottawa: Statistics Canada.

Mehlum, L., K. Hytten, and F. Gjertsen. 1999. "Epidemiological Trends of Youth Suicide in Norway." *Archives of Suicide Research* 5, 3: 193-205.

Miles-Doan, R., and S. Kelly. 1995. "Inequities in Health Care and Survival after Injury among Pedestrians: Explaining the Urban/Rural Differential." *Journal of Rural Health* 11, 3: 177-84.

Mitura, V., and R.D. Bollman. 2003. "The Health of Rural Canadians: A Rural-Urban Comparison of Health Indicators." *Rural and Small Town Canada Analysis Bulletin* 4, 6: 1-23.

—. 2004. "Health Status and Behaviours of Canada's Youth: A Rural-Urban Comparison." *Rural and Small Town Canada Analysis Bulletin* 5, 3: 1-22.

Ostry, A., S. Maggi, J. Tansey, J. Dunn, R. Hershler, L. Chen, A. Louie, and C. Hertzman. 2006. "The Impact of Father's Physical and Psychosocial Work Experience on Attempted and Completed Suicide among Their Children." *Bio-Medical Central Public Health* 6: 77-89.

Pitblado, J.R. 2005. "So, What Do We Mean by 'Rural,' 'Remote,' and 'Northern?'" *Canadian Journal of Nursing Research* 37, 1: 163-68.

Pong, R.W., and J.R. Pitblado. 2001. "Don't Take 'Geography' for Granted! Some Methodological Issues in Measuring Geographic Distribution of Physicians." *Canadian Journal of Rural Medicine* 6, 2: 103-13.

Statistics Canada. 2000. *Rural and Small Town Canada: An Overview.* Ottawa: Statistics Canada.

Chapter 4   **Health Services Utilization in Rural Canada: Are There Distinct Rural Patterns?**

R.W. Pong, M. DesMeules, J. Read Guernsey, D. Manuel, A. Kazanjian, and F. Wang

Key Points

- Place is an important factor in understanding both population health status and health services utilization. Rural Canadians use health care differently than their urban counterparts, and within rural Canada there is marked heterogeneity with regard to the utilization of health services.
- Rural residents do not necessarily use fewer health services, but they might use a different range of services. For example, rural Canadians are more reliant on family physicians, more likely to be hospitalized but for shorter lengths of stay, more likely to use services provided by nurses, but less likely to use dental services or access community-based care.
- Extensive and enduring health status disparities can be signs that some people in some places have a disproportionate disease burden and/or do not receive the care that they need.

A fundamental objective of the Canada Health Act, which sets out the conditions under which health care is provided in this country, is to facilitate reasonable access to health services without financial or other barriers. In 2002, two comprehensive federal policy documents – the "Kirby Report" (Kirby and LeBreton 2002) and the "Romanow Report" (Romanow 2002) – underscored this principle by emphasizing the importance of timely access to health care. Both reports also highlighted concerns about the accessibility and adequacy of health care in rural Canada. It is estimated that $148 billion was spent on health care in Canada in 2006. The three largest categories of spending were hospitals (about 30 percent of all health expenditures), retail drugs (about 17 percent), and physician services (about 13 percent) (Canadian Institute for Health Information [CIHI] 2007). Other services, such as dental care, homecare, and allied health services, are not covered under the Canada Health Act.

Two questions are frequently asked about rural health: "Are rural Canadians more or less healthy than their urban counterparts?" and "Do rural Canadians receive the kind of health care they need?" This chapter and Chapter 2 are based on a national research project titled Canada's Rural Communities: Understanding Rural Health and Its Determinants, funded by the Canadian Population Health Initiative and conducted by a consortium of researchers in 2003-6. Whereas Chapter 2 discusses the health status of rural Canadians, this chapter examines access to and use of health services by rural residents. The two chapters are therefore complementary.

Although health-care consumption by Canadians has been extensively examined, few studies describe patterns of utilization by rural Canadians, particularly at the national level. Most studies are regional in nature or target a specific community or population. Existing studies also tend to focus on a single mode or a limited range of services. Similarly, previous rural health studies have often treated the term "rural" as undifferentiated even though there is increasing evidence that rural communities are not homogeneous. Hence, it is problematic to assume that one rural region has the same health-care needs as another simply by being designated rural. The increasing attention paid to rural health reflects a growing interest in a broader issue – the relationship between place and health. Does where people live, work, and play affect their health status and health behaviours? Place is a shorthand way of describing a host of phenomena – geographical distance, population size, ecological and climatic conditions, socio-economic characteristics, occupational activities, community structure, ethnic composition, culture, and lifestyle – that can have health implications. It is now acknowledged that place should be seen as an important explanatory variable in population health (Curtis and Jones 1998; Fitzpatrick and LaGory 2000; MacIntyre, MacIver, and Soomans 1993).

Describing how rural Canadians use health services, this chapter has three objectives. First, since most people use a variety of health services to meet their health needs, it examines a broad range of services (limitations were imposed by lack of national data): family physician and specialist services, immediate health-care services, services provided by non-physician practitioners, community-based care, and hospital care. Second, intra-rural variations in utilization are documented, for such variations are just as important as knowing how rural differs from urban. This is done by using the four Metropolitan Influenced Zones (MIZ) categories. And third, while the national perspective is the focus of this study, the chapter also examines utilization patterns in two provinces – Ontario and Nova Scotia. The former represents a large and mostly urban province (87.0 percent of the population living in cities and less than 3.0 percent living in more remote areas), while the latter represents a smaller and relatively rural province (63.3 percent living in cities and 23.4 percent living in more remote areas). The intent is to examine the extent to which national and provincial utilization patterns converge or diverge.

It is beyond the scope of this chapter to examine the causes of regional variations in health services utilization. Suffice it to say that utilization is typically a function of a host of factors. In the case of health services utilization by rural residents, the determinants can include poorer socio-economic conditions and lower educational attainments (Alasia 2003; Alasia and Rothwell 2003; Mathers and Schofield 1998; Ronson and Rootman 2004; Xi et al. 2005); lack of health-care resources, including health human resources such as physicians (Pong and Pitblado 2005); inadequate public transportation (Arcury et al. 2005); and rural values and health beliefs (Casey, Call, and Klingner 2001; Dixon and Welch 2000; Humphreys, Mathews-Cowey, and Weinand 1997). According to Andersen (1995) and Andersen and Aday (1978), they can be grouped into three broad categories: predisposing, enabling, and needs-based factors. Thus, place can be seen as a predisposing factor since it helps to determine the health status of a population, which then translates into health-care needs. It can also be seen as an enabling factor since it can shape health-care delivery and affect how people access and consume services.

Data and Methods

This study used various kinds of data to ensure that the results were not an artifact of a single dataset. The following sources of data were used.

- Canadian Community Health Survey (CCHS) 2000-1 and Health Services Access Survey (HSAS) 2000-1. CCHS and HSAS data were based on a sample of all census subdivisions in Canada. Both surveys were administered to individuals twelve years of age and older.
- Physician claims files from Nova Scotia and Ontario (2001-2). Data from Nova Scotia and Ontario were used to examine physician services utilization patterns at the provincial level based on billing information. Physician visit rates (i.e., office visits, visits to outpatient departments, and emergency room visits) were calculated. A physician visit was defined as one patient-doctor encounter per day. Shadow billings, where available, were also included in the analysis to account for services delivered by non-fee-for-service physicians. The following indicators were calculated: (1) average number of visits to all physicians per 1,000 residents of the area; (2) average number of visits to family physicians per 1,000 residents; and (3) average number of visits to medical and surgical specialists per 1,000 residents.
- Hospital Morbidity Database (HMDB) 2000-1. The HMDB captures information on patient separations from hospitals. Data are reported based on the region of the patient's residence, not the region where the hospital is located. The figures thus reflect how frequently residents of a given area received hospital care. Discharge data from the HMDB were extracted for Nova Scotia and Ontario as well as for Canada as a whole but excluding Quebec. Discharge rates and length-of-stay figures were based on the number of discharges from a hospital in 2001-2. All indicators were sex and age standardized using the 1991 census population.

In Canada, there is no universally adopted or officially sanctioned definition of the term "rural." For this study, Statistics Canada's "Rural and Small Town" (RST) definition of rural and the four MIZ categories were adopted because it relied exclusively on the analysis of secondary data that were largely compatible with the RST definition and the MIZ categorization. The definition of rural and the differentiation of rural into four sub-categories were discussed in Chapter 2 and do not need to be repeated here. Although there might be important differences among cities of different sizes, it is not the purpose of this chapter to examine them, so the heterogeneity of Census Metropolitan Areas and Census Agglomerations (CMAs/CAs) is not analyzed. Data for all cities were grouped together and used as a reference point, against which different rural categories were compared. Statistical significance of rates was tested using Byar's method and based on the assumption of a Poisson distribution (Breslow and Day 1989). In the following, rates described as "significantly different" can be taken to mean statistically significant differences at the 95 percent level. Readers are referred to the report of the research project Canada's Rural Communities (CIHI 2006) for more detailed information on data sources and methodologies.

Results

Utilization of Physician Services

Over three-quarters of all male respondents to the CCHS 2000-1 reported having received care provided by family physicians and/or physician specialists in the twelve-month period before the survey. Lower proportions of men living in Moderate and Weak MIZ areas reported using physician services compared with urban residents (CMA/CA: 83.3 percent; Weak MIZ: 76.6 percent). As Figure 4.1 shows, there were no statistically significant differences between urban and all rural areas in the use of services provided by family physicians. However, among those who had received care from specialists, men in Moderate MIZ (8.6 percent) and Weak MIZ (7.6 percent) areas had significantly lower utilization rates than urban residents (13.1 percent).

Over 80 percent of women reported having received care from family physicians and/or specialists in the twelve months prior to the survey. However, lower proportions of women in Weak MIZ (86.9 percent) and No MIZ (81.8 percent) areas received physician care in the previous twelve months compared with their urban counterparts (89.7 percent). As Figure 4.1 shows, there were no statistically significant differences in the proportions of women who had visited family doctors, except for a higher proportion among those in Weak MIZ areas (CMA/CA: 74.6 percent; Weak MIZ: 78.5 percent). On the other hand, women living in Weak MIZ areas reported significantly lower specialist utilization rates compared with those in cities (CMA/CA: 15.1 percent; Weak MIZ: 8.4 percent).

According to the HSAS, men living in all rural areas were more likely than their urban counterparts to report that they had not seen a doctor in the previous twelve months (see Table 4.1). The highest proportions were in Strong MIZ and No MIZ areas (CMA/CA: 26.5 percent; Strong MIZ: 31.6 percent; No MIZ: 33.6 percent). Between

Figure 4.1 Age-standardized proportions of men and women fifteen years of age or over who reported using physician services in the past twelve months, by type of physician and place of residence, Canada, 2000-1

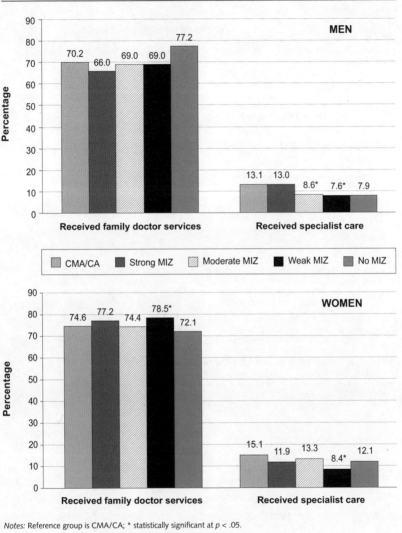

Notes: Reference group is CMA/CA; * statistically significant at $p < .05$.
Source: Statistics Canada, Canadian Community Health Survey, 2000-1.

21.1 percent and 24.1 percent of men reported four or more consultations with a family physician, and the differences between urban and rural areas were not statistically significant. Consultation with "other medical doctors" was reported by between 24.0 percent of men living in CMA/CA and 16.1 percent of men in No MIZ areas. Differences among

Table 4.1 Age-standardized proportions of Canadians twelve years of age or over who reported having consulted with a physician, by place of residence, Canada, 2000-1

Consultations to health services providers	Proportion (95% CI)				
	CMA/CA	Strong MIZ	Moderate MIZ	Weak MIZ	No MIZ
People who reported 0 consultations with family doctor					
Men	26.5 (25.9-27.2)	31.6 (29.7-33.4)*	29.4 (27.9-30.8)*	29.2 (28.0-30.5)*	33.6 (29.8-37.5)*
Women	15.3 (14.8-15.8)	16.5 (15.0-17.9)	17.4 (16.2-18.6)*	17.3 (16.3-18.3)*	20.3 (17.2-23.4)*
People who reported 4 or more consultations with family doctor					
Men	23.1 (22.5-23.7)	21.1 (19.6-22.6)	22.4 (21.2-23.6)	24.1 (23.0-25.2)	23.7 (20.8-26.6)
Women	34.4 (33.8-35.4)	33.2 (31.4-35.0)	34.9 (33.5-36.2)	37.2 (36.0-38.4)*	38.3 (34.9-41.6)
People who reported 1 or more consultations with other medical doctors					
Men	24.0 (23.4-24.6)	23.5 (21.8-25.1)	20.2 (18.9-21.4)*	19.0 (17.9-20.0)*	16.1 (13.4-18.9)*
Women	34.5 (33.9-35.1)	31.7 (29.9-33.4)*	29.5 (28.2-30.9)*	27.1 (26.0-28.3)*	30.4 (27.0-33.8)*

Notes: Reference group is CMA/CA; * statistically significant at $p < .05$.
Source: Statistics Canada, Health Services Access Survey, 2000-1.

CMA/CA and Moderate, Weak, and No MIZ areas were statistically significant.

Table 4.1 also shows that women living in Moderate, Weak, and No MIZ areas reported not having seen a family doctor in the previous twelve months in significantly greater proportions than their urban counterparts (CMA/CA: 15.3 percent; No MIZ: 20.3 percent). Over one-third of the female respondents reported having seen a family doctor four or more times. However, significant differences were found only between urban and Weak MIZ areas (CMA/CA: 34.4 percent; Weak MIZ: 37.2 percent). Residents in all MIZ areas also reported lower consultation rates with "other medical doctors" than those in urban areas, with the lowest proportions in Weak MIZ areas (CMA/CA: 34.5 percent; Weak MIZ: 27.1 percent).

Figure 4.2   Age-standardized percentages of individuals twelve years of age or over who reported requiring access to emergency health-care services, by place of residence, Canada, 2000-1

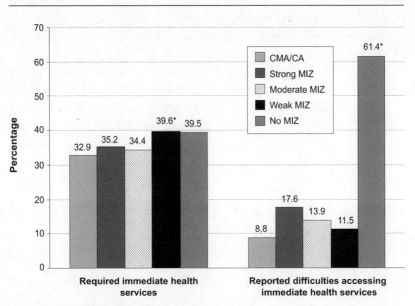

Notes: Reference group is CMA/CA; * statistically significant at *p* < .05.
Source: Statistics Canada, Health Services Access Survey, 2000-1.

Access to Immediate Health Care Services

As HSAS data in Figure 4.2 show, compared with their urban counterparts, a significantly higher proportion of residents in Weak MIZ areas reported needing immediate health-care services for minor health problems during the twelve-month period before the survey. At the same time, a significantly higher proportion of respondents living in No MIZ areas experienced difficulties accessing immediate health care because it was not available in the area or at the time required or due to transportation problems (CMA/CA: 8.8 percent; No MIZ: 61.4 percent).

Consultations with Other Practitioners

CCHS 2000-1 data suggest that consultations by Canadians with non-physician practitioners, such as nurses, dentists, complementary/alternative medicine (CAM) practitioners, and other providers, varied by place of residence. Consultations with a nurse were more frequent among rural than urban residents. Men and women living in Moderate, Weak, and No MIZ areas were more likely than those in cities to have one or more consultations with a nurse, with the highest proportion reported by individuals living in No MIZ areas (men, CMA/CA: 7.8 percent; No MIZ: 10.5 percent; women, CMA/CA: 11.6 percent; No MIZ: 20.3 percent).

Rural residents were less likely to have seen a dentist than urban residents. Whereas 59.8 percent of men living in CMAs/CAs reported having seen a dentist, only 44.1 percent of men living in No MIZ areas reported having at least one dental visit. Similarly, 64.2 percent of women living in CMAs/CAs reported having at least one dental visit compared with 45.4 percent of women in No MIZ areas. No substantial variations were found for consultations with CAM or other practitioners, but significantly lower proportions of men living in Moderate and No MIZ areas consulted with CAM providers compared with urban men.

Use of Community-Based Care

"Community-based care" is defined by the CCHS as any health care received outside a hospital or a doctor's office, such as home nursing care, home-based therapy, and personal care. Rural men and women in Strong, Moderate, and Weak MIZ areas were significantly less likely than their urban counterparts to use such services. But the difference between No MIZ residents and those in cities was not statistically significant.

Hospitalization

HMDB 2001-2 data were used to examine the utilization of hospital services at the national level. Data in Table 4.2 show that higher hospitalization rates were observed for all rural residents compared with urban residents, and the differences between urban and all rural areas were statistically significant. The highest hospitalization rates were reported in No MIZ areas among both men and women.

The average lengths of stay in hospitals increased with age but decreased with greater degree of rurality across all age groups and for both men and women. The length-of-stay patterns among men differed according to age. For those 20-44 years old, the average lengths of stay

Table 4.2   Age-standardized hospital discharge rates per 1,000 population, by place of residence and sex, Canada, Nova Scotia, and Ontario, 2001-2

	Rates (95% CI)				
	CMA/CA	Strong MIZ	Moderate MIZ	Weak MIZ	No MIZ
Canada					
Men	67.8 (67.7-68.0)	72.0 (71.4-72.7)*	83.8 (83.2-84.4)*	107.2 (106.5-107.8)*	116.6 (115.0-118.3)*
Women	88.2 (88.0-88.4)	98.6 (97.7-99.4)*	111.1 (110.3-111.8)*	140.0 (139.2-140.7)*	161.3 (159.2-163.4)*
Nova Scotia					
Men	89.5 (88.5-90.6)	108.1 (103.0-113.5)*	108.4 (105.5-111.3)*	100.6 (98.7-102.5)*	232.3 (213.4-252.8)*
Women	72.8 (71.8-73.8)	84.0 (79.4-88.8)*	87.3 (84.8-89.8)*	85.1 (83.4-86.8)*	171.8 (156.3-188.8)*
Ontario					
Men	66.4 (66.1-66.6)	74.2 (73.4-75.0)*	90.1 (89.0-91.2)*	114.4 (112.7-116.2)*	128.6 (123.5-133.9)*
Women	86.1 (85.8-86.3)	101.1 (100.1-102.1)*	119.6 (118.3-120.9)*	143.9 (141.8-146.0)*	178.8 (172.8-184.9)*

Notes: Pan-Canadian totals exclude Quebec due to insufficient geographical coding of source data; reference group is CMA/CA; * statistically significant at *p* < .05.
Source: CIHI, Hospital Morbidity Database, 2001-2.

were similar among rural and urban areas. Among those 45-64 years old, men living in Weak and No MIZ areas had significantly shorter hospital stays than their urban counterparts (CMA/CA: 8.24 days; No MIZ: 6.15 days). The average lengths of stay among rural men 65-74 years old were shorter compared with their urban counterparts. Finally, the average lengths of stay for men 75 years old or older living in Moderate, Weak, and No MIZ areas were shorter than for urban men in the same age group. Average lengths of stay among rural women were significantly shorter than among urban women, with the shortest lengths of stay reported by those in No MIZ areas. But there was one exception to this pattern: no significant difference was found between women 65-74 years old living in Moderate MIZ areas and those in CMAs/CAs.

Rural/Urban Differences in Physician Visits and Hospitalization:
Provincial Patterns

The following presents a descriptive analysis of all-cause physician visit
rates and all-cause hospital discharge rates derived from provincial
physician billing and hospital data from Nova Scotia and Ontario.

Nova Scotia

Physician Visits
In general, men and women living in Nova Scotia cities visited a family
physician or physician specialist more often than some of their rural
counterparts and less often than others in 2001-2 (see Figure 4.3). Men
living in Strong MIZ areas and women living in Strong and Moderate
MIZ areas had physician visit rates that were higher than those of urban
residents. In contrast, men living in Moderate, Weak, and No MIZ
areas and women living in Weak and No MIZ areas had visit rates that
were lower than the rates of those residing in cities.

In 2001-2, higher family physician visit rates were observed for both
men and women living in rural areas compared with their urban
counterparts. Men living in Strong, Moderate, and No MIZ areas had
visit rates that were higher than those for men in urban areas (CMA/
CA: 3,319 per 1,000; Strong MIZ: 3,639 per 1,000). Visit rates were
generally higher for rural women compared with those for their urban
counterparts. The highest visit rates were observed among women living in Strong MIZ areas (CMA/CA: 4,729 per 1,000; Strong MIZ:
5,412 per 1,000), and the lowest visit rates were observed among women
living in No MIZ areas (4,516 per 1,000).

The pattern of specialist visits in Nova Scotia differed between medical and surgical specialists. For visits to medical specialists, a significant
decreasing gradient by extent of rurality was observed for both men
and women. Urban residents had between 1.3 and 2.2 times the number of visits compared with residents in Weak or No MIZ areas.
Similarly, lower visit rates to surgical specialists were observed for all
rural areas, except among men in No MIZ areas and among women in
No MIZ areas.

Hospitalization
As Table 4.2 shows, compared with their urban counterparts, rural
Nova Scotians, regardless of sex, had higher all-cause hospital discharge

Figure 4.3 Average annual age-standardized physician visit rates per 1,000 population to all physicians, by place of residence and sex, Nova Scotia and Ontario, 2001-2

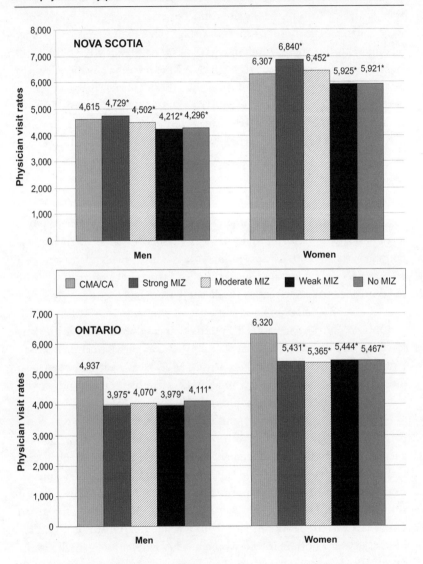

Notes: Reference group is CMA/CA; * statistically significant at *p* < .05.
Source: Nova Scotia and Ontario physicians claims files, 2001-2.

rates. Generally speaking, the discharge rates increased with increasing rurality. In 2001-2, the average lengths of stay in hospital for men of all ages living in Strong, Moderate, and No MIZ areas in Nova Scotia were shorter than those for men in urban areas (CMA/CA: 9.01 days; Strong MIZ: 7.00 days; Moderate MIZ: 7.09 days; No MIZ: 6.39 days). Among women, only those living in No MIZ areas had average lengths of stay that were significantly shorter than those for their urban counterparts (CMA/CA: 9.43 days; No MIZ: 6.92 days). The average lengths of stay for women in other MIZ areas were also shorter than those for urban women, but the differences were not statistically significant.

Ontario

Physician Visits
In Ontario, both men and women living in urban areas had more physician visits (i.e., family physicians and/or specialists) than their rural counterparts in 2001-2 (see Figure 4.3). Rural men's physician visit rates were lower compared with those of urban men, regardless of the MIZ area. Similarly, women in all rural areas had significantly lower visit rates in 2001-2 compared with urban women.

Ontario's physician claims data show that rural men had significantly lower family physician visit rates in 2001-2 compared with their urban counterparts, and men living in Strong MIZ areas had the lowest visit rates. Similarly, women living in all MIZ areas had significantly lower family physician visit rates than those in CMAs/CAs.

Specialist visit rates were significantly lower in all rural areas compared with urban areas, for both men and women in 2001-2, but the patterns differed between medical and surgical specialists. Medical specialist visit rates generally decreased with increasing rurality. Visit rates to medical specialists for urban residents were at least twice the rates for rural residents. Likewise, the visit rate to surgical specialists for urban Ontarians was higher than that for rural residents. But surgical specialist visit rates for both men and women in No MIZ areas were the highest of all rural areas in Ontario.

Hospitalization
According to the HMDB, all-cause hospital discharge rates were higher among women than men in Ontario in 2001-2. Table 4.2 shows that, compared with their urban counterparts, Ontarians living in all rural

areas – both males and females – had higher overall hospital discharge rates, and they increased with increasing rurality.

Ontario men living in all MIZ areas had shorter average lengths of stay than their urban counterparts, but none of the differences was statistically significant. Similarly, women living in all MIZ areas had shorter average lengths of stay than women in urban areas, but only some of the differences were statistically significant (CMA/CA: 7.06 days; Strong MIZ: 5.87 days; Moderate MIZ: 6.00 days).

Discussion

Using national data and data from two provinces, the research reported in this chapter investigated the relationships between place of residence and health services utilization at the national level and from the provincial perspective. This is the first national study that has examined patterns of health services utilization by rural Canadians, using the MIZ rural categorization. As such, it has gone beyond a simplistic representation of rural Canada as amorphous and undifferentiated. To enhance validity, the investigation was based on data from a variety of sources, including both survey and administrative data. Although slightly different results were obtained, depending on how questions were asked and how data were collected, the data were generally consistent, thus lending credence to the findings of the research.

Are there distinct patterns of health services utilization by rural Canadians? This question cannot be answered by a simple yes or no. Our findings have shown that differences between rural and urban Canadians with regard to utilization exist for some health services but not others. But several broad patterns are discernible. First, there are no major differences between rural and urban residents with regard to use of family physician services (except in the case of Ontario), but there are substantial differences in rates of utilization of services provided by physician specialists – rural residents are much less likely to see specialists. Second, while rural residents are more likely to see a nurse and visit an emergency department, they are less likely to use community-based care and services provided by other practitioners such as dentists. Third, rural Canadians are more likely than their urban counterparts to be hospitalized, but they tend to have shorter lengths of stay once they are admitted. Fourth, with regard to the use of physician and hospital services, provincial data from Nova Scotia and Ontario are generally consistent with national data. In addition, three important issues are discussed as follows.

"Rural" Is Not a Unitary Concept

This study has shown that rural is not homogeneous with regard to health services utilization. There are intra-rural differences, just as there are differences between rural and urban. Strong MIZ areas appear to be quite different from other rural areas with regard to various measures of health status and health services utilization. People living in Strong MIZ areas enjoy long average life expectancy (men: 77.4 years; women: 81.5 years) and long average health-adjusted life expectancy (men: 68.7 years; women: 71.3 years), compared with the average Canadian (CIHI et al. 2006). Strong MIZ residents, relative to other rural residents, might have fewer health-care needs, experience fewer access barriers, or be in a better position to overcome barriers if they do exist. Conversely, No MIZ residents have the shortest average life expectancy (men: 74.0 years; women: 81.4 years) and the shortest average health-adjusted life expectancy (men: 65.5 years; women: 69.9 years). They also tend to face major challenges in accessing care due to, among other things, geographical distances and lack of health-care resources in remote locations. From a health equity perspective, people in No MIZ areas (and, to some extent, in Weak MIZ areas) might have the greatest need for support. From a health-care planning perspective, a generic rural health strategy might be just as inappropriate as a one-size-fits-all health policy for the entire nation.

Different Patterns of Service Delivery

Rural residents do not necessarily use fewer services, but they might use a different range of services. For instance, hospitalization rates increase, but lengths of stay decrease, with increasing rurality. These findings might reflect dissimilarities in how health care is organized and delivered in non-urban areas or suggest that rural residents use hospitals for different reasons or in different ways. Differences between rural and urban family physicians with regard to practice profile have been noted (Pong and Pitblado 2005). Given the relative absence of specialists in rural areas, some rural family doctors expand their scope of practice to fill some of the service gaps. More so than their urban counterparts, rural family physicians work in emergency departments, admit patients to hospitals, attend to patients in hospitals and during follow-up care, and deliver babies. It is not surprising, therefore, to find considerable differences in how rural and urban residents use physician services. Compared with urban residents, rural Canadians are more reliant on family physicians but much less likely to use specialist services.

The greater use of hospitals and emergency departments by rural residents could be due to the lack of community-based ambulatory care facilities such as walk-in clinics and community health centres in many smaller communities (Haggerty et al. 2007). This might have implications for health-care planning. For instance, "ambulatory care sensitive conditions" are commonly used to gauge the effectiveness of community-based chronic disease management on the assumption that, if chronic diseases such as diabetes and congestive heart failure are not well managed in community settings, patients are more likely to be treated in emergency departments or hospitalized. But given that emergency department visits and hospitalizations are more prevalent in rural areas for reasons noted above, ambulatory care sensitive conditions as an indicator of effectiveness need to be used with caution in rural settings.

Rural residents are more likely than urban residents to have one or more consultations with a nurse. This might be due to the fact that physicians are unlikely to be found in remote or very small communities. Some of these communities have nursing stations or clinics staffed by outpost nurses or nurse practitioners who offer a broader range of health services, including diagnosis and treatment of minor or common diseases, with physicians, often family doctors, providing secondary care at a distance (e.g., by means of telemedicine) and/or periodic outreach visits (Humphreys, Mathews-Cowey, and Rolley 1996; MacLeod 1999; Pong 2002). This shows that differences in how health services are delivered and used in rural and urban areas are not necessarily undesirable but might reflect different conditions, needs, and health services delivery mechanisms (see Chapters 9, 11, and 13, this volume). What works in big cities might not work in smaller or more remote communities.

Health-Care System and Health Services Utilization

The Canadian Medicare system and the Canada Health Act aim to eliminate financial wherewithal as a condition for accessing necessary medical and hospital care. But universal access is meaningless if facilities, practitioners, and services are not available or very difficult to find in certain regions of the country. As a result, nearly all provincial and territorial governments have established special programs, such as the Underserviced Area Program in Ontario (Pong 2008) and the Travel Assistance Program in British Columbia (Ministry of Health 2006), to bring health services to residents in rural or more remote regions or to assist those who have to travel great distances to receive care. Such measures have helped to improve service access in rural areas.

This study has focused mostly on insured health services such as those provided by physicians and in hospitals. Services not covered under Medicare, such as rehabilitation therapy, homecare, and community mental health, have not been examined extensively, mostly because data are not available except from surveys such as the CCHS and HSAS. As a result, whether rural Canadians use such services at levels similar to urban residents remains largely unknown, though there are indications that such services are less available in rural areas (Cott et al. 2007; Kitchen et al. 2011; Mitchell, Strain, and Blandford 2007). Further investigations are needed, but they are not possible unless data on what nurses and other practitioners do in different geographical settings are captured and made available to researchers.

Whether urban and rural residents experience similar ease or difficulty accessing care is also largely unknown, again mostly because of data unavailability. For instance, although residents in remote communities have the same right to specialist care as those in metropolitan centres, they might have to travel great distances to see a specialist. This might require them to take time off work, suffer income loss, incur substantial travel costs, and endure greater emotional distress. In other words, the right to care is one thing; the costs entailed – both material and psychological – are another. This aspect also deserves further discussion.

Conclusion: The Role of Place in Health

Does place matter? Does where people live, work, and play make a difference in terms of access to and utilization of health services? Based on our findings, the answer to these questions is, yes, place does matter – in some cases. But what is it about place that makes it an important factor to consider in examining use of health services? This is a more difficult question to answer. As noted earlier, place, as a concept, embodies much more than locality. Thus, when we talk about the role of place in health, we are in fact talking about how health status and health behaviours, including health services utilization, are shaped by an aggregate of interacting factors in specific geographical locations. Now that this study, as well as others, has determined that there is a place for place in our understanding of health, it behooves us to go beyond locality and look at how these interacting factors affect, and are affected by, health in the context of rural Canada. A series of multivariate regression analyses in the original Canada's Rural Communities research project (not reported in this chapter) has shown that, after controlling for some socio-demographic, disease, and health behaviour variables, place of residence still has an independent effect on many aspects of health services utilization.

This chapter, together with Chapter 2, suggests that place is an important factor in understanding both population health status and health services utilization. Place should also figure prominently in the health policy discourse. One of the policy implications arising from these two chapters is that differences in how services are delivered and used across Canada – a vast country with considerable diversities – might be acceptable, but substantial and persistent regional variations in population health status should not be tolerated. This is because extensive and enduring health status disparities could be signs that some people in some places have a disproportionate disease burden and/or do not receive the care that they need. The interface between place and health could tell us where attention should be paid and where actions should be taken. But our understanding of the complex relationships between place and health is still limited, and there is considerable room for further exploration.

References

Alasia, A. 2003. "Rural and Urban Educational Attainment: An Investigation of Patterns and Trends, 1981-1996." *Rural and Small Town Canada Analysis Bulletin* 4, 5: 1-22.

Alasia, A., and N. Rothwell. 2003. "The Rural/Urban Divide Is Not Changing: Income Disparities Persist." *Rural and Small Town Canada Analysis Bulletin* 4, 4: 1-17.

Andersen, R.M. 1995. "Revisiting the Behavioral Model and Access to Medical Care: Does It Matter?" *Journal of Health and Social Behaviour* 36, 1: 1-10.

Andersen, R.M., and L.A. Aday. 1978. "Access to Medical Care in the U.S.: Realized and Potential." *Medical Care* 16, 4: 533-46.

Arcury, T.A., J.S. Preisser, W.M. Gesler, and J.M. Powers. 2005. "Access to Transportation and Health Care Utilization in a Rural Region." *Journal of Rural Health* 21, 1: 31-38.

Breslow, N.E., and N.E. Day. 1989. "Design Considerations." In *The Design and Analysis of Cohort Studies.* Vol. 2 of *Statistical Methods in Cancer Research,* edited by E. Heseltine, 272-315. Lyons: Oxford University Press.

Canadian Institute for Health Information (CIHI). 2006. *How Healthy Are Rural Canadians? An Assessment of Their Health Status and Health Determinants.* M. DesMeules and R. Pong, principal investigators. Ottawa: CIHI.

–. 2007. *Health Care in Canada 2007.* Ottawa: CIHI.

Casey, M.M., K.T. Call, and J.M. Klingner. 2001. "Are Rural Residents Less Likely to Obtain Recommended Preventive Healthcare Services?" *American Journal of Preventive Medicine* 21, 3: 182-88.

Cott, C.A., R.M.A. Devitt, L-B. Falter, L.J. Soever, and L.A. Passalant. 2007. "Barriers to Rehabilitation in Primary Health Care in Ontario: Funding and Wait Time for Physical Therapy Services." *Physiotherapy Canada* 59, 3: 173-83.

Curtis, S., and I.R. Jones. 1998. "Is There a Place for Geography in the Analysis of Health Inequality?" *Sociology of Health and Illness* 20, 5: 645-72.

Dixon, J., and N. Welch. 2000. "Researching the Rural-Metropolitan Health Differential Using the Social Determinants of Health." *Australian Journal of Rural Health* 8, 5: 254-60.

Fitzpatrick, K., and M. LaGory. 2000. *Unhealthy Places: The Ecology of Risk in the Urban Landscape.* New York: Routledge.

Haggerty, J.L., D. Roberge, R. Pineault, D. Larouche, and N. Touati. 2007. "Features of Primary Healthcare Clinics Associated with Patients' Utilization of Emergency Rooms: Urban-Rural Differences." *Healthcare Policy* 3, 2: 72-85.

Humphreys, J.S., S. Mathews-Cowey, and F. Rolley. 1996. *Health Service Frameworks for Small Rural and Remote Communities: Issues and Options.* Armidale, Australia: Department of Geography and Planning, University of New England.

Humphreys, J.S., S. Mathews-Cowey, and H.C. Weinand. 1997. "Factors in Accessibility of General Practice in Rural Australia." *Medical Journal of Australia* 166, 11: 557-80.

Kirby, M.J.L., and M. LeBreton. 2002. *Recommendations for Reform.* Vol. 6 of *The Health of Canadians: The Federal Role.* Ottawa: Standing Senate Committee on Social Affairs.

Kitchen, P., A. Williams, R.W. Pong, and D. Wilson. 2011. "Socio-Spatial Patterns of Home Care Use in Ontario, Canada: A Case Study." *Health and Place* 17: 195-206.

MacIntyre, S., S. MacIver, and A. Soomans. 1993. "Area, Class, and Health: Should We Be Focusing on Places or People?" *International Social Policy* 22, 2: 213-34.

MacLeod, M. 1999. "'We're It': Issues and Realities in Rural Nursing Practice." In *Health in Rural Settings: Contexts for Action,* edited by W. Ramp et al., 165-78. Lethbridge: University of Lethbridge.

Mathers, C.D., and D.J. Schofield. 1998. "The Health Consequences of Unemployment: The Evidence." *Medical Journal of Australia* 168, 4: 178-82.

Ministry of Health. 2006. *Travel Assistance Program Patients: Rural Health.* Victoria: Ministry of Health, http://www.health.gov.bc.ca/.

Mitchell, L.A., L.A. Strain, and A.A. Blandford. 2007. "Indicators of Home Care Use in Urban and Rural Settings." *Canadian Journal on Aging* 26, 3: 275-80.

Pong, R.W. 2002. *The Health Transition Fund Synthesis Series: Rural Health/Telehealth.* Ottawa: Health Canada, http://www.hc-sc.gc.ca/.

–. 2008. "Strategies to Overcome Physician Shortages in Northern Ontario: A Study of Policy Implementation over 35 Years." *Human Resources for Health* 6, 24: 9 pp. + appendix, http://www.human-resources-health.com/.

Pong, R.W., and J.R. Pitblado. 2005. *Geographic Distribution of Physicians in Canada: Beyond How Many and Where.* Ottawa: CIHI.

Romanow, R. 2002. *Building on Values: The Future of Health Care in Canada.* Saskatoon: Commission on the Future of Health Care in Canada.

Ronson, B., and I. Rootman. 2004. "Literacy: One of the Most Important Determinants of Health Today." In *Social Determinants of Health: Canadian Perspective,* edited by D. Raphael, 155-69. Toronto: Canadian Scholars' Press.

Xi, G., I. McDowell, R. Nair, and R. Spasoff. 2005. "Income Inequality and Health in Ontario." *Canadian Journal of Public Health* 96, 3: 206-11.

Part 2: Rural Health Human Resources

Chapter 5   Geographical Distribution of Rural Health Human Resources

J. Roger Pitblado

Key Points

- In Canada, the overall supply of health-care providers is increasing. However, this observation does not apply equally to all health occupational groups, nor does it take into consideration the supply differences between rural and urban areas of the country.
- The absolute numbers of health-care workers in rural Canada have increased in only 40 percent of the twenty-seven occupational groups discussed in this chapter. Those increases were insufficient to bring health-care provider-to-population ratios or percentages to levels enjoyed in urban areas of the country.
- Demographic characteristics differ significantly between rural and urban health-care occupational groups. Rural health-care workers tend to be older, and there are fewer men compared with their urban counterparts.
- Health-care workers are generally more mobile than the general population, and significant decreases in the numbers of rural health-care providers can be associated with rural-to-urban migration patterns.
- For many health-care occupational groups, basic supply-side planning and monitoring of internal migration patterns are inhibited due to the lack of adequate databases.

The need to pay special attention to health human resources (HHR) issues appears to have been recognized in Canada. That impression would be gained by listing the reports that have been published in this country over many decades by numerous commissions and task forces. These reports would include the relatively recent work of the Commission on the Future of Health Care in Canada (the "Romanow Report"; Romanow 2002) and the Standing Committee on Social Affairs, Science, and Technology (the "Kirby Report"; Kirby 2002). As well, the Health Council of Canada was established to monitor and report on the implementation of the 2003 First Ministers' Accord on Health Care Renewal. The accord (Health Canada 2003) declared that "appropriate planning and management of health human resources is key to ensuring that Canadians have access to the health providers they need." In a broader context, when the World Health Organization (WHO 2006, xv) released its annual report on World Health Day in April 2006, it stated that, "at the heart of each and every health system, the workforce is central to advancing health."

On closer inspection, the state of HHR planning might not be all that healthy. This is reflected in the joint call by the Canadian Medical Association and the Canadian Nurses Association (2005) for a pan-Canadian planning framework. Furthermore, in a review of the country's modelling capacity, Kazanjian and Apland (2004, 24) concluded that, "given the breadth of HHR research in universities, research institutes, professional associations, and other organizations across Canada and the fact that health human resources planning is a high priority component activity of ministries of health in each jurisdiction of Canada's federal system, the number of robust HHR models identified and discussed [in this report] can be described as meagre."

The need for improved HHR planning models and results is particularly relevant to rural and remote areas of Canada, where access to health-care providers is often very limited. Although the health-care workforce is relatively large (Canadian Institute for Health Information [CIHI] 2007a), it is unevenly distributed geographically in relationship to the distribution of Canadians as a whole (Pitblado 2007; Pitblado et al. 2002; Pong and Pitblado 2005). As well, that geographical distribution is constantly being modified by internal migration (movements within provinces or territories or from one province or territory to another) and external or international migration (movements from one country to another).

Although HHR planning is known to be a complex enterprise that requires multiple inputs and considerations (O'Brien-Pallas et al. 2007), there is often a paucity of national-level data for even basic supply-side modelling. This stems primarily from the fact that there are limited sources of data upon which to base such analyses. In this chapter, the objective is to provide a summative, empirical overview of the stock of health human resources in Canada. Although the focus is on the health-care workforces in rural areas of the country (see Chapter 1, this volume, for the "Rural and Small Town" [RST] definition of rural), selected comparisons with their urban counterparts are also provided.

Definitions and Data Issues

Health-Care Occupations

The provision of health care relies on the skills and efforts of many individuals in a wide variety of roles. One might expect to find, then, detailed databases to assist HHR planning in Canada. That is not the case. Although there are many good databases, particularly those held by the Canadian Medical Association, the provincial colleges or registrars of nurses, and the Canadian Institute for Health Information, they do not represent the full spectrum of health-care providers. Many of the databases that do exist are not national in scope and, in the context of this chapter, do not indicate where these individuals practise or their mobility characteristics. The lack of national, occupation-specific databases in which health-care workers are uniquely identified makes enumeration and mobility monitoring extremely problematic. Perhaps the only truly national databases that provide this information are based on the Canadian Census of Population.

The census is administered every five years using two questionnaires. The *short form* is completed by 80 percent of all households, while the *long form* is completed by the remaining 20 percent. The long form is the most relevant here as it is used to collect detailed socio-demographic and -economic information, including occupation and mobility.

With regard to occupations, 2001 census responses from persons fifteen years of age and older are coded into one of the categories of the *National Occupational Classification for Statistics* (Statistics Canada 2001). The 1991 and 1996 census responses were grouped using the

1991 *Standard Occupational Classification*. The equivalencies between these two classification systems are outlined on the Statistics Canada website (www.statcan.ca). Data from the 2006 census were not available at the time of writing (see the acknowledgments at the end of this chapter for additional data release information).

This chapter deals with twenty-seven workforce groups listed under the broad occupational category of "health occupations" using the Statistics Canada classification systems. These workforce groups include physicians, nurses, technical occupations, dental occupations, among others listed in later sections of the chapter.

There are difficulties associated with HHR planning if based solely on the census. The latter is based on the self-reporting of occupations, and responses might thereby be misinterpreted by Statistics Canada coders; information is provided about where people live and not necessarily where they work; and there is little else within the census that is reported about many of the characteristics (e.g., job position, responsibilities, education or training background, etc.) of the individuals within the occupations. Users of the census must also take into consideration that the enumeration is based on a 20 percent household sample adjusted using regression weighting to represent the whole population of health-care workers in the country. Also, the health occupation category does not include professionals who might well be considered as health-care providers, such as psychologists and social workers (CIHI 2001, 2007a). In spite of these known limitations, the census does provide us with adequate information to create an overview of rural and urban differences, geographical distribution, and mobility patterns of the majority of health occupational groups.

Geographical Distribution and Mobility

The primary interest in geographical distribution for HHR planning is in the spatial distribution of health-care providers relative to the distribution of the general population. It is the mismatch between these spatial distributions that captures the attention of the public, mass media, policy makers, health-care administrators, and researchers (Pitblado and Pong 1999). It is this mismatch, in Canada and elsewhere, that has generated a substantial literature dealing with "shortages" (see, e.g., Canadian Society for Medical Laboratory Science 2000; Gilbert 2004; Konieczna 2004; and Sobel et al. 2000) and "imbalances" (Dussault and Franceschini 2006; Zurn et al. 2004). Rural/urban differences and the general geographical distribution of physicians and registered nurses are reasonably well known. However, there is very little discussion of these important planning topics for any of the remaining health-care workforce groups (Pitblado 2007).

Migration can be viewed as the dynamic component of geographical distribution as people move from source to destination regions. It is also a reflection of a major HHR planning issue: namely, recruitment and retention (see also Chapter 7, this volume), with recruitment implying an increase in mobility and retention implying a decrease in mobility. In- or out-migration can affect source and destination regions in many different ways. In the context of remote rural communities in the United Kingdom, for example, it has been argued that "health professionals, working and residing locally, make a valuable contribution to the social structure of remote communities, in addition to health care, social care and economic contributions" (Farmer et al. 2003). Similar comments have been made in the context of the migration of rural nurses in Canada (Pitblado, Medves, and Stewart 2005).

One of the questions included in a recent WHO guide to the assessment of human resources for health (HRH) is this: "To what extent does internal migration of staff create distributional imbalance of HRH?" (2004, 10). Similarly, in a review of Canada's health-care providers, almost the same question was posed: "How many regulated and unregulated health care providers move each year and what is the impact of their migration on health care services?" (CIHI 2001, xi).

But once again there are only limited discussions of the migration patterns of Canada's health-care providers. Concern has been expressed about a "brain drain" of health-care workers moving out of the country, especially to the United States. However, "the interprovincial flow of physicians is far larger than the flow to the U.S. Maldistribution is as much or more of a problem than migration southward" (Helliwell, as quoted by Gray 1999, 1028). There are many studies of interprovincial migration of physicians (Basu and Rajbhandary 2006; Benarroch and Grant 2004; Rajbhandary and Basu 2006; Sempowski, Godwin, and Sequin 2002) and of nurses (Baumann et al. 2004; Pitblado, Medves, and Stewart 2005). And interprovincial migration statistics are a regular component of the many annual HHR publications of CIHI (e.g., 2007b, 2007c, 2007d). Rarely do these studies provide information about the movements of health personnel to or from rural areas of the country, nor do they deal with workforces other than physicians or nurses. One must turn again to the census to acquire data that would assist with such analyses.

The long form census questionnaire asks, among other questions, where all individuals fifteen years of age and older in a household lived one year ago and five years ago. Based on the results of the latter question, the five-year mobility status of Canadians can be determined (Statistics Canada 2002). These include results for non–movers and non-migrants, intraprovincial migrants, interprovincial migrants, and international migrants. As space is limited, this chapter is restricted to a discussion of only one form of *internal* migration, Canadian rural–urban mobility patterns. More detailed discussions of provincial/territorial distributions as well as international, interprovincial, and intraprovincial mobility characteristics can be found in Pitblado (2007).

Health Workforce Numbers and Demographics

In 2001, using the *National Occupational Classification for Statistics,* the Census of Population recorded a total of close to 750,000 persons in the category of health occupations. This represents an increase of 7.8 percent in this broad occupational classification since 1991. But that figure is not very representative of the changes that occurred for individual health-care occupational groups when split into rural and urban categories. Not all occupational groups experienced the same rate of growth (see Table 5.1).

Among the technical occupations, for example, the numbers of medical lab technologists and technicians decreased in both rural and urban areas. The largest increases, in both rural and urban areas of the country, were experienced by medical sonographers and electroencephalographic technologists. With the exception of rural audiologists/speech-language pathologists, all three of the rehabilitative workforces experienced substantial percentage increases in numbers in this ten-year period. Most of the other occupational groups included in Table 5.1 experienced relatively large percentage increases as well. Notable exceptions were the decreases in the numbers of registered nurses and licensed practical nurses. Although both urban and rural areas of the country experienced these decreases, the proportional losses in numbers of nurses (for both registered nurses and licensed practical nurses) were greatest in rural Canada.

Table 5.1 Percentage change in workforce numbers by health occupation for urban and rural areas of Canada, 1991-2001

Health occupation	Percentage change	
	Urban	Rural
Medical laboratory technologists and pathologists' assistants	-5.7	-6.3
Medical laboratory technicians	-20.0	-6.2
Respiratory therapists and clinical perfusionists	41.0	81.2
Medical radiation technologists	-2.6	2.9
Medical sonographers	93.8	108.3
Cardiology technologists	11.6	-25.0
Electroencephalographic and other diagnostic technologists	76.4	214.3
Audiologists and speech-language pathologists	60.9	3.4
Physiotherapists	42.0	66.3
Occupational therapists	65.6	89.7
Dentists	36.0	23.4
Denturists	19.5	-7.6
Dental hygienists and dental therapists	47.7	75.4
Dental technicians and laboratory bench workers	-5.7	101.6
Dental assistants	15.8	6.8
Pharmacists	37.9	21.6
Optometrists	31.0	-14.5
Opticians	55.1	36.4
Chiropractors	58.2	24.6
Dietitians and nutritionists	84.7	68.1
Ambulance attendants and other paramedical occupations	35.7	35.6
Registered nurses	-1.8	-5.8
Licensed practical nurses	-11.5	-13.4
Nurse aides, orderlies, and patient service associates	18.7	3.9
Specialist physicians	33.0	70.3
General practitioners and family physicians	11.7	5.1
All physicians	19.0	15.1

Source: Statistics Canada, Census of Population, 1991 and 2001.

As a general rule, large increases or decreases in the 1991-2001 percentages of health-care providers were associated with those occupations with relatively small absolute numbers. In these groups, the addition or loss of a few individuals had a comparatively large impact on the proportional changes over this decade. The relationships between the numbers of these health-care occupational groups and those of the general population are explored later in the chapter.

Many health-care workforces are composed predominantly of either males or females. Changes in workforce male-female mix are increasingly included in HHR discussions since the processes of masculinization and feminization can have significant impacts on the supply of health-care providers and on professional practice patterns (Evans 2004; Incitti et al. 2003).

Although there was little change in the male-female proportional composition of most health occupational groups from 1991 to 2001, there were some significant differences between rural and urban areas of the country. These differences are illustrated in Figure 5.1, where the 2001 proportions of males in each occupational group are shown for both rural and urban areas of the country. With few exceptions, there were higher proportions of male health workers in urban Canada compared with rural Canada. To illustrate, approximately 36 percent (210 of 585) of rural dental technologists in 2001 were male compared with about 55 percent (3,190 of 6,780) of their urban colleagues. The difference between the two is shown as -19.3 percent in Figure 5.1.

One might argue that having a male-female proportional composition similar to that of the general population is not appropriate for each health occupational group. However, in times of so-called shortages, it seems that we are missing out by not recruiting or making professions such as dentistry more attractive to females or cardiology technology more attractive to males, especially in rural areas of the country.

Based on numerous observations and various analytical scenarios, Canada's population is known to be aging, and it is expected to age more rapidly in the coming years with decreasing proportions of children, increasing proportions of seniors, and climbing median and average ages (Bélanger, Martel, and Caron-Malenfant 2005). How this trend will affect the health-care systems of the country is subject to considerable debate (Denton, Gafni, and Spencer 2003; Evans et al. 2001). Not debated is the fact that, along with the overall population, health-care workforces are also aging. And, generally, these workforces are aging faster than the general workforce. Among others, pharmacists are projecting shortfalls in their numbers that will grow as the workforce continues to age (Canadian Pharmacists Association 2005).

In 2001, the average ages of health occupational groups in rural Canada ranged from thirty-five years for dental assistants to forty-nine years for specialist physicians. Average ages for the same occupational groups in urban areas of the country ranged from thirty-four years to

Figure 5.1   Percentage of males by health occupation in rural Canada, 2001

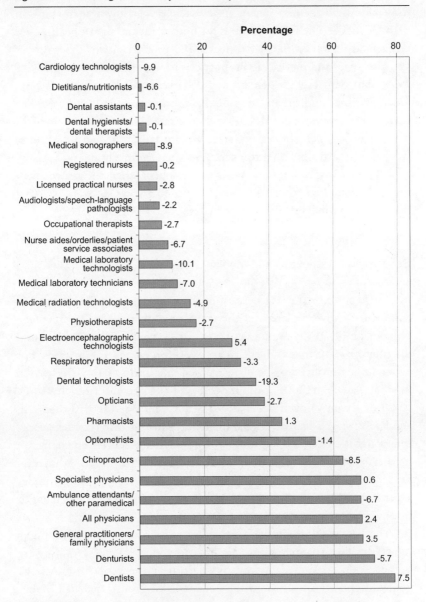

Note: Figures at the ends of the bars show the absolute percentage differences in the proportion of males in the respective health occupations in urban Canada in 2001.
Source: Statistics Canada, Census of Population, 2001.

forty-five years respectively. Few rural occupational groups among those discussed in this chapter have average ages lower than those in urban Canada. The general trends for both rural and urban health-care workers are very similar, with decreasing proportions in the younger age categories and increasing proportions in the older age categories. In 1991, approximately 23 percent and 25 percent of all health-care providers in rural and urban areas of the country, respectively, were less than thirty years of age. By 2001, the equivalent percentages were 15 percent and 16 percent respectively. We are failing to recruit younger workers into the health professions, especially in rural areas of the country. If early retirements become the norm, then the concerns of the Canadian Pharmacists Association cited earlier as well as many other occupational groups are justified (see also O'Brien-Pallas, Alksnis, and Wang 2003).

Geographical Distribution and Mobility Patterns

In 2001, approximately 21 percent of the Canadian population lived in rural and small-town areas of the country, a decrease of 2 percentage points from 1991. These percentages can be compared with the rural distribution of Canada's health-care workforces (see Figure 5.2). For example, just over 25 percent of licensed practical nurses were located in rural Canada in 2001, a slight decrease (-0.4 percent) from 1991.

Of the twenty-seven occupational groups included in that diagram, rural percentages decreased for sixteen of the health-care provider workforces and increased for another ten, and one experienced no change in its rural proportions from 1991 to 2001. Most of the increases in rural percentages for these workforces occurred within a range of just under 1 percent to just over 5 percent. Decreases ranged from -0.1 percent to just below 6 percent.

Whether or not there were decreases or increases, Figure 5.2 highlights the fact that very few health-care occupational groups were present in rural Canada with anywhere near the proportions of the general population. Of the three occupational groups that had higher rural proportions than the general population, two (nurse aides etc. and licensed practical nurses) experienced decreases in those proportions since 1991, while the third (ambulance attendants and other paramedical occupations) had no change over the ten-year period.

Another way to look at the relationship between the geographical distribution of health occupational groups and the general population is

Figure 5.2   Proportions of the general population and the health-care workforces located in rural Canada in 2001

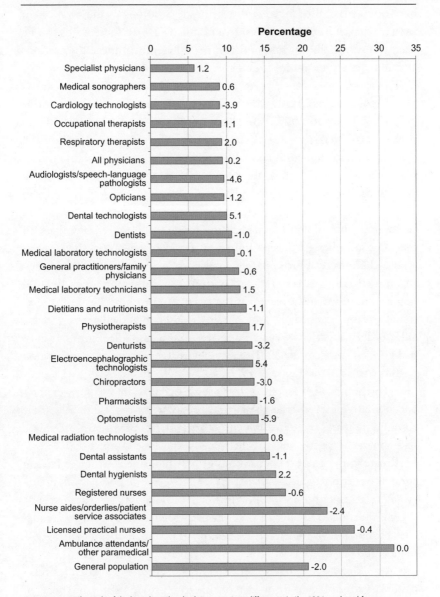

Note: Figures at the ends of the bars show the absolute percentage differences in the 1991 rural workforces for the respective health occupations.
Source: Statistics Canada, Census of Population, 1991 and 2001.

to examine the number of health-care providers per 100,000 persons. The nation-wide health-care-provider-to-population ratios presented here often mask provincial and territorial variations in these ratios. In spite of known limitations (Pong and Pitblado 2001), these ratios can be used to examine both temporal and spatial trends in these associations and continue to be useful if employed with caution.

The range in health-care-provider-to-population ratios by occupational group is graphically shown in many publications (see, e.g., CIHI 2007a, 57; Pitblado 2007, 10). Those illustrations provide national and perhaps provincial/territorial ratios at best. They do not highlight the differences between rural and urban areas of the country or differences within rural areas. In 2001, for example, there were approximately 100 physicians (family physicians plus specialist physicians) practising in rural Canada for every 100,000 persons in the general rural population. In comparison, urban areas had approximately 150 more physicians for the same number of people living in urban Canada. As another example, there were approximately 35 physiotherapists per 100,000 population in rural Canada compared with 61 physiotherapists per 100,000 population in urban Canada. Of the twenty-seven health-care occupational groups examined, only three (licensed practical nurses, nurse aides/orderlies/patient service associates, and paramedical professionals) had population ratios in 2001 that were greater in rural areas compared with urban areas of the country.

Even though 40 percent of the health occupational groups experienced relative increases in their rural proportions (see Table 5.1), their absolute increases were insufficient to bring their health-care-provider-to-population ratios up to the level experienced in urban areas. Fortunately, the three occupational groups described earlier as having rural proportions greater than that of the general population maintained relatively high ratios. Nurses, with various skill sets, are exceedingly important in the provision of health-care services in rural Canada. The proportion of registered nurses in rural Canada decreased by less than 1 percent from 1991 to 2001. However, given the overall size of this workforce, even that small percentage represents a loss of a relatively large number of front-line health-care providers in rural areas of the country.

The relative proportions and population ratios for rural and urban areas of the country can be useful as general guidelines for health human resources planning. In the United States, higher nurse-to-population and physician-to-population ratios are associated with higher overall state health rankings (Bigbee 2008). On the other hand, using physician distribution in the United States, Goodman and Grumbach (2008, 337) argue that, "if the goals for a health system are access, quality, better outcomes, and efficiency, indiscriminately aiming for more physicians per capita is unlikely to move the system toward better performance." This can be contrasted to the results of a Canadian study that found statistically significant positive impacts on self-reported general and mental health status with higher family physician-to-population ratios (Sarma and Peddigrew 2008). But what is the "right" ratio for each health occupational group? It would be very difficult to find a consensus on this question. As well, some health occupational groups are unlikely to be present in large numbers in rural Canada. Many of the health-care provider groups examined in this chapter require the use of specialized equipment or services often found only in clinics or hospitals in cities.

Little information is available that examines the detailed movements of Canadians to and from urban or rural areas of the country (Audas and McDonald 2004; Dupuy, Mayer, and Morissette 2000). And, until recently, there has been none at a national or provincial/territorial level for the majority of health-care providers (Pitblado 2007). The gap in information for the general Canadian population (aged fifteen years and older) has been filled, to some extent, by the recent work of Clemenson and Pitblado (2007) and Rothwell et al. (2002). Those studies indicate that for the general population there was a very small negative rural net migration over the period 1986-91 followed by a positive rate in 1991-96, when more Canadians moved from urban to rural areas of the country than the reverse. However, the rural net migration rate was again negative in the census migration period of 1996-2001. Similar rural-urban flow patterns were recorded for the same migration periods for the aggregate of all health-care providers. However, the net migration rates were higher. This is only partially explained by the smaller numbers of health-care workers relative to the general population. More importantly, it reflects the fact that the health workforce in Canada is highly mobile, more so than the general population.

The aggregate statistics briefly outlined above mask the wide variations in rural-urban mobility patterns of individual health occupational groups. Rural net migration rates for each of these workforces for the 1996-2001 migration period are shown in Figure 5.3. Sixty-five percent of Canada's health workforce groups had a negative rural net migration rate during that period of time. Those rates ranged from

-0.4 percent for licensed practical nurses to -12.5 percent for respiratory therapists. Excluding the one workforce (medical sonagraphers) that had a neutral rate, only 35 percent of the workforces shown in Figure 5.3 had positive rural net migration rates during 1996-2001. These

Figure 5.3   Rural net migration rates by health occupations for the 1996-2001 migration period

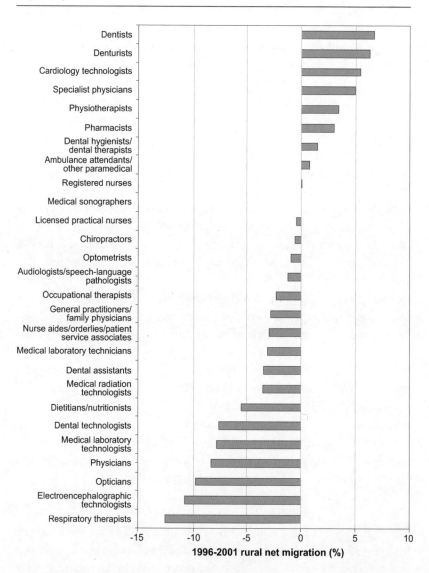

Source: Statistics Canada, Census of Population, 2001.

positive rates ranged from 0.1 percent for registered nurses to 6.7 percent for dentists.

Looking to the Future

The goal of HHR planning is often expressed as "having the right people with the right skills in the right place at the right time to provide the right services to the right people" (Birch 2002, 109). That task is especially difficult if we do not know some of the basic characteristics of our health-care workforces and who is working where and when and whether or not they are highly mobile. This chapter was designed to provide some of those basics within the limited space available. Interested readers should explore some of the many references provided and additional ones in Pitblado (2007).

As I was writing this chapter, the premiers of the provinces and territories met in July 2008 for their annual Council of the Federation. They signed a new Agreement on Internal Trade that will ease some of the current barriers to interprovincial labour mobility. Partially implemented in April 2009, the agreement will enable most citizens and permanent residents in regulated occupations who are accredited in one province or territory to move to another without requiring additional credentials. Although this agreement was not universally welcomed, the editorials in most of the major newspapers in the country hailed the move as a positive step. Such a move would acknowledge the long-held view that "migration is the main mechanism through which regional and local populations adjust to changing economic and social circumstances" (Bryant and Joseph 2001, 133).

This new mobility agreement will likely have a significant impact on the distribution of Canada's rural health-care workers. Rural areas of the country are now in a deficit position with regard to the complements of most health occupational groups. Access to health facilities and services will become even more difficult if increasing numbers of health-care workers move out of those areas (see Chapter 4, this volume). It will be incumbent on planners, governments, and employers of those rural health-care providers to increase their recruitment and retention efforts just to maintain those complements. Nation-wide, occupation-specific databases that uniquely identify and describe the professional and mobility characteristics of Canada's health-care providers are needed to assist with these important tasks.

Acknowledgments

Much of this chapter is based on my work in preparing a series of reports for the Canadian Institute for Health Information under the banner Distribution and Internal Migration of Canada's Health Care Workforce. A summary and fifteen occupation-specific reports (although only one is included in the references list here [Pitblado 2007]) were prepared for that series and are freely available on the CIHI website (http://www.cihi.ca). I am currently collaborating with CIHI to update that work using more recent census data.

References

Audas, R., and T. McDonald. 2004. "Rural-Urban Migration in the 1990s." *Canadian Social Trends* 73 (summer): 17-24. Statistics Canada Catalogue No. 11-008.

Basu, K., and S. Rajbhandary. 2006. "Interprovincial Migration of Physicians in Canada: What Are the Determinants?" *Health Policy* 76: 186-93.

Baumann, A., J. Blythe, C. Kolotylo, and J. Underwood. 2004. *Mobility of Nurses in Canada.* Ottawa: Nursing Sector Study Corporation.

Bélanger, A., L. Martel, and É. Caron-Malenfant. 2005. *Population Projections for Canada, Provinces, and Territories 2005-2031.* Catalogue No. 91-520-XIE. Ottawa: Minister of Industry.

Benarroch, M., and H. Grant. 2004. "The Interprovincial Migration of Canadian Physicians: Does Income Matter?" *Applied Economics* 36: 2335-45.

Bigbee, J.L. 2008. "Relationships between Nurse- and Physician-to-Population Ratios and State Health Rankings." *Public Health Nursing* 25: 244-52.

Birch, S. 2002. "Health Human Resource Planning for the New Millennium: Inputs in the Production of Health, Illness, and Recovery in Populations." *Canadian Journal of Nursing Research* 33: 109-14.

Bryant, C., and A.E. Joseph. 2001. "Canada's Rural Population: Trends in Space and Implications in Place." *Canadian Geographer* 45: 132-37.

Canadian Institute for Health Information (CIHI). 2001. *Canada's Health Care Providers.* Ottawa: CIHI.

—. 2007a. *Canada's Health Care Providers, 2007.* Ottawa: CIHI.

—. 2007b. *Supply, Distribution, and Migration of Canadian Physicians, 2006.* Ottawa: CIHI.

—. 2007c. *Workforce Trends of Registered Nurses in Canada, 2006.* Ottawa: CIHI.

—. 2007d. *Workforce Trends of Licensed Practical Nurses in Canada, 2006.* Ottawa: CIHI.

Canadian Medical Association and Canadian Nurses Association. 2005. *Toward a Pan-Canadian Planning Framework for Health Human Resources.* Ottawa: Canadian Medical Association, http://www.cma.ca/.

Canadian Pharmacists Association. 2005. *Pharmacy Human Resources in Canada: A Study of Pharmacists and Pharmacy Technicians: Project Summary.* Ottawa: Canadian Pharmacists Association, http://www.pharmacists.ca/.

Canadian Society for Medical Laboratory Science. 2000. "Survey Reveals Shortage of Medical Laboratory Technologists Approaching Faster than Anticipated." News release, 10 April. Hamilton: Canadian Society for Medical Laboratory Science, http://www.csmls.org/.

Clemenson, H.A., and J.R. Pitblado. 2007. "Recent Trends in Rural-Urban Migration." *Our Diverse Cities* 3: 25-29.

Denton, F.T., A. Gafni, and B.G. Spencer. 2003. "Requirements for Physicians in 2030: Why Population Aging Matters Less than You Think." *Canadian Medical Association Journal* 168: 1545-47.

Dupuy, R., F. Mayer, and R. Morissette. 2000. *Rural Youth: Stayers, Leavers, and Return Migrants.* Catalogue No. 11F0019MPE, Issue No. 152. Ottawa: Statistics Canada.

Dussault, G., and M.C. Franceschini. 2006. "Not Enough There, Too Many Here: Understanding Geographical Imbalances in the Distribution of the Health Workforce." *Human Resources for Health* 4, 12, http://www.human-resources-health.com/.

Evans, J. 2004. "Men Nurses: A Historical and Feminist Perspective." *Journal of Advanced Nursing* 47: 321-28.

Evans, R.G., K.M. McGrail, S.G. Morgan, M.L. Barer, and C. Hertman. 2001. "Apocalypse No: Population Aging and the Future of Health Care Systems." *Canadian Journal of Aging* 20, Supplement 1: 160-91.

Farmer, J., W. Lauder, H. Richards, and S. Sharkey. 2003. "Dr. John Has Gone: Assessing Health Professionals' Contribution to Remote Rural Community Sustainability in the UK." *Social Science and Medicine* 57: 673-86.

Gilbert, C. 2004. "OMA President Says Its Crucial Doctor Shortage Issue Addressed: Many Physicians Deciding to Leave Ontario." *Northern Life* [Sudbury], 7 March, 6.

Goodman, D.C., and K. Grumbach. 2008. "Does Having More Physicians Lead to Better Health System Performance?" *Journal of the American Medical Association* 299: 335-37.

Gray, C. 1999. "How Bad Is the Brain Drain?" *Canadian Medical Association Journal* 161: 1028-29.

Health Canada. 2003. First Ministers' Accord on Health Care Renewal. Ottawa: Health Canada, http://www.hc-sc.gc.ca/.

Incitti, F., J. Rourke, L.L. Rourke, and M-A. Kennard. 2003. "Rural Women Family Physicians: Are They Unique?" *Canadian Family Physician* 49: 320-27.

Kazanjian, A., and L. Apland. 2004. *Estimating National Health Human Resources Modeling Capacity.* Vancouver: Department of Health Care and Epidemiology, Faculty of Medicine, University of British Columbia.

Kirby, M.J.L. (chair). 2002. *The Health of Canadians: The Federal Role. Final Report. Volume Six: Recommendations for Reform.* Ottawa: Standing Senate Committee on Social Affairs, Science and Technology.

Konieczna, M. 2004. "Prescription Needed for Pharmacist Shortage." *Globe and Mail,* 21 May, C1.

O'Brien-Pallas, L., C. Alksnis, and S. Wang. 2003. *Bringing the Future into Focus: Projecting RN Retirement in Canada.* Ottawa: CIHI.

O'Brien-Pallas, L., G. Tomblin Murphy, S. Birch, G. Kephart, R. Meyer, K. Eisler, L. Lethbridge, and A. Cook. 2007. *Health Human Resources Modelling: Challenging the Past, Creating the Future.* Ottawa: Canadian Health Services Research Foundation.

Pitblado, J.R. 2007. *Summary Report: Distribution and Internal Migration of Canada's Health Care Workforce.* Ottawa: CIHI.

Pitblado, J.R., J.M. Medves, M.L.P. MacLeod, N.J. Stewart, and J.C. Kulig. 2002. *Supply and Distribution of Registered Nurses in Rural and Small Town Canada, 2000.* Ottawa: CIHI.

Pitblado, J.R., J.M. Medves, and N.J. Stewart. 2005. "For Work and for School: Internal Migration of Canada's Rural Nurses." *Canadian Journal of Nursing Research* 37: 102-21.

Pitblado, J.R., and R.W. Pong. 1999. *Geographic Distribution of Physicians in Canada.* Report prepared for Health Canada. Sudbury: Centre for Rural and Northern Health Research, Laurentian University.

Pong, R.W., and J.R. Pitblado. 2001. "Don't Take 'Geography' for Granted! Some Methodological Issues in Measuring Geographic Distribution of Physicians." *Canadian Journal of Rural Medicine* 6: 103-12.

–. 2005. *Geographic Distribution of Physicians in Canada: Beyond How Many and Where.* Ottawa: CIHI.

Rajbhandary, S., and K. Basu. 2006. "Interprovincial Migration of Physicians in Canada: Where Are They Moving and Why?" *Health Policy* 79: 265-73.

Romanow, R.J. (commissioner). 2002. *Building on Values: The Future of Health Care in Canada.* Saskatoon: Commission on the Future of Health Care in Canada.

Rothwell, N., R.D. Bollman, J. Tremblay, and J. Marshall. 2002. "Migration to and from Rural and Small Town Canada." *Rural and Small Town Canada Analysis Bulletin* 3, 6: 1-24. Statistics Canada Catalogue No. 21-006-XIE.

Sarma, S., and C. Peddigrew. 2008. "The Relationship between Family Physician Density and Health Related Outcomes: The Canadian Evidence." *Cahiers de sociologie et de démographie médicales* 48: 61-105.

Sempowski, I.P., M. Godwin, and R. Seguin. 2002. "Physicians Who Stay versus Physicians Who Go: Results of a Cross-Sectional Survey of Ontario Rural Physicians." *Canadian Journal of Rural Medicine* 7: 173-79.

Sobel, M., P. Litwin, C. Seville, and C. Homuth. 2000. "The Coming RT Shortage." *Revue canadienne de la thérapie respiratoire* 36 (winter): 38-42.

Statistics Canada. 2001. *National Occupational Classification for Statistics.* Catalogue No. 12-583-XPE. Ottawa: Ministry of Industry.

–. 2002. *Profile of the Canadian Population by Mobility Status: Canada, a Nation on the Move.* 2001 Census Analysis Series. Catalogue No. 96F0030XIE2001006. Ottawa: Industry Canada.

World Health Organization (WHO). 2004. *A Guide to Rapid Assessment of Human Resources for Health.* Geneva: WHO, http://www.who.int/.

–. 2006. *The World Health Report: Working Together for Health.* Geneva: WHO.

Zurn, P., M.R. Dal Poz, B. Stilwell, and O. Adams. 2004. "Imbalance in the Health Workforce." *Human Resources for Health* 2, 13, http://www.human-resources-health.com/.

Chapter 6   Rural Health Training Institute

P. Goodman

Key Points

- The Rural Health Training Institute can be described as a "branding" depiction of an innovative model comprised of four key components: collaborative partnerships between academia and health care; multi-disciplinary students; multi-sector placements; and multi-dimensional focus spanning the career spectrum for rural practice.
- Given the uniqueness of rural health, each component in isolation will not have as powerful an impact on rural health services delivery.
- Rather, a synthesis of these components serves to attract students and health-care professionals to rural communities; increase training opportunities for students in rural communities; and adequately prepare students for the uniqueness of rural and primary care practice.
- This case study provides steps for the implementation of an innovative rural health training model that could be considered for replication in other similar rural communities.

Lakeridge Health is a publicly funded community hospital providing services that range from primary care to tertiary care to both urban and rural communities of Durham Region in central-eastern Ontario (rural as per the "Rural and Small Town" definition [du Plessis et al. 2001]). The Rural Health Training Institute (RHTI) was conceptualized as a means to address the unique needs of rural health, particularly in the training of health-care professionals for rural practice. Although a search of the literature identified international initiatives that addressed the encouragement of health-care professionals to rural practice, it did not uncover any published Canadian models that addressed the gaps specific to rural health training. These gaps, and a synthesis of the key components to address them, became the basis upon which the conceptual framework for the RHTI initiative was formed.

The goal of the RHTI is to enhance health service delivery to patients and their families living in rural communities of Durham Region. The objectives for the RHTI are to brand an innovative rural health-training model that highlights the uniqueness of rural health needs; to attract students and health-care professionals to rural communities; to adequately prepare students for the uniqueness of rural and primary care practice; to increase training opportunities for students in the health professions in rural communities; and to strengthen partnerships between academic centres and community health-care providers. The most important element for consideration and implementation of the RHTI is to fund or extend a position whose role is to identify, facilitate, and coordinate existing resources in participating organizations.

The cost of the initiative was $20,000, primarily to offset student accommodation and transportation. Operational costs did not include the human resources required to develop and manage the RHTI since these responsibilities were added to existing roles in participating organizations. Similarly, capital and operational costs were not necessary for physical space since the RHTI is not located in a separate building. In this sense, the RHTI is a virtual institute in which an existing office at Lakeridge Health centralizes the administration of various placement sites, and once the schedule is finalized the students are physically located at each of the selected sites. Thus, the RHTI can be described as a branding depiction of an innovative model that synthesizes the four elements unique to rural health training. This case study outlines the planning and sequential steps for implementation of an RHTI model that could be considered for replication in other similar rural communities.

Step 1: Review of Evidence

A literature review was conducted to compare the rural and urban contexts of health-care delivery for the purpose of identifying gaps in meeting rural health-training needs. The literature noted that the urban context of clinical practice is characterized by a high-density population in which health care is accessed for isolated medical conditions (Kamien

1996; Probst et al. 2002). Practitioners tend to be specialists working in secondary or tertiary care facilities; the referral base consists of a wide range of specialists and other health-care professionals in hospitals and/ or communities (Romanow 2002). This critical mass of health-care professionals enhances accessibility both for patient care and for inter-professional networking and support (McNair et al. 2001).

In comparison, the rural context of clinical practice is characterized by a low-density population in which health care is accessed for comprehensive care, including non-medical conditions (Kamien 1996; Probst et al. 2002). Health-care practitioners tend to be generalists working in a primary care approach; the referral base in rural practice has a limited range of health-care professionals and few or no specialists available in the community (Romanow 2002). This situation necessitates multi-tasking, service coordination, and referrals outside the community, so treatment is further impeded by time, distance, and availability (Kamien 1996). Limited access to interprofessional networking and support exacerbates professional isolation, thereby compromising retention efforts (McNair et al. 2001). Recruitment efforts are further jeopardized if health-care professional students are ill prepared for rural practice (Paterson, McColl, and Paterson 2004).

This contrast in clinical practice between urban and rural contexts highlights the need for a training model that adequately prepares health-care professional students for the realities of rural practice. The unique characteristics of rural practice cannot simply adapt generic or urban-centric models that do not meet rural health-care needs. Rather, the very nature of generalist rural practice necessitates a training model that emphasizes the sharing of clinical, education, and research activities by disciplines across the spectrum of health-care and academic sectors (Medves et al. 2006).

A rural health-training model that encompasses rural-centric clinical, education, and research opportunities can increase exposure, experience, and socialization in rural settings (Christianson and Grogan 1990; Tepper 1999). In turn, a synergy of these opportunities can maximize both health-care professional students' and professionals' confidence and inclination for rural practice. Such an innovative model can strengthen the linkages between academic centres, hospitals, and community health-care providers, thereby narrowing the gaps currently experienced by rural patients and professionals alike (Romanow 2002). Students would be adequately prepared for the uniqueness of rural practice, characterized by a generalist knowledge and skill base;

collaborative interprofessional teamwork; integrated practice among health-care providers in the community; and comprehensive patient-/family-centred care (Medves et al. 2006).

Based on the literature review, four key components were identified as critical to addressing the gaps in rural health training: collaborative partnerships, multi-disciplinary students, multi-sector placements, and multi-dimensional focus. Several international initiatives have been implemented to address some of these gaps, such as the establishment of Rural Health Training Units across Australia (Degn 1993; National Association of Rural Health Training Units 1999) and Area Health Education Centers throughout the United States (National Rural Association 2006).

The Commonwealth government's establishment of six university Departments of Rural Health in Australia is aimed at increasing the rural and remote health workforce through multi-disciplinary education and training centres in rural and remote settings, encouraging rural rotations of undergraduate and postgraduate trainees in a range of disciplines, and promoting professional support, education, and training for rural health workers (Humphreys et al. 2000; Humphreys and Nichols 2009). Such initiatives are successful in meeting some of the identified gaps in rural health training, in which partnerships between the university and health-care providers are forged, multi-disciplinary placements are developed, and rural-centric curriculum, professional development, and research are emphasized.

Area Health Education Centers (AHECs) are government-funded centres established by an act of the US Congress in 1971. In 2009, fifty-four AHECs served their communities through 208 centres in forty-seven states. The main purpose of the AHECs is to connect students to health career professionals and to communities to improve health-care outcomes. The AHECs focus on developing community-based health-care education programs, specifically to meet the health-care needs of rural and under-served areas, and promoting health careers (National Rural Health Association 2006). The website for the National Area Health Center Organization, http://www.nationalahec.org, outlines the successes of each of the established AHECs. The typical AHEC's functions are to enhance access to quality primary and preventive health care, provide information on health careers exploration for students, arrange health professional student placements in an under-served population, offer accredited continuing education opportunities, and link resources and connections to health professionals in under-served areas. An example is the Western Maryland AHEC, which used the following four-prong approach to prepare allied health students to be interdisciplinary team members in rural areas: in-class instruction, web-based modules, service-learning programs, and faculty development workshops (Fertman et al. 2005).

The RHTI model is a case study in Canada that builds on the success of these initiatives through a further synthesis of the four key components.

Collaborative Partnerships

Collaborative partnerships between academic centres and health-care providers are essential for sharing resources, specifically in the areas of human resources, technology infrastructure, and funds. Human resources are a challenge since a critical mass of students and preceptors is required, as is sufficient administrative and faculty support to coordinate the logistics of a training model. Technology infrastructure is required for video-conferencing capability to enable students to continue their classroom instruction while off-site, multi-sector sites to communicate and share clinical consultations, and faculty development sessions to be held across all sites. Funds are essential not only for human and technology infrastructure but also for student accommodation and transportation, which are often cited as pivotal factors in the choice of a rural placement.

Multi-Disciplinary Focus

There is inadequate emphasis on collaborative training for health-care professionals across the spectrum of disciplines. Traditional training models tend to isolate training to a single discipline at a time; few if any appear to integrate the training of a set of health-care professionals in rural settings. Yet rural practice necessitates interprofessional collaboration, which fosters the efficient use of scarce human health professional resources by augmenting roles while shaping best practices in adhering to patient-centred care (D'Eon 2005; McNair et al. 2001). Thus, a rural training model that emphasizes the immersion of a range of health-care students into interprofessional teams might fill the gap of traditional mono-discipline training models. In this case, the RHTI would have multiple occupations work together, such as physiotherapy and nursing students placed in the same setting at the same time.

Multi-Sector Placements

There is insufficient emphasis on integrated training for health-care professionals across a range of health-care settings. Traditional training models tend to isolate placement to one setting only, such as a health professional student's practicum consisting of only a hospital setting. Yet primary health care in rural settings necessitates the coordination of health-care providers across the continuum of health service delivery (Gordon et al. 1996). Thus, a rural training model that integrates the training of health-care professionals across relevant health-care sectors might fill the gap of traditional mono-sector training models. In this case, the RHTI would consist of a single practicum placement – held at a sequential range of health-care agencies – that parallels the trajectory of patient care across the continuum of health service delivery. For example, a single physiotherapy placement would consist of acute care hospital, outpatient, homecare, and long-term care settings.

Multi-Dimensional Focus

There is insufficient emphasis on the comprehensive nature of training. Traditional training models tend to isolate training to field placement only. Rural health care, however, needs to encompass the comprehensive nature of training whereby students are exposed to the full spectrum of career pathways for rural practice. The context of training must also include influential factors that both precede training (e.g., a rural-centric curriculum that affects choice of and preparation for a rural training placement) and follow training (e.g., rural-centric continuing education and professional development [CE/PD]) and research activities that substantiate the choice to remain in rural practice. Thus, a training model that incorporates rural-centric dimensions throughout the career pathway for rural practice might fill the gap of traditional mono-dimensional training models. In this case, the RHTI would focus on the synergy of rural-centric curriculum, field training, CE/ PD, and research, as outlined below.

Rural-Centric Curriculum
Research consistently indicates that substantial exposure to rural content in a curriculum has a positive influence on students' choice of and preparation for training and practice in a rural setting (LaSala et al. 1997). Yet the standard curriculum in health sciences programs embraces an

urban-centric educational paradigm in which the theoretical focus is on sub-specialization with an emphasis on solo practice. Few programs offer a rural-centric curriculum that focuses on the twin foundations of generalist and interprofessional collaborative practice that are essential preparation for rural training and practice.

Accordingly, the literature suggests that, in addition to a solid foundation in the specific discipline, students should be exposed to core topics in rural health within an interprofessional education format (McNair et al. 2001). Such courses might focus on the primary health-care approach to preventive, acute, and chronic care; the bio-psycho-social framework; and the roles and functions of various professionals in the health-care team. A rural-centric curriculum can be achieved through joint appointments in which rural practitioners can develop curriculum, teach courses, and/or be guest lecturers, with students marketing and promoting rural training and practice opportunities (D'Eon 2005). The success of a rural-centric curriculum can lead to an advanced certificate or degree in rural health. Furthermore, since the literature identifies one's rural background as a key indicator of returning to rural practice, it would be worthwhile to consider devising a student enrolment selection process that provides recognition of and credit for students' rural backgrounds, experiences, and interests and to include rural practitioners in the selection process (Easterbrook et al. 1999; Rolfe et al. 1995).

Field Placements
Training for rural settings tends to be adapted from urban-centric models. The standard training for health-care students in urban settings tends to be characterized by placements in secondary or tertiary care settings, supervision by one preceptor in one specialized unit, and emphasis on specialized care and solo practice. In contrast, rural training tends to be characterized by placements in primary care settings, supervision shared by multiple preceptors in multiple settings, emphasis on a broader range of care, and active participation in a collaborative interprofessional team. Thus, to ensure a positive training experience in a rural setting, students need to be adequately prepared for the demands of rural practice (Medves et al. 2006), especially if they have not been exposed to a rural-centric curriculum. Preparation for rural training can be achieved through guest lectures by rural practitioners and by current students, specifically on the clinical and social expectations and realities of rural practice (Paterson, McColl, and Paterson 2004).

CE/PD

Factors that follow training, such as rural-centric CE/PD and research activities, are critical to the spectrum of rural training, for they affect the choices of rural practitioners to become preceptors to students as well as to remain in rural practice. Yet the literature indicates that, like the adaptation of urban-centric curriculum and training models, relevant CE/PD activities remain elusive to the rural practitioner in several ways (Solomon, Salvatori, and Berry 2001; also see Chapter 7, this volume). Urban practitioners enjoy a strong collegial critical mass of support, networking, and maintenance of professional practice activities as well as financial and clinical coverage to enable attendance at offered activities. The locale, time, format, and specialized content of CE/PD activities are customized to the convenience and relevance of urban practitioners (Gordon et al. 1996).

In contrast, due to the limited range of health-care professionals in rural settings, rural practitioners experience professional isolation, fewer opportunities for professional support and networking, inconvenient times and locations for CE/PD activities, and limited financial and clinical coverage (Solomon, Salvatori, and Berry 2001). Moreover, the format is not based on case reviews, and the content does not consider the context of generalist primary care or multi-disciplinary care, which are the most relevant education methods for rural practitioners (Gordon et al. 1996).

The literature suggests that, to meet the CE/PD needs of rural practitioners, professional practice activities should be located in a rural regional centre and centrally coordinated. This arrangement would facilitate rural-centric CE/PD activities such as collaboration of rural practitioners with disciplines across all sectors; educational needs assessment for rural practitioners to identify relevant content, timing, and format of CE/PD activities; rural CE/PD programs developed and conducted by and for rural practitioners; and CE/PD topics focused on interprofessional, primary health care, and rural health issues (Gordon et al. 1996).

Research in Rural Health

Interrelated with continuing education and the need to enhance student experiences, research electives in undergraduate and postgraduate programs should include a rural focus. During their training, students should be exposed to and included in program evaluations or research projects related to primary health-care and rural health issues (Kelly and Rourke 2002). Health-care professionals need to develop and participate in rural-centric research and presentations that promote rural health and rural practice. Such research can be collaborative and integrated with academic and health-care providers in the community. Attending to these issues will negate the challenges of conducting rural health research: the few rural health researchers are spread across the country, and the paucity of information about rural health issues often leads to descriptive research. There is a dearth of literature specific to rural issues, notably health (Kulig, Minore, and Stewart 2004). To increase the profile of rural health, the successes of rural health-training and delivery models need to be documented and published.

Overall, the literature review revealed common gaps in traditional urban-centric training models that were not conducive to meeting the unique needs of rural health care. Simply adapting these generic models would not do rural health service delivery justice. Rather, an innovative training model geared specifically to rural health care is required. The four key components absent in traditional training models, yet absolutely critical to rural practice, became the foundation for the RHTI: collaborative partnerships and multi-disciplinary, multi-sector, and multi-dimensional foci.

Step 2: Interviews

Based on the four key components identified from the literature review, interviews were conducted by Lakeridge Health to determine the viability and sustainability of local rural health-training opportunities. A letter of interest was sent to the administrators of community agencies and hospitals, to physicians in the Durham Region, and to the deans and field practicum coordinators of colleges and universities with health sciences programs. Eleven health-care providers and six academic centres accepted scheduled meeting times, ranging from sixty to ninety minutes, in their offices.

Semi-structured interviews consisted of a series of questions on (1) the organization's current training model and its successes and gaps in relation to rural health training; (2) a proposed training model in relation to a rural-centric curriculum, field placements, CE/PD activities, and research components; and (3) resources required to sustain these components. Data gathered from the interviews were transcribed verbatim and analyzed using the constant comparative method of content analysis (Glaser and Strauss 1967). To ensure reliability, two staff members worked independently on the chosen dataset to identify codes and themes for the responses to the questions.

The findings indicated that the schools of health sciences eagerly sought alternative placements particularly since increased enrolment had exhausted the limited supply of conventional placements. They pointed to a noticeable shift in students' interest from urban to rural and community placements. Rehabilitation therapy students in the newly initiated graduate programs tend to come with more experience, maturity, and confidence, and they are likely keen to choose alternative placements and non-traditional training models in which their autonomy and experience are not only valued but also required. Nursing students increasingly favour rural and community placements due to the requisite two-year primary care placements during their undergraduate studies if they wish to be admitted to the coveted Primary Care Nurse Practitioner program in Ontario. Participation in undergraduate rural placements was viewed by students as increasing their chances for graduate admission and/or obtaining employment in rural communities.

In a similar vein, the findings indicated that community health-care providers and hospitals expressed strong support for a collaborative and integrated training model. Factors that had impeded them from accepting more students in the past were an overwhelming workload; a perception of not having a wide-ranging clinical caseload or sufficient patient volume to meet students' learning objectives; and minimal health-care professionals on-site to provide full-time supervision. These limitations, however, can be overcome by the ability to share students across sectors and disciplines. Agencies welcomed the opportunity to expose students to an integrated rural experience and to help meet the increased demand for placements. Rural training opportunities with a mixed group of health-care students can maximize early assimilation into interprofessional collaboration and minimize social and professional isolation.

Although a proposed collaborative and integrated training model was met with general enthusiasm from both the academic and the health-care sectors, they acknowledged the challenge of coordinating the complex logistics. It was agreed that the choice of agencies and disciplines is heavily, if not solely, dependent on the central objective to meet the individual student's learning plan. Revolving around this premise were five key themes identified from the interviews – trajectory of service, training level, administrative lead, preceptor coordinator, and partnership – that were further developed in the next step.

Step 3: Outcome of the Interviews

A report on the study – outlining the literature review and results of the interviews – was circulated to all interviewees, and interested parties were invited to form an RHTI Advisory Council. The purpose of the council was to develop the logistics of a rural health-training model by implementing the five key themes identified from the interviews.

Trajectory of Service

Since the RHTI model consists of a variety of health sectors, it is ideal if each placement follows the trajectory of a service through the health-care system. For example, if the student's goal is to work in the mental health field, then the training would parallel the continuum of health service delivery that a mental health patient typically accesses. The student's learning plan would clearly identify learning objectives, the respective agency and discipline that are most suitable to help achieve these learning outcomes, and the role and function of each preceptor.

Training Level

Given that the RHTI model involves a variety of health-care students, having all the students at a similar training level – preferably during their final placement requirements – would enrich their practicum experience. By sharing similar cognitive knowledge, general maturity, and clinical experience, this set of multi-disciplinary students would be more likely to have common themes in their learning goals. In turn, they can enhance their interprofessional teamwork by complementing the diverse health-care needs of the patient, thereby adhering to patient-centred care. In this case, students and preceptors would identify core learning objectives that are cross-disciplined as well as learning objectives that are specific to each student's discipline. For example, a common learning objective might be determining how the role and function of each discipline complement the needs of the stroke patient, and a discipline-specific objective might be creating a treatment program that meets the criteria of the student's own discipline.

Administrative Lead

Since the RHTI model encompasses multiple partners, it is paramount that a central office is responsible for administering standardized documents between academic centres and health-care providers (e.g., affiliation agreements, insurance, orientation packages for preceptors and students) and takes the lead in research and presentations related to the RHTI.

Preceptor Coordinator

In view of the fact that the RHTI model comprises multiple sectors, it is ideal if a central person is responsible for coordinating the logistics of each placement schedule between applicable academic and health-care partners. This includes arranging local accommodation and transportation and compiling the final student evaluation with input from site preceptors.

Academic and Health-Care Partners

Each student has a faculty member responsible for interpreting curriculum requirements, developing learning goals and objectives, and participating in student evaluations. Each placement site identifies preceptors who can deliver site-specific student learning objectives and has regular contact with the faculty member to monitor the student's progress. Ongoing communication between these key roles – administrative lead, preceptor coordinator, faculty, and site preceptors – is essential to ensuring that each placement successfully meets the multi-sector trajectory of service and multi-disciplinary training-level criteria of RHTI placements.

Step 4: Pilot Projects

Pilot projects – incorporating the four key components identified from the literature review and the five key themes identified from the interviews – were initiated. Objectives of the pilot projects were to review successes and challenges in implementation of the RHTI and to determine its sustainability.

The four pilot projects consisted of two physiotherapy students in their final year of the master's program; two nursing students in their final year of the baccalaureate's program; two universities; and four health-care sectors (emergency, acute hospital, post-acute community care, and long-term care). Descriptions of the pilot placements were marketed at the universities, and a final schedule was prepared for each student. At the end of each pilot project, face-to-face, semi-structured interviews reviewed the process, content, and outcome evaluation of the project. Students, faculty, and health-care providers cited the strengths, gaps, and areas for improvement at each phase of the placement. They are outlined within three categories reflecting the training trajectory.

Pre-Placement

Preceptor recruitment is critical at each of the multi-sector sites. Important factors in the encouragement and preparation of staff to become preceptors were preceptor workshops, a preceptor general orientation handbook, and strong support from management and colleagues. Similarly, student recruitment was necessary due to the novelty of the RHTI placements. Practicum coordinators marketed the pilot projects by emphasizing the breadth of experience to be gained from the uniqueness of a multi-disciplinary and multi-sector placement, the advanced training-level criteria, free accommodation and transportation, and a student general orientation handbook describing the RHTI and the community.

Synchronization of a multi-sector schedule was a challenge since the key was to ensure that preceptors at each practicum site that paralleled the trajectory of a service were actually available for the specified dates. Schedules were modified based on whether each site maximized the student's learning objectives. For example, the original schedule for a mental health placement followed the typical trajectory of an emergency/ crisis unit, acute in-patient care, homecare, and long-term care. However, students identified that they would have felt more adequately prepared for the intensity of the emergency/crisis unit if they had first been exposed to the homecare/long-term sites. Based on this feedback, subsequent RHTI placements were rescheduled to reflect this revised trajectory of care.

During Placement

Transportation was a challenge: students usually do not have access to a car; public transportation in rural communities typically does not run at regular intervals, thereby severely limiting students' arrival and departure times; and frequent travel was required between multi-sector sites. To mitigate some of these challenges, accessibility to a car was mentioned as an asset but not required, site preceptors provided transportation and used this time for supervision, transportation costs were absorbed by the RHTI, and liability issues regarding transportation were referenced in the affiliation agreements and in each organization's insurance policy. Since recruitment of health-care professionals benefits the community as a whole, the RHTI can partner with community volunteers to extend the usual client transportation services to RHTI students. Communication and flexibility are critical; despite all efforts to synchronize a final placement schedule, last-minute adaptations to the schedule are inevitable due to changes in preceptors or transportation arrangements.

Post-Placement

Student evaluations were completed among the student, faculty member, and site preceptors. The Advisory Council held annual evaluations to assess the successes, gaps, and areas for improvement of the RHTI. Ongoing appreciation of preceptors was critical, including soliciting feedback on areas for improvement, hosting an annual RHTI appreciation dinner, and ensuring that all partners are cited in any presentations related to the RHTI.

Step 5: RHTI Sustainability

The RHTI Advisory Council convened to evaluate the outcome of the pilot projects and to determine whether sufficient human capital could sustain the RHTI. Overall, key stakeholders indicated satisfaction with the RHTI pilot placements. Students confirmed that the breadth of the multi-disciplinary and multi-sector RHTI placements adequately prepared them for rural practice. Academic centres confirmed the RHTI increased placement opportunities while being aligned with an increasing emphasis on interprofessional curriculum and multi-disciplinary clinical placements. Health-care providers confirmed that the RHTI created an increase in otherwise scarce supervisory opportunities at their individual organizations. This increased both recruitment and retention potential since staff expressed pride that their sharing of professional skills, knowledge, and experiences could have an impact on shaping the careers of future health-care practitioners. Factors critical to the success of the RHTI are strong endorsement from both students and preceptors to their peers, support from senior directors and managers at each practicum site, and ongoing monitoring of the progress of the RHTI.

Summary

The success of this case study has led to continuation of the RHTI in the Durham Region. As the RHTI expands, however, operational costs are expected to increase. Of significance is that human resource costs have been kept to a minimum since the development and ongoing management of the RHTI continue to be absorbed by existing staff. The growth of the RHTI might necessitate funding a position solely dedicated to this initiative. This position would enable further development in the multi-dimensional component of the RHTI, such as establishing regular rural-centric interprofessional development activities, developing rural-centric curricula, conducting rural research, creating an RHTI website, and producing an RHTI "how-to" manual or video. These means of knowledge dissemination can promote rural placements and rural practice while highlighting the unique needs of rural health across Canada.

The RHTI model could be considered for implementation by similar rural communities across Canada. Given the uniqueness of rural health, each component in isolation will not have as powerful an impact on rural health service delivery. Rather, the sustainability of such a model is contingent on the synthesis of the four key components: academic and health-care partnerships, multi-disciplinary students, multi-sector placements, and multi-dimensional focus spanning the career spectrum for rural practice.

Moreover, since primary health care is an inherent aspect of rural health-care delivery, the RHTI model can be considered in urban settings. Romanow (2002) emphasizes that primary health care is a cornerstone of an efficient and robust health-care system. As the initial entry point to the health system for many patients and families, an integrated and comprehensive primary health-care system acts as a mechanism to ensure continuity of care throughout the system. As such, not only can the RHTI be a blueprint for replication in other rural communities across Canada, but it can also help to shape the development of primary health-care reform in urban settings.

Acknowledgments

The concept of the Rural Health Training Institute could not have been transformed into reality without its founding academic and health-care partners: Dr. Pansy Goodman and Tina Demmers from Lakeridge Health Corporation; Elizabeth Tata from Queen's University; Judith Robinson from Durham College; Dr. Carolyn Byrne and Dr. Wendy Stanyon from the University of Ontario Institute of Technology; Sally Davis from Central East Community Care Access Centre; Linda Coles from Durham Region Lakeview Manor; and Heather Cooper from Community Nursing Home Port Perry.

References

Christianson, J., and C. Grogan. 1990. "Alternative Models for the Delivery of Rural Health Services." *Journal of Rural Health* 6, 4: 419-36.

Degn, D. 1993. "Rural Health Training Units." Armidale, New South Wales: 2nd National Rural Health Conference, http://www.nrha.ruralhealth.org.au/.

D'Eon, M. 2005. "A Blueprint for Interprofessional Learning." *Journal of Interprofessional Care* 19: 39-48.

du Plessis, V., R. Beshiri, R.D. Bollman, and H. Clemenson. 2001. "Definitions of Rural." *Rural and Small Town Canada Analysis Bulletin* 3, 3: 1-17. Statistics Canada Catalogue No. 21-006-XIE.

Easterbrook, M., M. Godwin, R. Wilson, G. Hodgetts, G. Brown, R. Pong, and E. Najgebauer. 1999. "Rural Background and Clinical Rural Rotations during Medical Training: Effect on Practice and Location." *Canadian Medical Association Journal* 160, 8: 1159-63.

Fertman, C.I., S. Dotson, G.O. Mazzocco, and S. Maggie Reitz. 2005. "Challenges of Preparing Allied Health Professionals for Interdisciplinary Practice in Rural Areas." *Journal of Allied Health* 34, 3: 163-68.

Glaser, B., and A. Strauss. 1967. *The Discovery of Grounded Theory: Strategies for Qualitative Research*. Chicago: Aldine Publications.

Gordon, P., L. Carlson, A. Chessman, M. Kundrat, P. Morahan, and L. Headrick. 1996. "A Multisite Collaborative for the Development of Interdisciplinary Education in Continuous Improvement for Health Professions." *Academic Medicine* 71: 973-78.

Humphreys, J.S., D. Lyle, J. Wakerman, E. Chalmers, D. Wilkinson, J. Walker, D. Simmons, and A. Larson. 2000. "Roles and Activities of the Commonwealth Government University Departments of Rural Health." *Australian Journal of Rural Health* 8: 120-33.

Humphreys, J.S., and A. Nichols. 2009. "Education and Training: Role of Rural Health Training Units." *Australian Journal of Rural Health* 3, 2: 80-86.

Kamien, M. 1996. "A Comparison of Medical Student Experiences in Rural Specialty and Metropolitan Teaching Hospital Practice." *Australian Journal of Rural Health* 4: 151-58.

Kelly, L., and J. Rourke. 2002. "Research Electives in Rural Health Care." *Canadian Family Physician* 48: 1476-80.

Kulig, J., B. Minore, and N. Stewart. 2004. "Capacity Building in Rural Health Research: A Canadian Perspective." *Rural and Remote Health* 4: 1-7.

LaSala, K., S. Hopper, D. Rissmeyer, and D. Shipe. 1997. "Rural Health Care and Interdisciplinary Education." *Nursing and Health Care Perspectives* 18, 6: 292-98.

McNair, R., R. Brown, N. Stone, and J. Sims. 2001. "Rural Interprofessional Education: Promoting Teamwork in Primary Health Care Education and Practice." *Australian Journal of Rural Health* 9: 19-26.

Medves, J., P. Paterson, J. Young, B. McAndrews, D. Bowes, and E. Smith. 2006. "Preparing Professionals from a Wide Range of Disciplines for Life and Work in Rural and Small Communities." *Australian Journal of Rural Health* 14: 225-26.

National Association of Rural Health Training Units. 1999. "Ten Years in the Making: The Evolution of Rural Health Training Units." Toowoomba, Queensland: National Association of Rural Health Training Units.

National Rural Health Association. 2006. "Effective Partnerships for the Recruitment of Health Professionals." Kansas City, MO: National Area Health Education Center Organization, http://www.nationalahec.org/.

Paterson, M., M. McColl, and H. Paterson. 2004. "Preparing Allied Health Students for Fieldwork in Small Communities." *Australian Journal of Rural Health* 12: 32-33.

Probst, J., C. Moore, E. Baxley, and J. Lammie. 2002. "Rural-Urban Differences in Visits to Primary Care Physicians." *Family Medicine* 34, 8: 609-15.

Rolfe, I., S. Pearson, D. O'Connell, and J. Dickinson. 1995. "Finding Solutions to the Rural Doctor Shortage: The Roles of Selection versus Undergraduate Medical Education at Newcastle." *Australian and New Zealand Journal of Medicine* 25, 5: 512-17.

Romanow, R. 2002. *Building on Values: The Future of Health Care in Canada.* Saskatoon: Commission on the Future of Health Care in Canada.

Solomon, P., P. Salvatori, and S. Berry. 2001. "Perceptions of Important Retention and Recruitment Factors by Therapists in Northwestern Ontario." *Journal of Rural Health* 17: 278-85.

Tepper, J. 1999. "Changing the Norm: Ten Suggestions to Redress the Rural Crisis." *Canadian Family Physician* 45: 2935-37.

Chapter 7   **Building Capacity in Rural Health Services: The Effect of Continuing Education**

S. Habjan, K. Kortes-Miller, M.L. Kelley, H. Sullivan, and L. Pisco

Key Points

- Continuing education (CE) of rural health professionals is an effective strategy for building capacity within the rural health system.
- An effective CE model has been developed, guided by the principles of collaboration, capacity building, accessibility, interprofessional format, and responsiveness (CCAIR).
- Use of the CCAIR model can increase an individual's expertise, promote organizational change, strengthen social support across the rural region, and promote interprofessional collaboration.

Capacity building is gaining recognition as a strategy for program development and increasing health human resources, especially in rural locations (Hawe et al. 2000). Capacity includes those abilities, skills, understandings, attitudes, values, relationships, behaviours, motivations, resources, or conditions that are essential in enabling individuals, organizations, and communities to carry out functions and achieve their developmental objectives (Bolger 2000). In rural areas, where health-care providers frequently work with limited interaction and support from specialists in urban areas, capacity-building initiatives are most effectively targeted at the whole rural community and local interdisciplinary health-care providers (Kelley 2007). The desired outcome of these initiatives is to improve quality and availability of rural health services.

Education can play an important role in increasing health service capacity and the uptake of new knowledge, especially in rural and remote areas. Rural health-care providers are faced with significant barriers to access and integrate new information into their practice. One such barrier is professional isolation, a consequence of physical distance from larger urban areas, separation from a learning environment, and detachment from a peer support network (Jukkala, Henly, and Lindeke 2008; Molinari and Berry 1999). Heavy workloads, travel times, and financial constraints also represent barriers to attaining new information (Penz et al. 2007). Continuing education can be instrumental in enhancing the knowledge base of rural health-care providers by offering a direct means of increasing a community's capacity to deliver optimal care. However, this education needs to be planned and delivered in ways that recognize the realities of rural health practice.

Developing Capacity

The term "community capacity development" began to appear in the literature in the early 1990s (Craig 2007). Definitions of community capacity development vary; however, they consistently draw on the ideals of strengthening society through changes in social, cultural, and community engagements (Dressendorfer et al. 2005). The definition of community can also vary, describing an area contained by geographical boundaries, a cultural group, or a specific group of interest. As Dressendorfer and colleagues note, capacity development encompasses the idea of empowering a community to change, allowing for the skill set of the community to expand and become self-supportive.

According to Hawe et al. (1998), capacity development can be seen as a process in action that includes different levels and strategies, leading to a number of outcomes. The level of capacity building takes place not only within individuals, health-care teams, and organizations but also across organizations and within communities. Diverse strategies can be used to build capacity, from engaging people, challenging them on how they think or act, and using the right language to building new networks, ensuring that people receive recognition for actions taken, and working invisibly. Some of the outcomes of capacity building include positive attitudes, more skill acquisition, greater confidence and knowledge, and more action and organization put toward the issue at hand (see Table 7.1).

Table 7.1 Strategies and outcomes of capacity development

Levels of capacity building	Strategies used in capacity building	Outcomes of capacity building
Within individuals	Engaging people	Positive attitudes
Within health-care teams	Challenging the way people think or act	More skill acquisition
Within health organizations	Responding to their needs/issues first	Greater confidence and knowledge
Across organizations	Using the right language	More action and organizational effort put toward the issue
Within communities	Building personal credibility	The issue appears in the mission and policy documents of organizations
	Building local skills	
	Building new networks	Promotion becomes part of the routine activity of providers
	Structuring rewards and incentives for others to do promotion, such as seeding grants	
	Ensuring other people get credit and recognition for actions taken	
	Working invisibly	

Source: Hawe et al. (1998).

There is a general consensus in the literature that community capacity development is a collaborative social process that occurs as people develop their assets and abilities to foster social change (Chaskin 2001; Kretzmann and McKnight 1993; Minkler 2000). Capacity development allows communities to solve problems through informal methods and partnerships (Craig 2007; Dressendorfer et al. 2005). Seven dimensions are involved in community capacity: the level of knowledge, skills, and resources; the nature of social relationships; structures, mechanisms, and spaces for community dialogue; the quality of leadership and its development; the extent of civic participation; a value system; and a learning culture (Norton et al. 2002). Capacity development requires broad participation, building on local capacities, ongoing learning and adaptation, and long-term investment in and integration of activities at various levels to address complex problems (Lusthaus et al. 1999). The method of change is to enhance existing capacities and not to impose solutions from outside. The approach is strengths based rather than needs or deficit oriented (Horton and MacLeod 2008; Raeburn et al. 2006).

Capacity development in rural regions faces obstacles not present in urban areas, including location, economics, isolation, lack of transportation, and shortage of human resources. In rural and remote Canada, these factors often result in limited interactions among communities or members within a single community. For example, Moss et al. (Chapter 9, this volume) report that staff shortages and high turnover rates create difficulties in developing trusting relationships among residents, health-care providers, and community leaders.

In addition, rural communities might not have access to the same resources as urban regions, often lacking specific programs that might be common in urban areas (Kelley 2007). For instance, Moss et al. (Chapter 9, this volume) describe the concerns of rural residents regarding the availability of dental services, sustainability of homecare, and provision of health promotion programs. Some communities might experience obstacles relating to economics, such as the expenses of operating programs and hiring personnel or the financial ability of community members to participate in available programs (Curran, Fleet, and Kirby 2006).

A major issue in rural areas is the problem of recruiting and retaining health-care professionals (see Chapter 6, this volume). Although the Canadian health-care system currently employs more than 1 million people, consisting of over thirty different health professions and occupations (North West LHIN 2006), there are shortages of physicians, nurses, nurse practitioners, physician assistants, dentists, pharmacists, and many allied health professionals (O'Toole et al. 2008). In addition to the lack of health-care providers, Pitblado (Chapter 5, this volume) points out that the workforce is unevenly distributed geographically. For instance, in 2001, there were approximately 100 physicians practising in rural communities for every 100,000 persons compared with the urban areas, which had approximately 150 more physicians available for the same number of people.

For communities located in rural areas, there is great difficulty not only in recruiting health professionals but also in retaining an essential local workforce (Daniels et al. 2007; Penz et al. 2008). Pitblado (Chapter 5, this volume) points out that, out of twenty-seven health professional and occupational groups studied, rural percentages of the workforce have decreased for sixteen of them from 1991 to 2001. For the groups that have shown relative increases in the rural percentages, their absolute numbers are still well below the ratio of health-care provider to population observed in urban areas.

Studies have found that overall recruitment of health professionals can be achieved through financial and educational incentives and by focusing on rural students (Chan et al. 2005; Curran and Rourke 2004). However, retention of these recruited individuals has proven to be a harder task. On a day-to-day basis, professional satisfaction is a key factor in retention of rural health-care providers (Kelley et al. 2008; Pathman et al. 2004).

The literature indicates numerous rationales offered by health professionals for leaving a rural community. As noted by others in this volume (see Chapter 6), rural practitioners experience professional isolation, fewer opportunities for professional support and networking, and inconvenient times and locations for continuing education. A study by Levett-Jones (2005) found that a key factor associated with retention of nurses is professional and personal satisfaction and recognition, while Kramer and Schmalenberg (2004) suggest that educational access and ongoing support are important to nurses in terms of job satisfaction. Gillham and Ristevski (2007) discuss the importance of access to professional development in relation to retention of allied health professionals and a need to provide opportunities for professional development. Also identified as a need is the recognition of advanced skills and the opportunity to perform extra duties. Solomon, Salvatori, and Berry (2001) found that rural physical and occupational therapists listed professional isolation and lack of educational activities as one of the top three causes of job dissatisfaction.

When continuing education is provided and supported, there are increases in staff satisfaction, self-esteem, and self-confidence. These increases are found not only among health-care providers attending CE programs but also among colleagues with whom the new knowledge and skills are shared (Robertson et al. 1999). Yet, while the importance of professional development is evident, providing education to health-care providers in rural areas remains challenging. Geographical location and the shortage of locally accessible professional educational programs impact a community's ability to provide up-to-date resources to support professional health-care practice. Curran, Fleet, and Kirby (2006) highlight common barriers to continuing education in rural areas, including geographical distance, inability of workers to leave their practice, lack of access to appropriate educational events, and cost of courses.

Technological advances have led to the decrease in the resource gap between urban and rural health professionals. Technology can link providers to resources and rural areas to each other or to urban areas, effectively decreasing professional isolation (Meyer 2006). However, even with advances in communication technology, Curran, Fleet, and Kirby (2006) found a lack of meaningful educational opportunities available to rural health professionals.

Educational initiatives not only improve professional and personal satisfaction and retention of rural health-care providers but also represent a key way to develop health service capacity in a community. Research by Kelley (2007) found that, within the capacity-building model developed for rural palliative care delivery, education and staff support were the most important factors in community engagement.

Continuing Education as a Means to Build Capacity

In northwestern Ontario, Canada, the Centre for Education and Research on Aging and Health (CERAH) at Lakehead University, Thunder Bay, has the mission to advance health and social care for an aging population and to promote the health and well-being of older people (see http://cerah.lakeheadu.ca). Continuing education and research are used to accomplish this mission. A major objective of CERAH is to contribute to building capacity in local health services by delivering CE to rural health-care providers.

The northwestern region of Ontario, CERAH's catchment area, can be defined as rural and remote as per DesMeules et al. (Chapter 2, this volume). Northwestern Ontario is comprised of the districts of Kenora, Rainy River, and Thunder Bay (see Figure 7.1). It covers an area (525,193 square kilometres) that is approximately 60 percent of the landmass of the province but contains only 2 percent of its population. The rural and remote areas include numerous small towns and First Nations communities. The distance between eastern and western boundaries is slightly over 1,000 kilometres, with a population density of 0.5 persons per square kilometre. The area extends from White River on the east to the Manitoba border on the west, to James Bay and Hudson Bay on the north, and to the US border on the south. The only major urban community in the region, Thunder Bay, has a population of 109,000 and is considered remote in relation to southern Ontario's major population areas. Thunder Bay is 1,374 kilometres by road from Toronto, the provincial capital (Northwestern Ontario District Health Council 2001).

Educational Model

Since 1993, CERAH has been developing and delivering continuing education in aging and health to health-care providers across northwestern Ontario, with funding assistance from the Ontario Ministry of

Figure 7.1   Map showing districts in northwestern Ontario

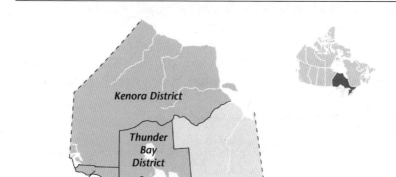

Health and Long-Term Care and more recently from the North West Local Health Integration Network (LHIN). Due to the flexibility of its programs, CERAH can respond to the educational needs of health providers in a timely manner and in an appropriate format and provide education on the topics most pertinent to care providers. With extensive dialogue and guidance from different sectors of care providers, CERAH can learn which educational format is the most appropriate and effective at a given time.

CERAH continuously evaluates and measures the impacts of curricula, educational approaches, methods, and formats. From 1993 to 2007, CERAH conducted evaluations of close to 200 separate educational initiatives and completed a number of mixed-methods studies (Kelley, Habjan, and Aegard 2004; Kelley and MacLean 1997; Kortes-Miller et al. 2007; Sellick et al. 1996) to learn the effectiveness of its educational initiatives. Based on the obtained data, in 2007 CERAH developed an educational model that has demonstrated success in capacity development of rural health services.

Table 7.2   CERAH's principles of education model (CCAIR)

Collaboration	Education planned and delivered in partnership with local and regional service providers
Capacity building	Development of interprofessional experts to be local resource people Ongoing consultation and accessibility of educational materials
Accessibility	Education delivered centrally (Thunder Bay), on site in agencies throughout northwestern Ontario, and via telehealth Distributed learning model
Interprofessional format	Inclusiveness of family physicians, long-term-care and interdisciplinary community care professionals, paraprofessionals, and volunteers Interdisciplinary and discipline specific
Responsiveness	Curriculum designed to meet needs of primary care and generalist providers Timely program reaction using appropriate formats

Five principles (CCAIR) guide CERAH's educational model: collaboration, capacity building, accessibility, interprofessional format, and responsiveness (see Table 7.2).

This unique model was developed by CERAH's researchers and educators through a systematic analysis of fifteen years of educational experience. The strength of the model lies in the description of the methods of working with rural health communities; it offers an approach to practice and not necessarily techniques and strategies. The review of the literature points to a number of different approaches to delivering quality continuing education for rural care providers. However, most writers discuss learning format preferences, modes of delivery, strategies to meet CE needs, or guiding principles from the perspective of the organization (Booth and Lawrance 2001; Hays 2006; Hill and Alexander 1996; Hoyal 1999). CERAH's model of education focuses on the principles of practice that contribute to capacity building in rural health services.

The model draws on multiple formats to provide educational initiatives, including short seminars and videoconferences, half-day and full-day workshops, a two- to three-day regional conference, and multi-day programs that can stretch over a period of several weeks. The educational format used depends to a large extent on the topic, the format preferred by the targeted health-care providers, and the complexity of the program offered. CERAH utilizes the principles of its model in every educational initiative, regardless of the format used or the topic delivered. Since palliative/end-of-life care has been a major focus in CERAH's CE program, it will be used as an example of the model application. However, the approach can be generalized to other educational topics since it is about the process of development and delivery of continuing education and is not content specific. The quotations used to illustrate the validity of five principles have been extracted from evaluation data such as surveys, focus groups, and written comments that measured the impacts of the educational model on capacity building.

Collaboration

The first principle is that of collaboration. In rural communities, collaboration among providers is partly motivated by the shortage of health human resources and the consequent need to work cooperatively to get the job done (Lightfoot et al. 2008). To be consistent with the rural collaborative culture, collaboration in the planning and delivery of education occurs with the service providers who will be the recipients of the education. Due to the nature and challenges of rural and remote areas, Moss et al. (Chapter 9, this volume) also endorse the need for partnerships by using creative planning among university educational programs, health authorities, and communities to achieve better health-care access in these regions.

Front-line providers in rural areas know what their educational needs are and which kind of delivery is most effective. Negotiating timing is a key factor since rural providers are frequently on call and have little backup to attend sessions. They value teamwork and forming strong and ongoing relationships with their educators. Through careful assessment and communication with care providers about their learning needs and preferences, an educational program can be designed that supports collaboration.

The following quotations, taken from focus groups conducted with rural health-care providers who participated in CERAH's continuing education, illustrate participants' perceptions of the importance of collaboration.

That initial contact [with the trainers] was the most important for us so they know who we are, and we know who they are, so it feels easier now to ask for [follow-up] help.

What we have been doing here, within our small group, is actually beginning to look at our collaborative practice. Doing that piece of work has highlighted our awareness of what collaborative practice truly is.

One example of a collaborative project is the Palliative Care in Long-Term Care educational program developed by CERAH for long-term-care facilities in Thunder Bay and the region. This approach involves an educational needs assessment in the long-term-care homes where the education is to be delivered, curriculum development to address the perceived needs, and delivery of the curriculum in a manner that reduces most of the identified barriers, such as cost, time, and location. The outcome of this approach is the educational initiative that is accessible and relevant and targeted to a group of health-care providers who often have little formal palliative care training. Furthermore, this approach builds capacity within the facility for future education. The use of in-house care providers as facilitators of education both empowers the staff and develops them as local resources for future education and mentorship (Kortes-Miller et al. 2007).

Capacity Building

The second principle is capacity building. Effective capacity building occurs from a strengths perspective, does not impose solutions from the outside, and strongly values the idea of collective problem solving (Horton and MacLeod 2008; Norton et al. 2002; Raeburn et al. 2006). From an educational perspective, the value and wisdom (capacity) of clinicians who are practising in a rural context is well regarded. Therefore, local health-care practitioners are identified as experts and subsequently supported to develop their skills and knowledge to strengthen their roles as educators within their peer group. Capacity building extends to the development and nurturing of local interprofessional experts, who can serve as a resource to local health-care providers and to educators in planning local educational initiatives (Kelley 2007).

Using the example given above (Palliative Care in Long-Term Care), the in-house facilitators of the curriculum are provided with a guide to the delivery of the education along with a variety of resources. However, the facilitators are also encouraged to incorporate their own clinical experiences and teaching styles. In addition, they receive ongoing support, including an introduction to the course by the curriculum developer. They are offered face-to-face meetings as needed and telephone or email support throughout delivery of the course. There is also an opportunity for facilitators to self-evaluate and debrief their experiences at the end of the course. Once the educational initiative is complete, the facilitators are encouraged to undertake the role of a mentor for the staff.

Recruitment of health-care providers to serve as local resource persons is part of CERAH's educational initiatives. Many individuals undertake this challenge enthusiastically, contributing to capacity building within their community. The following quotations taken from questionnaires completed by participants describe their future plans to share what they learned with others.

> *[I plan to] be a "resource person" in a facility for residents, family, and staff ... help provide information needed ... [and] put into practice what was learned.*

> *First, [I will] do a series of presentations to colleagues with a short synopsis of certain topics. Second, meet with people in leadership to ascertain what exists, what is needed, perceptions of palliative care.*

Accessibility

The third principle of CERAH's educational model is accessibility. As in any rural and remote area, isolation, cost of travel, and vast distances within northwestern Ontario are recognized barriers to health-care clinicians to obtain the continuing education necessary for the delivery of optimal care (Kortes-Miller et al. 2007). Therefore, education needs to be accessible, including being delivered on site in the health-care providers' community or place of employment. Through utilization of a distributed learning model, CERAH accesses technology such as telehealth, web streaming, and online learning to overcome some of the barriers to accessibility. If needed and requested by health-care providers, CERAH also travels to communities in northwestern Ontario to deliver education face to face.

CERAH's support of rural health professionals to deliver education in their home community increases accessibility to new information for the entire community over a long period of time. The following quotations, taken from participant surveys, describe how these professionals intend to make what has been learned accessible to their colleagues.

[I] will give in-service to staff at our facility. Make this binder [of information provided at the educational session] available for staff to view.

[I] will mentor colleagues and try to offer in-services for colleagues: awareness of burnout and palliative care teamwork.

Rural CE also needs to be delivered in a regional urban centre to tap into expert resources (Shipman et al. 2001) and to provide the opportunities for networking among health-care providers from different communities (Kelley et al. 2004). The opportunity for rural generalists to learn from and interact with experts is an important element in making contacts, exchanging ideas, and developing skill capacities. In addition, networking with others is perceived by rural health-care providers as an important process since it helps them to deal with the professional isolation associated with working in a rural setting.

The following quotations, taken from participant surveys about the benefits of attending the regional conference, illustrate how the participants valued access to new information, clinical experts, and networking opportunities with their rural colleagues.

This was my first conference, and the information I received was great! The networking was even more important. Knowing that people are just a phone call away is very helpful to people/organizations.

Incredible amount of knowledge; an opportunity to meet and learn from people from other communities.

Interprofessional Format

The fourth educational principle recognizes the important role of interprofessional formats and approaches when educating rural health professionals. Rural health-care practice can be described as generalist, collaborative, and community focused, with rural health-care providers carrying a higher level of clinical responsibility and enjoying less professional backup than their urban counterparts (MacLellan 2002). As described by Goodman (Chapter 6, this volume), the emphasis on collaborative training for health professionals across the spectrum of disciplines and a range of health-care settings is required in any educational programs offered in rural areas.

Interprofessional practice and teamwork are well established in rural health services (Strasser 1999). To support this rural teamwork approach, the majority of educational initiatives should be delivered using an interprofessional format. This approach also supports team building and interprofessional practice within the community or a workplace.

To illustrate, palliative care education through CERAH is primarily delivered with an interprofessional focus and includes rural family physicians, nurses, social workers, spiritual care providers, occupational therapists, physiotherapists, speech pathologists, and others. These participants come from a variety of settings, including acute care, long-term care, and community care. The following quotations, taken from participant questionnaires, illustrate the perceived value of taking an interprofessional approach to continuing education.

The feeling of equality felt by everyone involved at the [educational event] – whether it's between physicians, social workers, registered nurses ... We all felt we could share together with no sense of intimidation or labels.

I got a stronger sense of the value of interdisciplinary teamwork and need for mutual support. Need to keep learning together.

[I plan] to have interdisciplinary training in our agency. I've learned the importance of different job titles. I see things differently.

Within the context of CERAH's interdisciplinary educational approach, however, there is a need for some educational events that are discipline specific since they relate to a particular skill set that is within the scope of practice of an individual profession or discipline. An example is an educational session on the use of methadone for palliation, designed and delivered specifically for physicians. Rural generalist practitioners must have enhanced knowledge and skills in their profession since they work with minimal specialist support.

Responsiveness

The fifth and final principle of the educational model used by CERAH to build capacity is responsiveness. The continuing education in rural areas should be responsive to local needs, delivered in a timely manner, and be both proactive and reactive. Goodman (Chapter 6, this volume) echoes the importance of rural-centric continuing education since it is perceived to be critical to the spectrum of rural training.

Part of the principle of responsiveness also means that the curriculum has to meet the needs of the individual community, practice setting, or learner's skill level. In addition, an appropriate educational format that works for a specific community needs to be utilized. Responsiveness is viewed not only as a factor of time but also in the recognition that tried and tested methods of delivering education in an urban setting might not always be as well received in a rural one.

To achieve responsiveness, the other four principles of the educational model mentioned above need to be in place and fully utilized. Only through collaboration with local and regional service providers and a history of joint, regionally relevant educational projects will local needs be identified and brought forward to the education provider. Local experts, developed through capacity building, can facilitate needed consultation or mentoring in a crisis situation or on short notice. With accessibility in place, the education required can be delivered, when and where needed, without a major reorganization of educational format or time delays. And finally, by receiving the education in an interprofessional format, health-care providers are likely more able and willing to approach providers from other disciplines when a situation requires collaboration.

The following educational projects are the examples of CERAH's timely responsiveness to emerging educational needs. The first situation involved a community homecare agency with a client approaching the final stages of amyotrophic lateral sclerosis (ALS) who wished to die at home. Portable home ventilation was essential; however, agency staff were not prepared for this task since they had never provided homecare for a client with this condition. CERAH was contacted with the request for education. Within a few weeks, CERAH was able to deliver a learning module for home ventilation by recruiting specialists to develop a protocol for home ventilation, offer a hands-on workshop for agency staff, and disseminate this information across the region for other health-care providers who might require this knowledge in the future. This initiative not only provided the requested in-depth knowledge of and skills for home ventilation but also produced a protocol that can be utilized as needed.

Another example of responsiveness is a pediatric palliative care educational initiative. The practice of rural health-care providers does not often include pediatric palliative cases, so many do not feel confident about their knowledge regarding this subject. At one time, several children in northwestern Ontario were in different stages of terminal diseases, and a request for more in-depth education and information regarding pediatric palliative care was brought forward to educational planners at CERAH. Within weeks, CERAH recruited a nationally recognized pediatric palliative care practitioner who delivered three-part educational sessions to northwestern Ontario communities by videoconference. As a result of this initiative, rural health services have been enhanced, local health-care providers have developed a capacity to provide pediatric palliative care, and children do not have to leave their homes and communities in the last weeks of their lives.

The final example of the principle of responsiveness in capacity building involves a situation in a long-term care home. This home had experienced more than the usual number of residents' deaths over a short period of time, and the staff were experiencing difficulty coping with these deaths. The home approached CERAH, asking for interventional education to address this issue. A compassion fatigue educational initiative was not only developed and delivered to the staff of the home but also offered to other long-term-care homes in the region. A resource binder on compassion fatigue was also developed. This binder was given to every home so that a local resource person could utilize the information and provide in-house education and support when required.

The preceding examples illustrate the importance of responsiveness when utilizing education as a means of building capacity. However, responsiveness alone could not produce desired results. Only when used in conjunction with the other principles of education could a timely reaction to a pressing educational need be achieved. Since collaborative relationships had already been established, the partnerships and working relationships were in place to support a quick response. Through the capacity-building educational principles, the local resources had been developed, and they supported and built on existing capacities. Based on the accessibility principle, a practice and method of education had been established, leading to a short time frame between the request for education and its delivery. Finally, the interprofessional format of CERAH's educational model allowed the health-care providers to learn from each other in order to provide optimal care.

Capacity-Building Outcomes of Continuing Education

Utilizing CERAH's educational model not only addresses educational needs of rural health-care providers but also offers social support across the rural region to implement changes in health services. An extensive evaluation of CERAH's educational program indicates the model's contribution to the improvement of knowledge and skills of individual providers, the development of programs in rural communities, and the growth of local resource people who are able to educate their co-workers (Kelley, Habjan, and Aegard 2004). The following quotations illustrate how participants in educational initiatives perceived positive outcomes for building capacity.

> *Our knowledge base has increased and enhanced to where we can probably meet the needs except for those very really complicated cases.*

> *My colleagues and I are going to work together to work with people in the community to revitalize what exists and create new ways of "doing" in bite-size pieces.*

> *[The] conference has brought a group of us from different agencies closer and more client directed as a group. To assist our community as a whole. We will grow in leaps and bounds – we have great networking and resources.*

> *[I want to] be a "resource person" for residents, family, and staff. Help provide information needed. Put into practice what was learned and help make changes.*

Education has long been recognized as a powerful tool for social mobilization (Nutbeam 2000). Using continuing education in an appropriate way can contribute to capacity building in rural health services. Capacity cannot be generated or delivered from the outside but must be developed locally by doing (Lavergne and Saxby 2001). CERAH's educational model enhances and supports local health-care providers' capacity to promote and sustain changes in rural health service delivery.

For rural health-care providers, continuing education can impact individual abilities, skills, understandings, attitudes, and values. Furthermore, education motivates individuals to make behavioural changes in practice. Changes, however, do not occur only at the individual level. Fifteen years of experience and evaluation of the model have shown that education provided by CERAH has enabled health-care practitioners to gather together and form the relationships needed to change and enhance delivery of health services in their organizations and communities. CERAH's educational model can act as a guide for other institutions and organizations when delivering educational initiatives to achieve capacity development in rural health services across Canada and beyond.

References

Bolger, J. 2000. *Capacity Development: Why, What, and How.* Capacity Development, Occasional Series, vol. 1 (1), Canadian International Developmental Agency (CIDA), Policy Branch. Gatineau, QC: CIDA.

Booth, B., and R. Lawrance. 2001. "Quality Assurance and Continuing Education Needs of Rural and Remote General Practitioners: How Are They Changing?" *Australian Journal of Rural Health* 9, 6: 265-74.

Chan, B.T.B., N. Degani, T. Crichton, R.W. Pong, J.T. Rourke, J. Goertzen, and B. McCready. 2005. "Factors Influencing Family Physicians to Enter Rural Practice." *Canadian Family Physician* 5: 1246-47.

Chaskin, R.J. 2001. "Building Community Capacity: A Definitional Framework and Case Studies from a Comprehensive Community Initiative." *Urban Affairs Review* 36, 3: 291-323.

Craig, G. 2007. "Community Capacity Building: Something Old, Something New?" *Critical Social Policy* 27, 3: 335-59.

Curran, V.R., L. Fleet, and F. Kirby. 2006. "Factors Influencing Rural Health Care Professionals' Access to Continuing Professional Education." *Australian Journal of Rural Health* 14, 2: 51-55.

Curran, V.R., and J. Rourke. 2004. "The Role of Medical Education in the Recruitment and Retention of Rural Physicians." *Medical Teacher* 26, 3: 265-72.

Daniels, Z.M., B.J. VanLeit, B.J. Skipper, M.L. Sanders, and R.L. Rhyne. 2007. "Factors in Recruiting and Retaining Health Professionals for Rural Practice." *Journal of Rural Health* 23, 1: 62-71.

Dressendorfer, R.H., K. Raine, R.J. Dyck, R.C. Plotnikoff, R.L. Collins-Nakai, W.K. McLaughlin, and K. Ness. 2005. "A Conceptual Model of Community Capacity Development for Health Promotion in the Alberta Heart Health Project." *Health Promotion Practice* 6, 1: 31-36.

Gillham, S., and E. Ristevski. 2007. "Where Do I Go from Here: We've Got Enough Seniors?" *Australian Journal of Rural Health* 15, 5: 313-20.

Hawe, P., L. King, M. Noort, C. Jordens, and B. Lloyd. 2000. "Indicators to Help with Capacity Building in Health Promotion." North Sydney: Australian Centre for Health Promotion, http://www.health.nsw.gov.au/.

Hawe, P., M. Noort, S.M. Gifford, and B. Lloyd. 1998. "Working Invisibly: Health Workers Talk about Capacity Building in Health Promotion." *Health Promotion International* 13, 4: 285-96.

Hays, R.B. 2006. "Guiding Principles for Successful Innovation in Regional Medical Education Development." *Rural and Remote Health* 516: 1-5, http://www.rrh.org/.

Hill, P., and T. Alexander. 1996. "Continuing Professional Education: A Challenge for Rural Health Practitioners." *Australian Journal of Rural Health* 4, 4: 275-79.

Horton, J.E., and M.L.P. MacLeod. 2008. "The Experience of Capacity Building among Health Education Workers in the Yukon." *Canadian Journal of Public Health* 99, 1: 69-72.

Hoyal, F.M.D. 1999. "'Swallowing the Medicine': Determining the Present and Desired Modes for Delivery of Continuing Medical Education to Rural Doctors." *Australian Journal of Rural Health* 7, 4: 212-15.

Jukkala, A.M., S.J. Henly, and L.L. Lindeke. 2008. "Rural Perceptions of Continuing Professional Education." *Journal of Continuing Education in Nursing* 39, 12: 555-63.

Kelley, M.L. 2007. "Developing Rural Communities' Capacity for Palliative Care: A Conceptual Model." *Journal of Palliative Care* 23, 3: 143-53.

Kelley, M.L., S. Habjan, and J. Aegard. 2004. "Building Capacity to Provide Palliative Care in Rural and Remote Communities: Does Education Make a Difference?" *Journal of Palliative Care* 20, 4: 308-15.

Kelley, M.L., K. Kuluski, K. Brownlee, and S. Snow. 2008. "Physician Satisfaction and Practice Intentions in Northwestern Ontario." *Canadian Journal of Rural Medicine* 13, 3: 129-35.

Kelley, M.L., and M.J. MacLean. 1997. "Interdisciplinary Continuing Education in a Rural and Remote Area: The Approach of the Northern Educational Centre for Aging and Health." *Educational Gerontology* 23, 7: 631-49.

Kortes-Miller, K., S. Habjan, M.L. Kelley, and M. Fortier. 2007. "Development of Palliative Care Education Program in Rural Long-Term Care Facilities." *Journal of Palliative Care* 23, 3: 154-62.

Kramer, M., and C. Schmalenberg. 2004. "Essentials of a Magnetic Work Environment." *Nursing* 34, 6: 50-54.

Kretzmann, J., and J. McKnight. 1993. *Building Communities from the Inside Out: A Path toward Finding and Mobilizing a Community's Assets*. Chicago: ACTA Publications.

Lavergne, R., and J. Saxby. 2001. *Capacity Development: Vision and Implications*. Capacity Development, Occasional Series No. 3, CIDA, Policy Branch. Gatineau, QC: CIDA.

Levett-Jones, T.L. 2005. "Continuing Education for Nurses: A Necessity or a Nicety?" *Journal of Continuing Education in Nursing* 36, 5: 229-33.

Lightfoot, N., R. Strasser, M. Maar, and K. Jacklin. 2008. "Challenges and Rewards of Health Research in Northern, Rural, and Remote Communities." *Annals of Epidemiology* 18, 6: 507-14.

Lusthaus, C., M.H. Adrien, G. Anderson, and F. Carden. 1999. *Enhancing Organizational Performance: A Toolbox for Self-Assessment*. Montreal: Universalia.

MacLellan, K. 2002. "A Primer on Rural Medical Politics." *Canadian Journal of Rural Medicine* 7, 3: 212-14.

Meyer, D. 2006. "Technology, Job Satisfaction, and Retention: Rural Mental Health Practitioners." *Journal of Rural Health* 22, 2: 158-63.

Minkler, M. 2000. "Using Participatory Action Research to Build Healthy Communities." *Public Health Reports* 115, 2-3: 191-97.

Molinari, D.L., and J. Berry. 1999. "Telehealth: The Promise and the Need to Overcome the Knowledge Deficit Barrier." *Home Health Care Management and Practice* 11, 6: 36-41.

North West LHIN. 2006. *New Directions, Emerging Opportunities: A Health Human Resources Forum in the North West LHIN*. Thunder Bay: North West LHIN.

Northwestern Ontario District Health Council. 2001. *Annual Long-Term Care Service Plan for Northwestern Ontario.* Thunder Bay: Northwestern Ontario District Health Council.

Norton, B.L., K.R. McLeroy, J.N. Burdine, M.R.J. Felix, and A.M. Dorsey. 2002. "Community Capacity: Concept, Theory, and Methods." In *Emerging Theories in Health Promotion Practice and Research,* edited by R.J. DiClemente, R.A. Crosby, and M. Kegler, 194-227. San Francisco: Jossey-Bass.

Nutbeam, D. 2000. "Health Literacy as a Public Health Goal: A Challenge for Contemporary Health Education and Communication Strategies into the 21st Century." *Health Promotion International* 15, 3: 259-67.

O'Toole, K., A. Schoo, K. Stagnitti, and K. Cuss. 2008. "Rethinking Policies for the Retention of Allied Health Professionals in Rural Areas: A Social Relations Approach." *Health Policy* 87, 3: 326-32.

Pathman, D.E., T.R. Konrad, R. Dann, and G. Koch. 2004. "Retention of Primary Care Physicians in Rural Health Professional Shortage Areas." *American Journal of Public Health* 94, 10: 1723-29.

Penz, K., C. D'Arcy, N. Stewart, J. Kosteniuk, D. Morgan, and B. Smith. 2007. "Barriers to Participation in Continuing Education Activities among Rural and Remote Nurses." *Journal of Continuing Education in Nursing* 38, 2: 58-66.

Penz, K., N.J. Stewart, C. D'Arcy, and D. Morgan. 2008. "Predictors of Job Satisfaction for Rural Acute Care Registered Nurses in Canada." *Western Journal of Nursing Research* 30, 7: 785-800.

Raeburn, J., M. Akerman, K. Chuengsatiansup, F. Mejia, and O. Oladepo. 2006. "Community Capacity Building and Health Promotion in a Globalized World." *Health Promotion International* 21, S1: 84-90.

Robertson, E.M., L. Higgins, C. Rozmus, and J.P. Robinson. 1999. "Association between Continuing Education and Job Satisfaction of Nurses Employed in Long-Term Care Facilities." *Journal of Continuing Education in Nursing* 30, 3: 108-13.

Sellick, S.M., K. Charles, J. Dagsvik, and M.L. Kelley. 1996. "Palliative Care Providers' Perspectives on Service and Education Needs." *Journal of Palliative Care* 12, 2: 34-38.

Shipman, C., J. Addington-Hall, S. Barclay, J. Briggs, I. Cox, L. Daniels, and D. Millar. 2001. "Educational Opportunities in Palliative Care: What Do General Practitioners Want?" *Palliative Medicine* 15, 3: 191-96.

Solomon, P., P. Salvatori, and S. Berry. 2001. "Perceptions of Important Retention and Recruitment Factors by Therapists in Northwestern Ontario." *Journal of Rural Health* 17, 3: 278-85.

Strasser, R. 1999. "Teams in Rural Health." *Health Care and Informatics Review Online* 4, 1, http://www.hinz.org.nz/.

Chapter 8　　**The Rural-Urban Continuum as Place: What Can Be Learned from the Canadian Community Health Survey (CCHS) – Mental Health and Well-Being?**

C.H. Nelson and J. Park

Key Points

- Place matters in mental health, with rural and non-metro areas having better mental health status compared with urban and metropolitan areas.
- Place effects arise from differences in social and psychological support even after controlling for socio-economic factors and prevalence of mental disease.
- Strengthening community belonging and social support seem to reduce stress and depression and enhance self-esteem.
- Effectiveness in addressing rural mental health issues can be strengthened by professional training appropriate to the diversity and uniqueness of rural environments.
- These findings suggest that mental health status cannot be improved merely by focusing on better therapeutic techniques but would benefit from a paradigmatic shift from the focus on individual mental health illness to the enhancement of social-psychological supports.

Place has traditionally been perceived as having transformative properties. "Place saturates social life; it is one medium through which social life happens ... Place attachment facilitates a sense of security and well-being" (Gieryn 2000, 467, 481). A place-based context encourages responsive practice that is sensitive to unique community strengths. This perspective has led to several decades of ongoing academic debates about whether practitioners should differentiate along the rural/urban dichotomy (Chenoweth and Stehlik 2001; Collier 1984; Davenport and Davenport 1984; Farley et al. 1982; Ginsberg 1976; Hann-Morrison 2003; Martinez-Brawley 1986; Nelson, Kelley, and McPherson 1985; Nelson, McPherson, and Kelley 1987; Rich 1990; Schmidt 2000; Waltman 1986; Zapf 1985). However, increasingly and consistently, research findings confirm that context should be an essential feature of intervention (Moos 2003; Romanow 2002). For example, the Romanow Report states that "geography is, in fact, a determinant of health" (2002, 159). The distinctiveness of rural from urban is acknowledged as well as the potential inappropriateness of urban-based services as a model for rural health and social services. Enhancement of the rural environment itself is given priority as a focus for addressing rural health and corroborated in Chapters 2, 3, and 13 in this volume.

Relying on original data from the Canadian Community Health Survey (CCHS) – Mental Health and Well-Being (Statistics Canada 2002), this research investigates rural/urban and metropolitan/non-metropolitan differences for self-perceived mental health, mental disorders, social and community support, and utilization of mental health professionals and services. Typical prior studies of rural/urban differences in mental and physical health have relied on cross-sectional surveys of selected communities (Lev-Wiesel 2003; Muburak 1997). More prevalent are cross-sectional studies of rural communities and health (Chenoweth and Stehlik 2001; Glendinning et al. 2003; Jacob, Bourke, and Luloff 1997; Meyer and Lobao 2003; Molinari, Ahern, and Hendryx 1998; Sharp 2001; Theodori 2001; Wagner et al. 2002). Other studies simply look at the role in communities of social-psychological factors labelled with a range of terms, such as "social capital," "social support networks," and "social cohesion" (Bramston, Pretty, and Chipuer 2002; Leipert and George 2008; Murray 2000; Virgilis and Sarkella 1997). All have been small-scale projects (Romanow 2002).

Previous research has speculated about whether or not inconsistencies in outcome that distinguish rural from urban result from differences in definitions of rural (Martinez-Brawley 1980b; Smailes, Argent, and Griffin 2002; Whitaker 1986; Willits, Bealer, and Timbers 1990; York, Denton, and Moran 1989). The variations embedded in these definitions affect the characteristics of the population being studied as well as the size of each category. Rural is often defined as the absence of population or a certain density of population. Currently, Canada utilizes six definitions of rural (du Plessis et al. 2002). The census definition is more sensitive to neighbourhood-level information, while the metropolitan definition is more responsive to service-level data. Since this research is interested in both neighbourhood and service types of data, the analysis includes the more commonly used census definition of rural versus urban as well as the metropolitan/non-metropolitan distinction. Statistics Canada has published census data for this definition of rural for more than a century. However, one-third of this "census rural" population lives within the boundaries of Census Metropolitan Areas (CMAs) and Census Agglomerations (CAs) (Statistics Canada 2002). The metropolitan/non-metropolitan comparison is based on 1996 census data that identify twenty-five CMAs in Canada that are large urban areas, and their contiguous rural areas, which have a high degree of economic and social integration with the urban areas. To the best of our knowledge, no study has compared two definitions of rural in investigating the incidence of mental health issues. The use of these spatial definitions of rural/urban supports the need for a policy shift in Canada from a focus on sectoral policies (e.g., agriculture, fishing, mining, and forestry) to spatial, regional policies of rural/non-metropolitan and urban/metropolitan.

Methods

Data Source

The CCHS Cycle 1.2 on Mental Health and Well-Being provides national and provincial estimates of major mental disorders and problems and illuminates the issues associated with disabilities and the need for and provision of health care. The target population of the CCHS 1.2 excludes those living in the three territories, individuals living on reserves or crown land, residents of institutions, full-time members of the Armed Forces, and residents of some remote regions.

Analytical Techniques

Weighted cross-tabulations are used to estimate the average scores of mental health indicators (distress level) by place (urban versus rural and metropolitan versus non-metropolitan). Cross-tabulations by place are also used to estimate proportions of people reporting other mental health indicators (life satisfaction, perceived stress, self-rated mental health, and prevalence of mental diseases), social and psychological support, and utilization of mental health professionals and services. Multiple linear regression and logistic regression are used to model the relationship between place and mental health and illness as well as the relationship between place and mental health professional and service use. Socio-demographic characteristics and socio-psychological support variables are included in the models as control variables. To account for survey design effects, the variance used in the calculation of coefficients of variation and confidence limits is estimated with the bootstrap technique (Rao, Wu, and Yue 1992; Rust and Rao 1996; Yeo, Mantel, and Liu 1999).

Definitions

Mental Health Indicators

Distress measures the respondent's level of distress. Higher scores indicate more distress. It is based on the following six questions: "During the past month, about how often did you feel 1) nervous, 2) hopeless, 3) restless or fidgety, 4) so depressed that nothing could cheer you up, 5) that everything was an effort, and 6) worthless: all of the time, most of the time, some of the time, a little of the time, or none of the time?"

Life satisfaction is based on this question: "How satisfied are you with your life in general: very satisfied, satisfied, neither satisfied nor dissatisfied, dissatisfied, or very dissatisfied?" For this analysis, if respondents answer very satisfied or satisfied, they are considered to have life satisfaction.

Self-rated mental health is based on this question: "In general, would you say your mental health is: excellent, very good, good, fair, or poor?" For this study, if respondents answer excellent, very good, or good, they are considered to be in good mental health.

Self-perceived stress is determined from this question: "Thinking about the amount of stress in your life, would you say that most days are: not at all stressful, not very stressful, a bit stressful, quite a bit stressful, or extremely stressful?" In this study, respondents are considered to be under stress if they respond that most days are quite a bit or extremely stressful.

Mental disorder is stated to be present when a respondent is assessed by the CCHS 1.2 to have at least one of five selected mental disorders (depression, mania, panic episode, social phobia, and agoraphobia) or substance dependence (alcohol or illicit drug).

Social and Psychological Support Indicators

Tangible social support is configured from a number of questions that target specific kinds of tangible support. For example, the questions ask whether the respondent has someone to help if he or she is confined to bed, someone to take him or her to the doctor, someone to prepare meals, and someone to do daily chores. Higher scores indicate greater support.

Affection summarizes whether the respondent receives any affection. Questions about whether the respondent has someone who shows him or her love, someone to hug or someone to love, and someone to make him or her feel wanted are included. Higher scores indicate greater affection.

Emotional or informational support summarizes whether the respondent receives emotional or informational support. Questions ask whether the respondent has someone to listen and advise in a crisis, someone to give information and confide in and talk to, or someone to understand problems. Higher scores indicate greater support.

Positive social interaction summarizes whether the respondent is involved in positive social interaction. Questions ask whether the respondent has someone to have a good time with, get together with for relaxation, do things with to get his or her mind off things, or do something enjoyable with. Higher scores indicate greater interaction.

Community belonging is measured by asking respondents this question: "How would you describe your sense of belonging to your local community; would you say it is: very strong, somewhat strong, somewhat weak, or very weak?" Respondents are considered to have community belonging if they answer very strong or somewhat strong.

Self-esteem measurement is based on the well-being manifestations measure scale created by Masse and colleagues (1998a, 1998b) and is derived from four questions: "During the past month you felt 1) self-confident, 2) satisfied with what you were able to accomplish, proud of yourself, 3) loved and appreciated, and 4) useful: almost always (4 points), frequently (3 points), half the time (2 points), rarely (1 point), or never (0 points)?" Higher scores indicate greater self-esteem.

Control of self and events is based on the well-being manifestations measurement scale created by Masse and colleagues (1998a, 1998b) and is derived from four questions: "During the past month, you were 1) able to clearly sort things out when faced with complicated situations, 2) quite calm and level-headed, 3) able to easily find answers to your problems, and 4) able to face difficult situations in a positive way:

almost always (4 points), frequently (3 points), half the time (2 points), rarely (1 point), or never (0 points)?" Higher scores indicate greater control.

Limitations

The CCHS data are cross-sectional, and associations observed between variables cannot be inferred to be causal. For example, high association between low income and poor mental health does not necessarily mean that the former caused the latter. It can also mean that poor mental health resulted in a lower level of income. Furthermore, the data structure does not permit capturing all aspects of rurality. Philo, Parr, and Burns (2003) comment on unpacking the "rural" in rural mental health and becoming more sensitive to the diversity of human realities based on both history and geography. The data on utilization rates of types of professionals as resources for problems concerning emotions, mental health, or use of alcohol or drugs in the twelve months prior to the interview are limited by not being able to distinguish between utilization based on access to a particular type of professional and utilization based on the respondent's personal preferences.

Results

Table 8.1 shows differences in mental health by place and gender. For most indicators, urban and metropolitan residents seem to have poorer mental health compared with rural and non-metropolitan residents respectively. This finding is supported in Chapters 2 and 3 in this volume, where the more general discussions of rural health include indicators confirming that the prevalence of stress and all mental disorders is lower in rural areas. Moreover, Chapters 2 and 3 include data illustrating that almost all cancers are lower in rural areas, as is asthma.

More specific analysis of our findings reveals that, generally, women have poorer mental health than men, though such a gender difference does not exist in rural areas. These data demonstrate that a little over one-fifth of the population indicates high levels of self-perceived stress, with more stress in urban than rural areas. Furthermore, urban women have statistically higher odds than men of being stressed. In addition, approximately 10 percent of the population (or one out of ten persons) report some type of mental disease. In this case, the difference is only significant for women between rural and urban areas. In contrast,

Table 8.1   Mental health by urban and rural areas, and metropolitan and non-metropolitan areas, household population, aged fifteen or older, Canada, excluding territories, 2002

	Urban	Rural	Metropolitan	Non-metropolitan
Life satisfaction[1] *(%)*				
Men	85.1	89.3 *	84.7	88.0 †
Women	84.1	88.0 *	84.1	86.3 †‡
Self-rated mental health[2] *(%)*				
Men	94.0	93.7	94.4	93.3 †
Women	92.0 ‡	93.8 *	92.4 ‡	92.2 ‡
Distress (average score)				
Men	3.0	2.8 *	3.0	2.9
Women	3.2 ‡	3.0 *	3.2 ‡	3.1 ‡
Self-perceived stress[3] *(%)*				
Men	21.8	22.0	22.8	20.0 †
Women	24.9 ‡	22.1 *	25.8 ‡	22.0 †‡
Any mental disease[4] *(%)*				
Men	10.3	9.0	10.2	9.8
Women	12.1 ‡	9.4 *	11.9 ‡	11.2 ‡

Notes:
* Significantly different from estimate for urban ($p < .05$).
† Significantly different from estimate for metropolitan ($p < .05$).
‡ Significantly different from estimate for men ($p < .05$).
1 % of satisfied or very satisfied with life.
2 % of excellent, very good, or good mental health.
3 % of quite a bit or extremely stressful.
4 Having depression, mania, panic disorder, agoraphobia, social phobia, alcohol dependence,
   or illicit drug dependence.
Source: 2002 Canadian Community Health Survey Cycle 1.2.

gender differences are significant in urban, metropolitan, and non-metropolitan areas.

Philo, Parr, and Burns (2003) conclude that the findings of early research on mental health and place reveal more consistency on a gradient of urban core to suburbs to rural, where mental health was better in rural areas. More recent research has mixed outcomes, which are also reported in Chapter 13 in this volume. For example, Jacob, Bourke, and Luloff (1997), in their study of communities facing agricultural crisis, find no association between stress as an indicator of mental health and type of community. Wilkinson (1991) discusses at length lower individual well-being in rural communities experiencing boom growth and its accompanying structural changes. This inconsistency between

early research and more recent studies might indicate that the difference is caused by change itself: that is, rural agricultural crisis or boom
conditions associated with mining and pulp and paper. Likewise, studies in the past decade might reflect that rural communities are simply
more integrated into national and global economic and political systems that diffuse mental health status. However, there is a strong theme
in the literature that social and psychological factors are associated with
mental health status. For example, referring again to the Jacob, Bourke,
and Luloff research (1997), communities with higher levels of interaction show evidence of slightly lower stress.

Table 8.2 provides information for five different measures of social
and psychological support by place. For every indicator, rural and non-
metropolitan residents show higher levels of support. Women show
higher levels of affection, emotional support, and positive social interaction, while men have higher levels of tangible support, self-esteem,
and control of self and events. Rural/non-metropolitan residents show
a significantly higher percentage for both men and women of a strong
sense of community belonging. Chapter 3 supports this finding that
rural residents are found to have a stronger sense of community belonging. Moreover, Chapter 2 describes how the framework for indicating differences in health impacts between rural and urban is informed
by studies of social support networks that add credence to the position
that connections between health status and place can be direct, indirect,
and reciprocal.

Theodori (2001) found that in four communities in rural eastern
United States community belonging and community satisfaction are associated positively and independently with individual well-being, defined to include a measure of mental health. His analysis concludes that
rural residents have higher levels of both community belonging and
community satisfaction. From a study of three Midwestern rural communities, Sharp (2001) argues for connectedness between a strong social network and a positive subjective sense of community well-being.
Furthermore, within rural areas, social support is associated with lower
stress and depression (Meyer and Lobao 2003). Moreover, Meyer and
Lobao find that social support has a positive impact on mental health
even when such support cannot remove the distress caused by the structural crisis in rural farming. Moreover, social support is found to be a
significant factor in reducing stress, depression, and other mental disease. Such support is referred to as a "protective shield." Wagner et al.
(2002) find that drug use is lower in rural communities, where there is

Table 8.2 Social and community support by urban and rural areas, and metropolitan and non-metropolitan areas, household population, aged fifteen or older, Canada, excluding territories, 2002

	Urban	Rural	Metropolitan	Non-metropolitan
Tangible social support (average score)				
Men	13.7	14.1 *	13.7	14.0 †
Women	13.2 ‡	13.7 *‡	13.2 ‡	13.5 †‡
Affection (average score)				
Men	10.4	10.7 *	10.4	10.7 †
Women	10.6 ‡	10.9 *‡	10.6 ‡	10.8 ‡
Emotional or informational support (average score)				
Men	26.6	27.1 *	26.4	27.0 †
Women	27.1 ‡	27.6 *‡	27.1 ‡	27.4 †‡
Positive social interaction (average score)				
Men	13.7	14.0 *	13.6	14.0 †
Women	13.6	13.9 *‡	13.6	13.8 †‡
Strong community belonging[1] (%)				
Men	57.0	61.7 *	54.6	63.5 †
Women	57.8	61.1 *	55.2	64.0 †
Self-esteem (average score)				
Men	13.1	13.6 *	13.1	13.4 †
Women	12.9 ‡	13.2 *‡	12.9 ‡	13.1 †‡
Control of self and events (average score)				
Men	13.1	13.5 *	13.1	13.4 †
Women	12.8 ‡	13.2 *‡	12.8 ‡	13.2 †‡

Notes:
* Significantly different from estimate for urban ($p < .05$).
† Significantly different from estimate for metropolitan ($p < .05$).
‡ Significantly different from estimate for men ($p < .05$).
1 % of somewhat strong and very strong community belonging.
Source: 2002 Canadian Community Health Survey Cycle 1.2.

greater social cohesion and cultural identity as well as tighter community links. Moreover, subjective measures of community appear to have a stronger influence on mental health status than structural measures such as race, ethnicity, and socio-economic status (Aneshensel and Sucoff 1996). In addition, psychological support, such as self-esteem and control of self and events, has been found to be protective against stress and depression and to bring more constructive coping strategies (Longmore and DeMaris 1997; Pearlin and Schooler 1978; Spencer, Josephs, and Steele 1993; Thoits 1994).

Table 8.3 Adjusted odds ratios (OR) of mental health indicators, men and women aged fifteen or older, Canada, excluding territories, simple and extended models, 2002

| | Urban/rural | | | | Metro/non-metro | | | |
| | Simple model | | Extended model | | Simple model | | Extended model | |
Mental health indicators	Men	Women	Men	Women	Men	Women	Men	Women
Life satisfaction	0.71*	0.79*	0.85	0.92	0.75*	0.84*	0.87*	1.00
Self-rated positive mental health	1.07	0.80*	1.46*	0.97	1.19	0.98	1.47*	1.16
Distress†	0.15	0.13	-0.12	-0.07	0.10	0.08	-0.11	-0.18*
Self-perceived stress	0.98	1.12	0.88	1.04	1.17*	1.17*	1.11	1.09
Mental disorder	1.06	1.19*	0.88	1.08	0.98	1.00	0.87	0.87

Notes: Household income, education level, employment status, and marital status were adjusted for sample models; psychological support (emotional and informational support; positive social interaction; affection; tangible support; community belonging; self-esteem; and control of self and events) were additionally adjusted for extended models.
* Significantly different from rural (or non-metropolitan) areas ($p < .05$).
† Adjusted regression coefficients.
Source: 2002 Canadian Community Health Survey Cycle 1.2.

In summary, Table 8.1 provides evidence that place does have an impact on mental health status. Table 8.2 demonstrates that social and psychological factors also differ by place. However, these data alone do not provide proof that social and psychological factors have a substantive association with mental health status.

Table 8.3 displays the summary results[1] of several regression analyses of mental health indicators (life satisfaction, self-rated mental health, distress, self-perceived stress, and mental disorder). For each indicator, we conducted two regression analyses: simple and extended models. Simple models aimed to investigate the effect of place on mental health after controlling for socio-economic confounders such as household income, educational level, employment status, and marital status. Extended models aimed to see whether place had an effect on mental health even after controlling for social and psychological support factors (emotional and informational support, positive social interaction, affection, tangible social support, community belonging, self-esteem, and control of self and events) in addition to the socio-economic confounders. If a significant effect of place found in a simple model disappeared in its extended model, it could mean that place differences once observed were due to differing contexts of social and psychological supports.

Urban residents (both men and women) have a lower chance of life satisfaction than rural residents after controlling for socio-demographic factors. However, such rural/urban differences disappear when we control for factors of social and psychological support in addition to socio-demographic factors. It might mean that rural/urban differences in life satisfaction are associated with better conditions of social and psychological support in rural areas. Similarly, for women, differences in life satisfaction between metropolitan and non-metropolitan areas disappear after controlling for social and psychological support factors. Higher life satisfaction among non-metropolitan women compared with metropolitan women might be associated with their higher levels of social and psychological support. For example, Muburak (1997) discovers, in a survey of rural and urban Malaysian women, that there is a significant association between social cohesion and mental health of rural respondents. Furthermore, lack of social support is found to be a much more significant factor for rural women than urban women.

The results of logistic regressions on positive subjective mental health (see Table 8.3) suggest that urban men show no difference and that urban women show lower probability of positive subjective mental health compared with rural men and women respectively. Nevertheless, after controlling for factors of social and psychological support, urban men show higher subjective mental health, and urban women's previously higher level of mental health disappears. It might mean that rural/urban differences in subjective mental health are associated with differences in social and psychological supports between urban and rural areas. Similarly, after controlling for the support variables, metropolitan men seem to have higher odds of having subjective mental health. In other words, lower subjective mental health in urban and metropolitan areas is related to lower levels of social and psychological support.

According to the results of linear regressions on distress level, there are no statistically significant differences between distress levels of urban and rural residents. However, metropolitan men seem to have lower distress levels than men residing in other regions after controlling for factors of social and psychological support. This finding is contrasted with higher average scores of distress for men living in metropolitan areas (see Table 8.1). It might signify that the distress of men in big cities is related to their lower levels of social and psychological support.

Results of logistic regressions on self-perceived stress indicate that there are no statistically significant differences between perceived stress levels of urban and rural residents. However, metropolitan residents

(both men and women) seem to have higher odds of perceiving themselves as stressed than their non-metropolitan counterparts when we
control only for socio-demographic factors. When controlling for factors
of social and psychological support in addition to the socio-demographic
variables, we find that previously existing differences disappear. This
suggests that higher levels of self-perceived stress among metropolitan
residents are related to their lower levels of social and psychological
support.

Table 8.3 displays results of logistic regressions on having any mental
disorder or substance dependence. It indicates that there are no statistically significant differences between different places except for urban
women when we control for socio-demographic variables. As substan-
tiated in Chapters 2, 3, and 13, this might mean that differences in the
prevalence of mental disorders between different regions are related
mostly to socio-demographic conditions. Even urban women's high
prevalence disappears after we control for social and psychological support. The importance of socio-demographic factors on health is reported
in a study of acute coronary events in which both socio-economic factors and Aboriginal status explained primary effects of place (Beard et
al. 2008).

Table 8.4 displays mental health professional and service use by place
and gender. Generally, women use these services more than men; urban
men use them more than rural men, and, for psychiatrist/psychologist
use, urban and metropolitan residents show higher odds of use than
their rural and non-metropolitan counterparts. In all categories of professional use, women are significantly more likely than men to use services. For any service use, rural women are slightly more than twice as
likely as men to use services. Similarly, urban women are only slightly
less than twice as likely as men to use any service. This rate of differentiation of women to men continues for each specific category of professional service use. Similarly, metropolitan and non-metropolitan women
are significantly more likely to use services than men, with the exception of other service use that includes Internet support groups, self-help
groups, and telephone hotlines. For social worker use, the difference
between women and men is even greater. For all categories of service
use, there is no significant difference in utilization rates between rural
and urban women, except for urban residents' higher rates of consulting psychiatrists or psychologists. In contrast, rural men demonstrate
significantly less use of services than urban men in four of the six
categories. However, when using the metropolitan/non-metropolitan

Table 8.4   Mental health service use by urban and rural areas, and metropolitan and non-metropolitan areas, household population, aged fifteen or older, Canada, excluding territories, 2002

	Urban	Rural	Metropolitan	Non-metropolitan
Any service use (%)				
Men	7.1	5.3 *	6.8	6.6
Women	12.5 ‡	11.4 ‡	12.5 ‡	12.0 ‡
Psychiatrist or psychologist service use (%)				
Men	3.0	1.9 *	3.1	2.3 †
Women	4.5 ‡	3.0 ‡	4.8 ‡	3.3 †‡
Other MD service use[1] (%)				
Men	3.7	3.3	3.6	3.7
Women	7.4 ‡	6.3 ‡	7.2 ‡	7.2 ‡
Social worker use (%)				
Men	1.4	0.7 *E	1.2	1.4
Women	3.2 ‡	3.1 ‡	3.2 ‡	3.3 ‡
Other professional use[2] (%)				
Men	1.1	0.8 E	0.9	1.2
Women	2.2 ‡	1.9 ‡E	2.1 ‡	2.3 ‡
Other service use[3] (%)				
Men	1.8	0.7 *E	1.8	1.4
Women	2.3 ‡	1.9 ‡	2.1	2.5 ‡

Notes:
*   Significantly different from estimate for urban ($p < .05$).
†   Significantly different from estimate for metropolitan ($p < .05$).
‡   Significantly different from estimate for men ($p < .05$).
E   Coefficient of variation between 16.6% and 33.3%.
1   Including family doctor and other doctor.
2   Including nurse, religious adviser, and other professionals.
3   Including Internet support group, self-help group, and telephone helpline.
Source: 2002 Canadian Community Health Survey Cycle 1.2.

definition, men are only significantly different in their use of psychiatrists or psychologists, with non-metropolitan men using fewer services in this category.

After controlling for socio-demographic factors and the prevalence of mental disorders, we find that there still exists urban men's greater use of mental health-care services than rural men's use; similarly, metropolitan women have more visits to psychiatrists/psychologists than non-metropolitan women. Thus, those differences in professional utilization might not result merely from differences in economic conditions or prevalence of mental disorders.[2] They could be related to differences in availability of professionals and services (see Chapter 13, this volume) or differences in health behaviour between residents in different places.

Discussion

The 2002 CCHS 1.2 survey substantiates that rural areas are distinct from urban areas in the association between mental health and the amount of social and psychological support from all seven indexed measurements: tangible support, demonstrated affection, emotional and informational support, positive social interaction, strong community belonging, self-esteem, and control of self and events. There is substantial literature that confirms these findings, but there is no approach like this current research at a national level with results for two different place definitions (rural and metropolitan). The 2002 CCHS 1.2 findings support earlier and current community-based research that recognizes mutual aid systems and strong informal support networks as social-psychological factors that could be vital resources to practitioners serving rural areas (Davenport and Davenport 1984; Ginsberg 1976; Martinez-Brawley 1980a; Nelson, Kelley, and McPherson 1985; Nelson and McPherson 2004; Waltman 1989). These findings have implications for the approach taken by rural practitioners in addressing mental health issues.

First, the findings from the CCHS 1.2 suggest that practitioners should place more emphasis on sustaining social-psychological support in rural areas rather than individualized therapeutic intervention. Rural areas can take full advantage of better support networks in addressing mental health issues. Additionally, Chapter 13 in this volume advocates for the community-based approach as more cost effective and preventive in addressing mental health issues in these early stages. Moreover, urban areas can learn from rural areas about the importance of support networks. Even though the literature suggests that practitioners should practise differently in rural areas, York, Denton, and Moran (1989) find that, though practitioners did perceive their urban and rural work communities differently, they continued to practise similarly. In other words, though the rural practitioners perceived their communities as having more informal supports and paying more attention to community acceptance, compared with urban workers they made no distinguishable effort to view these informal networks as a resource to support individuals, groups, or the community itself. As an example, DeWeaver, Smith, and Hosang (1988) recognize that social work's return to a focus on the individual as a source of identifying and dealing with social problems is not productive for rural areas. Furthermore, imposed urban services carry the risk of nullifying existing natural support mechanisms. Other explanations include the urban influence on educational training and rural agencies that affect approaches taken by rural practitioners (Adams et al. 2006; Goldworthy 2002).

Second, these findings suggest that it might be prudent to curtail measuring rural/non-metropolitan in terms of its deficiencies compared with urban/metropolitan. We suggest a complete reversal in which, in terms of issues of mental health, urban/metropolitan is compared with rural/non-metropolitan in terms of the degree of social-psychological support and community belonging. The viability of urban communities might depend on shifting the emphasis from self-interest to greater responsibility to community (Glaser, Parker, and Payton 2001; Putnam 1993, 2000). Furthermore, these authors put forward a compelling argument that greater focus on social-psychological support can be successful in an urban community. Wagner et al. (2002) also suggest that social-psychological factors can be of benefit in urban areas.

The key roles of both social support and community belonging as potential buffers against higher prevalence of perceived mental health problems along with socio-demographic characteristics appear to have a strong association with perceptions of positive life satisfaction and lower prevalence of mental disease. Sustaining positive mental health might be more effective by bolstering social supports and perceived community well-being than relying on clinical intervention. Wolkow and Ferguson (2001) support this position when they note that child and family have remained the focus of programs of intervention even when community-level factors are highly represented in the literature as protective factors against adversity, including mental illness. They suggest that social-psychological support is a promising tool for community-level intervention. In addition, social support might lessen the need for more remedial therapeutic interventions that address problems after they are more firmly entrenched. Bramston, Pretty, and Chipuer (2002) corroborate this position through their finding that, though community factors might not directly affect quality of life, they do so indirectly through the impact of the individual variable loneliness. Thus, changes in social supports and perceptions of community belonging might change the individual's level of loneliness.

Moreover, Meyer and Lobao (2003) confirm that traditional individual coping strategies fail to affect positively either stress or depression. Furthermore, in all but one case, they have a negative impact: "All coping techniques, except direct action, were deleterious" (149). In terms of distress, individual coping efforts can exacerbate the condition (Mattlin, Wethington, and Kessler 1990; Pearlin 1989). Furthermore, Meyer and Lobao's (2003) findings, as well as their review of the literature, demonstrate that, for social support to be effective, it must be in place before the crisis occurs. Findings in Chapter 2 in this volume agree with this position and advocate for rural-specific prevention and promotion activities. What is more, seeking support at the time of crisis appears to increase mental health conditions such as depression and stress. Social supports appear to be a strong shield, not a remedial intervention approach. These findings suggest that programs aimed at personal challenges should be supplemented with initiatives addressing enhanced community belonging and social-psychological supports. Individualized clinical intervention typically addresses issues outside the community context, in which there is no opportunity to anchor outcome to sustaining community-level change. Chapter 9 in this volume adds to the discussion by advocating for "made-in-the-North" solutions and describing how decision making among multiple partners must be attentive to the context of community-based relationships.

Postsecondary institutions might need to guard against training only according to practice trends and preferences found in the curricula of urban-based accredited programs (Edwards 1987; Perry 2002). Instead, findings such as those in the CCHS 1.2 should be considered in determining training directions for rural practitioners. As supported in Chapters 9 and 13 in this volume, it is imperative for rural-oriented training programs to rethink their approaches so that curriculum has relevance to place (Florence et al. 2007).

Conclusion

Rural practitioners are embedded in community (Ungar 2002), where relationships can be key factors in helping (Ribner and Knei-Paz 2002). The CCHS 1.2 provides compelling evidence that social-psychological support is strongly associated with factors that affect mental health, and this support is more prevalent in rural and non-metropolitan areas.

Notes

1 Detailed results of each regression model are available on the website of the Food Security Research Network, http://www.foodsecurityresearch.ca/.
2 Results of multiple regression analyses on the use of mental health care are available on the website of the Food Security Research Network, http://www.foodsecurityresearch.ca/.

References

Adams, S.J., S. Xu, F. Dong, J. Fortney, and K. Rost. 2006. "Differential Effectiveness of Depression Disease Management for Rural and Urban Primary Care Patients." *Journal of Rural Health* 22, 4: 343-50.

Aneshensel, C.S., and C.A. Sucoff. 1996. "The Neighborhood Context of Adolescent Mental Health." *Journal of Health and Social Behavior* 37: 293-310.

Beard, J.R., A. Earnest, G. Morgan, H. Chan, R. Summerhayes, T.M. Dunn, N.A. Timaska, and L. Ryan. 2008. "Socioeconomic Disadvantage and Acute Coronary Events: A Spatiotemporal Analysis." *Epidemiology* 19, 3: 485-92.

Bramston, P., G. Pretty, and H. Chipuer. 2002. "Unravelling Subjective Quality of Life: An Investigation of Individual and Community Determinants." *Social Indicators Research* 59: 261-74.

Chenoweth, L., and D. Stehlik. 2001. "Building Resilient Communities: Social Work Practice and Rural Queensland." *Australian Social Work* 54, 2: 47-55.

Collier, K. 1984. *Social Work with Rural Peoples: Theory and Practice.* Vancouver: New Star Books.

Davenport, J., and J. Davenport. 1984. "Theoretical Perspectives of Rural/Urban Differences." *Human Services in the Rural Environment* 9, 1: 4-9.

DeWeaver, K.L., M.L. Smith, and M. Hosang. 1988. "Has Social Work Education Abandoned Preparation for Rural Practice?" *Human Services in the Rural Environment* 11, 4: 28-32.

du Plessis, V., R. Beshiri, and R.D. Bollman 2002. *Definitions of Rural.* Working Paper 61. Statistics Canada Catalogue No. 21-601-MIE.

Edwards, R.L. 1987. "Professional Social Work Organizations and Rural Poverty." *Human Services in the Rural Environment* 10, 4 and 11, 1: 66-75.

Farley, O.W., K.A. Griffiths, R.A. Skidmore, and M.G. Thackery. 1982. *Rural Social Work Practice.* New York: Free Press.

Florence, J.A., B. Goodrow, J. Wachs, S. Grover, and K.E. Olive. 2007. "Rural Health Professions Education at East Tennessee State University: Survey of Graduates from the First Decade of the Community Partnership Program." *Journal of Rural Health* 23, 1: 77-83.

Gieryn, T.F. 2000. "A Space for Place in Sociology." *Annual Review of Sociology* 26: 463-96.

Ginsberg, L., ed. 1976. *Social Work in Rural Communities: A Book of Readings.* New York: Council on Social Work Education.

Glaser, M.A., L.E. Parker, and S. Payton. 2001. "The Paradox between Community and Self-Interest: Local Government, Neighborhoods, and Media." *Journal of Urban Affairs* 23, 1: 87-102.

Glendinning, A., M. Nuttall, L. Hendry, M. Kloep, and S. Wood. 2003. "Rural Communities and Well-Being: A Good Place to Grow Up?" *Sociological Review* 51, 1: 129-56.

Goldworthy, J. 2002. "Resurrecting a Model of Integrating Individual Work with Community Development and Social Action." *Community Development Journal* 37, 4: 327-37.

Hann-Morrison, D. 2003. "An Alternative Approach to Rural Mental Health Service Delivery: A Case Study." *Rural Mental Health* (Winter): 4-7.

Jacob, S., L. Bourke, and A.E. Luloff. 1997. "Rural Community Stress, Distress, and Well-Being in Pennsylvania." *Journal of Rural Studies* 13, 3: 275-88.

Leipert, B.D., and J.A. George. 2008. "Determinants of Rural Women's Health: A Qualitative Study in Southwest Ontario." *Journal of Rural Health* 24, 2: 210-18.

Lev-Wiesel, R. 2003. "Indicators Constituting the Construct of 'Perceived Community Cohesion.'" *Community Development Journal* 38, 4: 332-43.

Longmore, M.A., and A. DeMaris. 1997. "Perceived Inequity and Depression in Intimate Relationships: The Moderating Effect of Self-Esteem." *Social Psychology Quarterly* 60: 172-84.

Martinez-Brawley, E., ed. 1980a. *Pioneer Efforts in Rural Social Work: First Hand Views since 1908.* University Park: Pennsylvania State University Press.

–. 1980b. "Identifying and Describing the Context of Rural in Social Work." *Arete* 6, 2: 21-32.

–. 1986. "Beyond Cracker-Barrel Images: The Rural Social Work Speciality." *Social Casework: The Journal of Contemporary Social Work* 67, 2: 101-7.

Masse, R., C. Poulin, C. Dassa, J. Lambert, S. Bélair, and M.A. Battaglini. 1998a. "Elaboration and Validation of a Tool to Measure Psychological Well-Being: WBMMS." *Canadian Journal of Public Health* 89, 5: 352-57.

–. 1998b. "The Structure of Mental Health Higher-Order Confirmatory Factor Analyses of Psychological Distress and Well-Being Measures." *Social Indicators Research* 45: 475-504.

Mattlin, J.A., F. Wethington, and R.C. Kessler. 1990. "Situational Determinants of Coping and Coping Effectiveness." *Journal of Health and Social Behavior* 31, 1: 103-22.

Meyer, K., and L. Lobao. 2003. "Economic Hardship, Religion, and Mental Health during the Midwestern Farm Crisis." *Journal of Rural Studies* 19: 139-55.

Molinari, C., M. Ahern, and M. Hendryx. 1998. "The Relationship of Community Quality to the Health of Women and Men." *Social Science and Medicine* 47, 8: 1113-20.

Moos, R.H. 2003. "Social Contexts: Transcending Their Power and Their Fragility." *American Journal of Community Psychology* 32, 1-2: 1-13.

Muburak, A.R. 1997. "A Comparative Study on Family, Social Supports, and Mental Health of Rural and Urban Malay Women." *Medical Journal of Malaysia* 52, 3: 274-84.

Murray, M. 2000. "Social Capital Formation and Healthy Communities: Insights from the Colorado Healthy Communities Initiative." *Community Development Journal* 35, 2: 99-108.

Nelson, C.H., M.L. Kelley, and D.H. McPherson. 1985. "Rediscovering Support in Social Work Practice." *Canadian Social Work Review* 1985: 231-48.

Nelson, C.H., and D.H. McPherson. 2004. "Contextual Fluidity: An Emerging Practice Model for Helping." *Rural Social Work* 9: 199-209.

Nelson, C.H., D.H. McPherson, and M.L. Kelley. 1987. "Contextual Patterning: A Key to Human Service Effectiveness in the North." In *Canada's Subarctic Universities,* edited by Peter Adams and Doug Parker, 66-82. Ottawa: Association of Canadian Universities for Northern Studies.

Pearlin, L. 1989. "The Sociological Study of Stress." *Journal of Health and Social Behavior* 30, 3: 241-56.

Pearlin, L.I., and C. Schooler. 1978. "The Structure of Coping." *Journal of Health and Social Behavior* 19: 2-21.

Perry, R. 2002. "The Classification, Intercorrelation, and Dynamic Nature of MSW Student Practice Preferences." *Journal of Social Work Education* 37, 3: 523-42.

Philo, C., H. Parr, and N. Burns. 2003. "Rural Madness: A Geographical Reading and Critique of the Rural Mental Health Literature." *Journal of Rural Studies* 19: 259-81.

Putnam, R. 1993. *Making Democracy Work: Civic Traditions in Modern Italy.* Princeton: Princeton University Press.

–. 2000. *Bowling Alone: The Collapse and Revival of American Community.* New York: Touchstone Books.

Rao, J.N.K., C.F.J. Wu, and K. Yue. 1992. "Some Recent Work on Resampling Methods for Complex Surveys." *Survey Methodology* 18, 2: 209-17. Statistics Canada Catalogue No. 12-001.

Ribner, D.S., and C. Knei-Paz. 2002. "Client's View of a Successful Helping Relationship." *Social Work* 47, 4: 379-87.

Rich, R.O. 1990. "The American Rural Metaphor: Myths and Realities in Rural Practice." *Human Services in the Rural Environment* 14, 1: 31-34.

Romanow, R. 2002. *Building on Values: The Future of Health Care in Canada.* Saskatoon: Commission on the Future of Health Care in Canada.

Rust, K.F., and J.N.K. Rao. 1996. "Variance Estimation for Complex Surveys Using Replication Techniques." *Statistical Methods in Medical Research* 5: 281-310.

Schmidt, G.G. 2000. "Remote, Northern Communities: Implications for Social Work Practice." *International Social Work* 43, 3: 337-49.

Sharp, J.S. 2001. "Locating the Community Field: A Study of Interorganizational Network Structure and Capacity for Community Action." *Rural Sociology* 66, 3: 403-24.

Smailes, P.J., N. Argent, and R.L.C. Griffin. 2002. "Rural Population Density: Its Impact on Social and Demographic Aspects of Rural Communities." *Journal of Rural Studies* 18: 385-404.

Spencer, S.J., R.A. Josephs, and C.M. Steele. 1993. "Low Self-Esteem: The Uphill Struggle for Self-Integrity." In *Self-Esteem: The Puzzle of Low Self-Regard,* edited by R.F. Baumeister, 21-36. New York: Plenum.

Statistics Canada. 2002. Canadian Community Health Survey (CCHS) – Mental Health and Well-Being 1.2.

Theodori, G.L. 2001. "Examining the Effects of Community Satisfaction and Attachment on Individual Well-Being." *Rural Sociology* 66, 4: 618-28.

Thoits, P.A. 1994. "Stressors and Problem Solving: The Individual as Psychological Activist." *Journal of Health and Social Behavior* 35: 143-59.

Ungar, M. 2002. "A Deeper, More Social Ecological Social Work Practice." *Social Service Review* 76, 3: 480-97.

Virgilis, E., and J. Sarkella. 1997. "Determinants and Indicators of Health and Well-Being: Tools for Educating Society." *Social Indicators Research* 40: 159-78.

Wagner, F., D.B. Diaz, A.L. Lopez, A.E. Collado, and E. Aldaz. 2002. "Social Cohesion, Cultural Identity, and Drug Use in Mexican Rural Communities." *Substance Use and Misuse* 37, 5-7: 715-47.

Waltman, G.J. 1986. "Main Street Revisited: Social Work Practice in Rural Areas." *Social Casework: The Journal of Contemporary Social Work* 67, 8: 466-74.

–. 1989. "Social Work in Consultation Services in Rural Areas." *Human Services in the Rural Environment* 12, 3: 17-21.

Whitaker, W.H. 1986. "A Survey of Perceptions of Social Work Practice in Rural and Urban Areas." *Human Services in the Rural Environment* 9, 3: 12-19.

Wilkinson, K.P. 1991. *The Community in Rural America*. New York: Greenwood Press.

Willits, F.K., R.C. Bealer, and V.L. Timbers. 1990. "Popular Images of 'Rurality': Data from a Pennsylvania Survey." *Rural Sociology* 55, 4: 559-78.

Wolkow, K.E., and H.B. Ferguson. 2001. "Community Factors in the Development of Resiliency: Considerations and Future Directions." *Community Mental Health Journal* 37, 6: 489-98.

Yeo, D., H. Mantel, and T.P. Liu. 1999. "Bootstrap Variance Estimation for the National Population Health Survey." In *American Statistical Association: Proceedings of the Survey Research Methods Section*. Baltimore: American Statistical Association.

York, R.O., R.T. Denton, and J.R. Moran. 1989. "Rural and Urban Social Work Practice: Is There a Difference?" *Social Casework: The Journal of Contemporary Social Work* 70, 4: 201-9.

Zapf, M.K. 1985. "Rural Social Work and Its Application to the Canadian North as a Practice Setting." Working Papers on Social Welfare in Canada 15. Toronto: Faculty of Social Work, University of Toronto.

Part 3: Rural Health Services Delivery

Chapter 9   **Transcending Boundaries:**
Collaborating to Improve Access
to Health Services in Northern
Manitoba and Saskatchewan

A. Moss, F. Racher, B. Jeffery, C. Hamilton,
M. Burles, and R.C. Annis

Key Points

- Multi-level and cross-jurisdictional partnerships and collaboration are crucial to ensure that policies and programs are well understood and altered at the right times for the right reasons. Partnerships and communication create understanding and foster balanced change and implementation.
- Understanding the unique circumstances of living in the North and respecting residents' desire to reside in the North are pivotal for government decision makers. Service providers and policy makers must have a meaningful knowledge of First Nations and northern culture, history, and tradition and a respect for differences that ensures service provision is appropriate and effective.
- Trust and relationship building are critical to effective service delivery. Open and sincere dialogue inform and support the principal argument that northerners and their communities need to be heard and involved in the process; workshop participants stressed the need to ensure that "northern health is in northern hands."

Access to health services is of particular concern to Canadians living in northern areas (Scott 2000) and the health professionals committed to providing care and services to them (MacLeod 1999). The challenges in accessing health services are coupled with the health-care needs related to the poor health status of northern residents (Fransoo et al. 2005;

Shields and Tremblay 2002); these issues are also noted among rural residents in southern locations of our country (see Chapter 16, this volume) and among Aboriginal peoples in general (see Chapters 20-22). To understand the range of issues and solutions, a multi-community collaborative effort addressed regional needs in northern rural and remote regions in Manitoba and Saskatchewan.

Participatory action research (PAR) was used to explore barriers to health-care access for northern residents and to find ways to dialogue with program planners and policy makers to effect change. PAR involves participation in the research by the people being studied; includes popular knowledge, personal experiences, and other ways of knowing; focuses on empowerment and power relations; and fosters awareness, education of the participants, and political action (Dickson 2000). PAR nurtures talent and leadership to enhance the quality of community life and tackle problems that threaten the community (Thurston, Scott, and Vollman 2004). PAR became a tool to help build community strength as northerners worked together to improve access to health services. This chapter describes the findings from the multi-year project and explores actions taken and lessons discovered throughout the participatory research processes.

Northern Health Status and Service Need

In health regions in northern Manitoba, life expectancy was 4.0 years less for males than the Manitoba average and 3.8 years less for females for the years 1999-2003 (Fransoo et al. 2005). The premature mortality rate in the North for men aged 0-74 years was 6.2 deaths per 1,000 residents, compared with the Manitoba rate of 4.4, and 4.1 among northern women, compared with the provincial rate of 2.6. The treatment prevalence for diabetes and hypertension was significantly higher in northern Manitoba than in Manitoba overall; early child immunization rates were significantly lower in the North (Fransoo et al. 2005); and treatment prevalence for substance abuse was significantly higher (Martens et al. 2004).

Similar to northern Manitoba, the relative poor health of northern Saskatchewan residents is reflected in the mortality and life expectancy statistics. For the years 1993-2002, life expectancy at birth for residents of Saskatchewan's Near and Far North was shorter than that for the average Saskatchewan resident by 5 years for men and close to 6 years for women. During this period, the annual age-adjusted mortality rate for northern Saskatchewan was 9 deaths per 1,000 residents for women and 10 per 1,000 for men, both higher than the provincial average of 6 per 1,000 for women and 7 per 1,000 for men. Infant mortality rates in the North were double the provincial average between 1998 and 2002, and early childhood immunization rates were lower in the North (Irvine, Stockdale, and Oliver 2004).

Interestingly, the prevalence of diabetes varies across both the province and the North. In 2000-1, the Mamawetan Churchill River Regional Health Authority reported the highest sex-age-adjusted diabetes prevalence rate in the province at 73 per 1,000, while the Athabasca Health Authority had the lowest rate at 30 per 1,000 (Irvine, Stockdale, and Oliver 2004).

Access to Health Services Theory

Access to health services and the various factors that contribute to access remain nebulous and obscure to consumers, health-care providers, and policy makers alike (Racher and Vollman 2002). Multiple understandings of access to health services impede progress in the development of policies, the creation of programs, and the transformation of health services. Historically, access to health care was assumed to exist if services were available. Donabedian (1972) posited that proof of access required use of a service, not merely presence of a facility. He distinguished between initiation and continuation in the use of service and emphasized that barriers to access are myriad, including financial, psychological, informational, social, organizational, spatial, and temporal factors. Mechanic (1972) agreed and stated that potential consumer willingness to seek care must be considered, dependent on one's health attitudes, knowledge about health care, and learned social and cultural definitions of illness.

The World Health Organization (WHO 1978, 28) identified access to health care as a principle of primary health care: "Accessibility implies the continuing and organized supply of care that is geographically, financially, culturally, and functionally within easy reach of the whole community. The care has to be appropriate and adequate in content and in amount to satisfy the needs of people and it has to be provided by methods acceptable to them."

Penchansky and Thomas (1981, 128) depicted access "as a concept representing the degree of fit between the clients and the system." Their taxonomy of access illustrated the variability and overlap of the concepts of availability, accessibility, affordability, accommodation, and acceptability, demonstrating the complexity of the issues and the need for creative planning to improve health-care access (Thomas and Penchansky 1984).

Participating Northern Communities

The three-year project, Community Collaboration to Improve Health Care Access of Northern Residents, began in 2005. The aim of the project was to use the information gathered during the study to influence programs and policies to improve northern residents' access to health services. Nor-Man Regional Health Authority (NRHA) and Burntwood Regional Health Authority (BRHA) in Manitoba, and Athabasca Health Authority (AHA) and Mamawetan Churchill River Regional Health Authority (MCRRHA) in Saskatchewan, agreed to partner in the project. Both First Nations and provincial communities agreed to partner with research institutes and participate in the project.

The northern Manitoba communities of Cormorant, Ilford, War Lake First Nation, Pikwitonei, Thicket Portage, and Wabowden ranged in size from 91 to 498 residents. The BRHA is located in the City of Thompson (population 13,446), the regional centre that provides acute hospital and medical care, diagnostics, long-term care, rehabilitation, and public health. Ilford, War Lake First Nation, Pikwitonei, and Thicket Portage are accessible by air, rail, and seasonal road; Wabowden and Cormorant have all-weather road access. Cormorant residents access primary health services in The Pas at the NRHA. Residents are required to travel from Thompson to Winnipeg or from The Pas to Winnipeg for specialist and tertiary care services.

Saskatchewan communities ranged in size from 6 to 3,757 residents; in the Far North, within the jurisdiction of the AHA, communities included Stony Rapids, Black Lake Denesuline First Nation, Fond du Lac Denesuline First Nation, Uranium City, and Camsell Portage. Black Lake and Stony Rapids are connected by an all-weather road; Fond du Lac, Uranium City, and Camsell Portage are accessible by air and seasonal road. AHA provides acute hospital and medical care, diagnostics, long-term care, rehabilitation, and public health services. In the Near North, communities included La Ronge and Pinehouse Lake. The MCRRHA, located in La Ronge, provides acute services,

**Table 9.1   Populations and travel distances of participating communities in
Manitoba and Saskatchewan**

Community	2006 population	Overland distance and time to larger centre	Transportation networks
Manitoba			
Cormorant	334	80 km to The Pas 1.5 hours	All-weather road, rail
Ilford/War Lake First Nation	116	207 km to Thompson 6 hours	Air, rail, seasonal road
Pikwitonei	91	65 km to Thompson 3 hours	Air, rail, seasonal road
Thicket Portage	156	70 km to Thompson 2 hours	Air, rail, seasonal road
Wabowden	498	105 km to Thompson 1.25 hours	All-weather road, air (float/ski), bus, rail, taxi
Thompson	13,446	761 km to Winnipeg 8 hours	All-weather road, air, bus, rail
The Pas	5,589	623 km to Winnipeg 7 hours	All-weather road, air, bus, rail
Saskatchewan			
Stony Rapids	255	872 km to Prince Albert 9-12 hours (road) 2.5 hours (air)	Air, seasonal road
Black Lake/ Denesuline Nation	1,155	22 km to Stony Rapids 0.5 hours	Air, all-weather road
Fond du Lac/ Denesuline Nation	801	82 km to Stony Rapids 0.5 hours (air)	Air, seasonal road
Uranium City	~ 100	175 km to Stony Rapids 45 minutes (air)	Air, seasonal road
Camsell Portage	~ 6	200 km to Stony Rapids 1 hour	Air
La Ronge (includes Air Ronge)	3,757	238 km to Prince Albert 2.5 hours	All-weather road
Pinehouse Lake	1,076	211 km to La Ronge 2 hours	All-weather road
Prince Albert	34,000	142 km to Saskatoon 1.5 hours	All-weather road, air, bus

emergency services, and some specialized services. Pinehouse Lake is connected to La Ronge by an all-weather road. Many northern residents travel to Prince Albert (population 34,000) or to Saskatoon for specialist services.

Findings

In Saskatchewan, Prince Albert provides a substantive array of health services in the community and to communities farther north. In Manitoba, services available in Thompson are more limited in scope and in human resources available for outreach. Modes of available transportation influence the ability of Regional Health Authorities (RHAs) to provide itinerant services and challenge residents travelling out of their communities for care. Many services available in Prince Albert, or an hour and a half south in Saskatoon, are available for northern Manitobans only in Winnipeg, eight hours south.

Manitoba Findings

Challenges to access faced by residents in Manitoba stem from a provincial system ill equipped to provide health services in a region defined by a dispersed population over a vast, rugged terrain with limited transportation networks. Issues abound provincially, regionally, and locally.

Provincial Health System

Resources and services in northern Manitoba were limited. The system did not meet the needs of northern residents. Policies and programs designed and implemented in southern Manitoba created an environment that was fundamentally incapable of fostering acceptable levels of access to health services in the North.

Residents and providers stated that the current provincial healthcare system was inconsistent and created confusion for those seeking care. The system was fraught with jurisdictional issues and a lack of clarity regarding eligibility for services. Individuals without treaty status experienced more limited access to services than those with treaty status. Some individuals reported access to health services through social assistance. Those employed yet living below the poverty line and without treaty status often were less well served by the system.

Northern residents complained of being stripped of their autonomy when they entered the health-care system. Northerners residing in small, isolated communities described a lack of opportunity for decision making. The bureaucratic system required health providers to arrange and coordinate appointments and travel. The system fostered dependence, leaving clients unable to plan according to their needs.

The Northern Patient Transport Program (NPTP) in Manitoba was designed to assist with health-care travel costs for residents north of the fifty-third parallel. NPTP uses funding rates and policies developed in the early 1990s that are unresponsive to growing costs associated with travel in the North. Inequitable access to NPTP funding, rigid policies on transportation options, and limited opportunities for the use and coverage of escorts were identified.

Local Access

Each of the six Manitoban communities involved had a health centre or nursing station. The level of service varied depending on availability and certification of local staff and frequency of travel by itinerants. Staff shortages and turnover created difficulties in the development of trusting relationships among residents, providers, community leaders, and health service administrations. Communities raised concerns about emergency services and runways unable to accommodate medical evacuation flights, particularly at night. Rail service every other day was the only other travel option in addition to winter roads.

Access to local health services and facilities, availability of dental services, sustainability of homecare, and provision of health promotion and education programs were raised. Participants talked about unequal and inequitable access to dental care related to treaty and/or financial status. Communication was a barrier; school administrators wondered why public health nurses did not provide prevention programs in the schools, and public health nurses wondered why school administrators did not call to seek prevention programs. School administrators and public health nurses cited respect for the other's role in not making initial contact.

When people believed that services were not available to them, or they were not eligible for them, they did not seek care. In one case, an individual did not seek to obtain dentures because a service provider indicated that denturists preferred not to take clients receiving social assistance. Others on social assistance reported being required to travel beyond Thompson for dental services. They believed that dentists in Thompson refused to provide services to those on social assistance because their rate of coverage was lower than that for those with insurance through employment plans, and social assistance programs had the reputation of being slow to reimburse dentists for services.

Access to homecare was a contentious issue across communities; participants suspected that services differed across communities. Local tensions seemed to occur with staff shortages and subsequent lack of continuity. Staff were typically required to have a high school diploma or equivalent; limited educational levels impacted their eligibility to work for homecare. Some residents saw the coordination of homecare by public health nurses as a secondary role, resulting in nurses having less commitment and time for the homecare program.

With the shortage of qualified health professionals, service providers reported plans to leave the community to prevent burnout. Some noted that funding formulas designed in southern Manitoba, even with northern allowances, were not sufficient to attract and retain health professionals in northern Manitoba.

Health-care providers reported that their focus was on acute and chronic care, with little time available for health promotion and education. Some suggested that community collaboration and partnerships held considerable potential to create education and prevention activities within communities.

Regional Access

Participants raised concerns about access to family physicians and specialists in referral centres. Waiting times for appointments reflected physician shortages across the North. Individuals thus went to the hospital emergency room, straining its resources. Clients did not seek follow-up care due to long waiting periods and provider turnover. Lack of coordination of appointments required residents to make numerous trips for physician and diagnostic appointments in addition to treatment requirements. Better organization could reduce time lost, travel costs, personal inconvenience, and emotional strain.

Mental health and addiction services were not seen as readily available, even within regional centres. Anxiety about confidentiality and stigma related to services inhibited some individuals from obtaining care.

Urban Access

Access to specialized services or treatment necessitated travel to Winnipeg. Apprehension about visiting the city compounded difficulties associated with navigating the health system. Coordination of services to minimize travel was perceived to be vital. Lack of communication hampered appointment scheduling; in some cases, by the time residents were informed of cancellations, they were already en route.

Transportation networks connecting the North were limited. Northern residents took the bus when they did not have access to a vehicle or were hesitant to drive the distances to the city or navigate city traffic. Individuals took the overnight bus to decrease accommodation costs and reduce time away from home.

Participants shared feelings of fear and anxiety when travelling alone to the city. One elderly participant described moving furniture to block the door to her room and related sleepless nights. Those on social assistance reported better access to health services in Winnipeg than those on pensions.

Saskatchewan Findings

Northern Saskatchewan residents face challenges in accessing health services related to local and regional services and facilities, service providers, costs, transportation, and service delivery.

Local and Regional Services and Facilities

Residents of both health authorities discussed their appreciation of local and regional health services because they eliminate many problems associated with travelling elsewhere. However, some gaps exist in communities, including prenatal care and birthing facilities, emergency medical equipment for Uranium City and Camsell Portage, homecare services and facilities in Uranium City and Black Lake, and long-term-care facilities in Black Lake and Fond du Lac. La Ronge and Pinehouse Lake residents suggested that services for elderly residents be expanded, along with cancer-related services. Participants proposed a chemotherapy out-patient service in La Ronge since several residents regularly travel to Prince Albert or Saskatoon for cancer treatments. Participants indicated that expansion of health-care facilities in the region would benefit residents and alleviate demand for services elsewhere in the province. Participants acknowledged that travel for advanced care and specialist services would always be necessary for some residents of the AHA and MCRRHA areas, and they were impressed by the availability of primary services in smaller communities, enabling access to health-care services.

Health-Care Service Providers

Several residents acknowledged the hard work and dedication of local health-care providers, recalling examples of exceptional service. However, participants noted that availability of staff was important to ensure the provision of high-quality services. High turnover contributed to difficulties for health-care providers in trying to implement programs or follow-up with clients. Delivery of health services was more efficient and effective when consistent providers were available, and familiarity allowed provider-client rapport to develop. MCRRHA participants indicated a need for improvements in wait times for medical appointments. Participants expressed desire to establish regular family doctors to obtain access to consistent health services, and they recognized that the shortage of health-care providers in the province increased the difficulty of attracting and retaining a sufficient number of providers in the region.

Costs

Travel-related costs posed problems for residents required to travel within and outside the regions to receive health services. The remote locations of the AHA communities in particular had profound influence on the affordability of accessing health services. For some residents, personal health insurance and other factors enabled them to travel for health services; however, participants indicated that not all AHA residents had access to these resources. Some residents were unable to access health services unless they received First Nations and Inuit Health (FNIH) coverage for travel costs, which did not necessarily cover all costs incurred while travelling for health services. Differential access to travel coverage existed among residents of the AHA region. Residents without First Nations treaty status received little travel coverage, whereas residents with treaty status had most travel expenses covered. Affordability of health-care services emerged as a barrier to MCRRHA residents' access to services. Costs of transportation and accommodation as a result of travelling elsewhere for health services were a barrier. Elderly individuals and others on fixed incomes were especially at risk. Participants noted that the costs of prescription drugs resulted in some residents going without them despite their necessity.

Transportation

In the AHA region, transportation is necessary to receive many health services, and problems are associated with transportation both within and outside the region. Access to automobiles for travel within the region and availability of emergency services to transport residents outside the region are of concern. Participants from La Ronge identified transportation issues arising from their need to travel to Prince Albert and Saskatoon, and participants from Pinehouse Lake discussed issues arising from travel to La Ronge and elsewhere in the province. Pinehouse Lake residents mentioned that transportation services for individuals with disabilities needed improvement. La Ronge residents needed transportation for advanced treatments or specialist services. Participants reported driving several hours for short appointments since service was not available within the region. Taking time off work or finding a driver to attend appointments was often problematic.

Service Delivery

Health-care providers raised the topic of jurisdiction. Divisions within the health-care system were reported to cause fragmented funding and service delivery and affect relationships among providers and within communities. For example, health-care providers might be employed by different authorities, making a team approach difficult and requiring providers to negotiate discrepancies in procedures. Jurisdictional differences led to lack of awareness and confusion over the availability of health services for residents.

Service delivery in these regions was negatively affected by poor communication and information sharing among some health-care providers. Efficient and quality care is dependent on accurate and timely sharing of health information among First Nations and provincial systems, local and out-of-region providers, and health centres and physicians. Clients missed follow-up appointments on occasion because information was not passed on to them or local providers. Miscommunication of discharge plans for individuals released from health-care facilities outside the region was problematic. Providers with the MCRRHA stated that they did not have easy access to First Nations immunization records, resulting in children being over- or under-immunized.

Participants thought that health service delivery was negatively affected by issues related to interactions with providers. Difficulties in communication between providers and clients could result in inaccurate or incomplete information being passed on. Difficulties with language or literacy, cultural differences, insufficient time with providers, and confidentiality issues had negative implications for clients' access to appropriate health services.

Discussion

Penchansky and Thomas' (1981) taxonomy of access illustrates the five concepts of availability, accessibility, affordability, accommodation, and acceptability. The five concepts are defined in Table 9.2.

Similarities across Saskatchewan and Manitoba have been synthesized to indicate key themes having impacts on northerners' access to health services. Concepts and themes interface, depicting unique challenges related to distance, jurisdiction, lack of critical population mass, communication, collaboration and cooperation, staff and resource shortages, physical infrastructure, client status, and transportation networks.

A lack of critical population mass across the North generated a health-care system under-resourced to fulfill the needs of residents, leaving many services unavailable in Manitoba and services requiring improvement in Saskatchewan. Centralization in regional and urban centres put northern residents at a disadvantage since services were

Table 9.2   Taxonomic definition of access

Term	Definition
Availability	The relationship between volume and type of existing resources and volume of clients and type of needs (i.e., the adequacy of supply of providers, facilities, programs, and services).
Accessibility	The relationship between the location of supply and the location of clients, taking into account client transportation resources, travel time, distance, and cost.
Accommodation	The relationship between the manner that supply resources are organized to accept clients (including appointment systems, hours of operation, walk-in facilities, and telephone services) and the clients' ability to fit with these factors.
Affordability	The relationship between prices of services and providers' insurance or deposit requirements and clients' income, ability to pay, and existing health insurance; client perception of worth relative to total cost, including client knowledge of price and possible credit arrangements.
Acceptability	The relationship between clients' attitudes about personal and practice characteristics of existing providers, including age, sex, location and type of facility, religious affiliation of provider or facility, as well as provider attitudes about acceptable personal characteristics of clients, including ethnicity and patient payment source.

Source: Thomas and Penchansky (1984).

inaccessible in their communities and often in Manitoba were not available in the regional centre. Services could be unaffordable for northern residents due to the high cost of travel, accommodation, and time spent away from families and employment. Personal costs were high, and residents were confronted with burdens associated with navigating the complex and unaccommodating system. The quality of client and provider interactions and relationships often was unacceptable due to high turnover of health professionals. Understanding the unique circumstances of living in the North and respecting residents' desire to reside in the North are pivotal for government decision makers. Service providers and policy makers must have a meaningful knowledge of First Nations and northern culture, history, and tradition and a respect for differences that ensures service provision is appropriate and effective. Shortages of health professionals and the resulting work environments were unacceptable to health-care providers, who suggested that service delivery could be improved by ensuring that all health-care staff are utilized to the full scope of their particular practice. Specifically, licensed practical nurses and homecare aides should use all their skills to relieve some of the demand for other providers. Clarifying and expanding the transfer of the medical function process could enhance service delivery, for current practice is inconsistent among health-care facilities within the regions, and few providers are certified to oversee the process. Participants indicated that funds should be used to support transfer-of-function certification for existing staff and to recruit certified staff to the regions.

Greater utilization of telehealth, a program that enables health-care staff to consult with patients using visual interactive technology, was recommended. Although insufficient technology currently limits use of telehealth in the AHA region, MCRRHA participants reported that telehealth was under-utilized because of the perceived reluctance of providers in southern Saskatchewan. Efforts could be made to implement telehealth in both regions, particularly for initial consultations and follow-up appointments with specialists, health promotion and education purposes, and communication between providers within and outside the regions.

Expansion of translation services at health centres and cultural awareness training for new staff to develop an understanding of the cultural backgrounds and values of residents were suggested. Greater efforts by health-care staff to ensure confidentiality for clients would help residents to overcome feelings of stigmatization associated with certain health conditions and increase the likelihood of their seeking health services.

Many issues were complex and demonstrated various challenges to be managed. Recommendations of residents and providers focused on the need for more partnerships to advocate for the North and participate in creative planning involving the strengths of the partners to generate made-in-the-North solutions. Some university medical and dental programs in the South currently work with health authorities and communities in the North. Expansion of these programs and development of similar programs hold promise for better health-care access in the North. Partnerships among service providers and programs from the South, local and regional providers in the North, and community leaders and residents hold potential for meaningful change.

Policy makers, service providers, and people of the North must work together to ensure that solutions are tailored to suit the unique nature and challenges of the North. Examples in both provinces illustrated new partnerships that are working to generate innovative and creative solutions. In Manitoba, communities along the Bayline Railway came together to form the Bayline Regional Round Table (BRRT), an organization based on shared identity and concern for creating a collective voice and demanding attention and response to issues. Similarly, in Saskatchewan, the Northern Health Strategy (NHS) and AHA represent creative organizational arrangements to improve northerners' access to health services and ensure that policy and program design reflects the unique needs of the North.

Actions

A key objective of this project was to foster discussion and share knowledge at various levels, across jurisdictions, in keeping with the fundamental principles of PAR and community development. Northern people guided the processes, and discussions were facilitated across sectors as community members and health authority representatives met to share their concerns and generate solutions. Over the three years, northern Manitoba and Saskatchewan residents and representatives from their health authorities met with provincial and federal policy makers to share concerns, exchange knowledge and ideas, gain insight, and develop relationships to foster change.

Manitoba Action

BRRT representatives met regularly with researchers from the Rural Development Institute (RDI), Brandon University. Community leaders offered advice and guidance to researchers and facilitated interviews and focus groups in their communities. BRRT representatives shared findings with their communities. The BRRT hosted a series of workshops during the final year of the project to discuss issues and generate solutions, initially among themselves, then with the RHAs, and finally with provincial and federal stakeholders. Building healthy and trusting relationships among community members, service providers, and government representatives was critical in order to move forward with actions proposed through project findings. Discussions focused on three questions. How can a healthy dialogue among the BRRT, RHAs, and provincial and federal sectors be maintained and further developed? How can the BRRT, RHAs, provincial and federal sectors, and other stakeholders work together to strengthen the health of northern communities? How can information from the research project contribute to healthy dialogue and subsequent action?

Workshop participants broke into working groups to focus on three key areas for action: (1) pathfinding in a complex system; (2) addressing local issues of access to care; and (3) facilitating relationships, dialogue, and action. The workshop fostered communication and encouraged inclusion of local knowledge in planning and implementing health services.

Saskatchewan Action

In Saskatchewan, research project steering committees were created from the AHA and the MCRRHA, with managers, health directors, and board members participating. Steering committees and researchers from the Saskatchewan Population Health and Evaluation Research Unit (SPHERU), University of Regina, met throughout the project to develop strategies for data collection, review and verify data analysis, and provide feedback and suggestions for actions to address issues identified. The committees were involved in planning the bi-provincial workshop and identified key participants from their provincial, federal, and First Nations partners. Existing partnerships among the province and regional health authorities are strong, and cross-jurisdictional partnering has been advanced by creation of the NHS, a coalition of service providers within the region encompassing federal, provincial, non-governmental, and First Nations organizations. The AHA delivers services to both First Nations and provincial communities under a unique partnership arrangement with provincial, federal, and First Nations governments. Recognizing the strength of these partnerships, Saskatchewan steering committees focused their discussions on using these links to find new ways of working together to share resources and streamline fragmented service delivery to address the issues raised.

Action Together

SPHERU and RDI hosted a final workshop in Saskatoon in the spring of 2008. Participants included community residents from northern Saskatchewan and northern Manitoba, AHA, BRRT, BRHA, First Nations and Inuit Health, Health Canada, MCRRHA, Manitoba Health and Healthy Living, NRHA, Northern Medical Services, Rural Secretariat, Saskatchewan Health, SPHERU, and RDI. The purpose of the workshop was to share and learn from research processes and findings across the two provinces. The workshop provided a unique forum that transcended provincial boundaries and drew from successes and challenges. Dialogue provided the opportunity to generate ideas for improving access to health services in the North.

Participants worked together in breakout sessions reflective of priorities developed at the onset of the workshop. Breakout session topics included community partnerships, federal-provincial partnerships, the concept of pathfinding to assist residents in navigating a complex health-care system, creating a vision for northern health services, staff recruitment to the North, and fostering cross-border cooperation and partnerships. Open and honest communication was critical to support meaningful change through partnership, and increased awareness and understanding of the unique nature of the North evolved. Existing partnerships were enhanced, and new partnerships were formed.

Multi-level and cross-jurisdictional partnerships and collaboration are crucial to ensure that policy and programming are well understood and altered at the right times for the right reasons. Partnerships and communication create understanding and foster balanced change and implementation. With community partnerships, the provision of care at the local level will be more successful. Trust and relationship building are critical in effective service delivery. Participants proclaimed joy in "comparing apples to apples instead of apples to oranges," as is often the case as the North relates to the South. Open and sincere dialogue inform and support the principal argument that northerners and their communities need to be heard and involved in the process; workshop participants stressed the need to ensure that "northern health is in northern hands."

Lessons Learned

Many lessons were learned during the project and upon reflection. Effective partnerships encourage participation and nurture a diversity of people and ideas, in generating meaningful change, by developing shared goals and moving to collective action. Community members have expert knowledge of their communities. Listening initially to understand and then speaking to be understood ensure that knowledge is shared and people are respected. People living in the North share some issues with those living in the South. However, many of their issues are unique to living in the North and require different approaches. Program and service planners require knowledge of the ways of life in the North and commitment to the people of the North. Made-in-the-North solutions have the greatest potential to resolve issues of access. Creativity and imagination are needed to devise new ways to tackle persistent barriers and problems. Relationships, social practices, and institutions must be restructured to empower service users. Working with multiple partners offers challenges in supporting and ensuring processes through which all groups are respected, involved, contributing as able, included in decision making, and benefiting equitably. Decision making should be attentive to the context of relationships, and an ethic of care should guide interaction. Conflict should be resolved in ways that preserve and strengthen connections.

Health professionals and health-care organizations need to reflect on their values and principles in working cross-culturally in the North, particularly with residents from Aboriginal cultures. There are four primary questions to be answered. (1) How do I and how does my organization demonstrate behaviours, attitudes, policies, and structures when working cross-culturally? (2) How do I and how does my organization value diversity, manage the dynamics of difference, acquire and institutionalize cultural knowledge, and adapt to diversity and the cultural contexts of the communities that we serve? (3) When does difference make a difference? (4) What do we need to do differently to be more inclusive and generate feelings of belonging among residents from all cultures?

Jurisdiction can be a huge barrier to progress in managing access to health services more competently in the North. Historically, local health providers, as well as those with provincial programs or federal services, have used the ambiguity around "who is responsible to deliver which services to whom" to justify their own lack of action. New partnerships such as the AHA provide opportunities for the development of trusting and committed relationships across jurisdictions to focus on the shared goal of providing quality health services in the most appropriate and effective ways to better meet the needs of all residents of the North. Issues of equity and fair access to services need to be improved. Some health services, such as prescriptions, dental services, and transportation to medical appointments, are insured for some populations. People with First Nations treaty status have access to insured services that are not available without costs for other residents of the North. The need and desire for equity are growing, and northerners recognize that availability of and access to services should be provided more equitably to all according to need rather than status.

Transportation networks are the lifeline of the North and need to be maintained and improved. The rail system in northern Manitoba is a deteriorating yet essential transportation network. Stakeholders across communities need to work together to ensure that transportation modes and routes are developed and sustained over time. Deterioration of seasonal roads due to climate change and the need to improve the all-weather road network bear further discussion and planning to meet current and future needs in the North.

The youth of the North are the future of the North. Northerners should be encouraged to enter into health professions. Partnerships need to be developed with local schools, colleges, and universities to encourage program entry and prepare students for success. Improving access to postsecondary education in the North (and in the South for northerners) and fostering preparation for successful completion of educational programs are keys to building the array of health professionals and support staff needed in the North, a group knowledgeable about and committed to the North and its people.

References

Dickson, G. 2000. "Participatory Action Research: Theory and Practice." In *Community Nursing: Promoting Canadians' Health,* edited by M. Stewart, 542-63. Toronto: W.B. Saunders Canada.

Donabedian, A. 1972. "Models for Organizing the Delivery of Personal Health Services and Criteria for Evaluating Them." *Milbank Memorial Fund Quarterly* 50: 103-54.

Fransoo, R., P. Martens, The Need to Know Team, E. Burland, H. Prior, C. Burchill, D. Chateau, and R. Walld. 2005. *Sex Differences in Health Status, Health Care Use, and Quality of Care: A Population-Based Analysis for Manitoba's Regional Health Authorities.* Winnipeg: Manitoba Centre for Health Policy.

Irvine, J., D. Stockdale, and R. Oliver. 2004. *Northern Saskatchewan Health Indicators Report, 2004.* La Ronge, SK: Population Health Unit.

MacLeod, M. 1999. "'We're It': Issues and Realities in Rural Nursing Practice." In *Health in Rural Settings: Context for Action,* edited by W. Ramp, J. Kulig, I. Townsend, and V. McGowan, 165-78. Lethbridge: University of Lethbridge.

Martens, P., R. Fransoo, N. McKeen, The Need to Know Team, E. Burland, L. Jabamani, C. Burchill, C. De Coster, O. Ekuma, and H. Prior. 2004. *Patterns of Regional Mental Illness Disorder Diagnoses and Service Use in Manitoba: A Population-Based Study.* Winnipeg: Manitoba Centre for Health Policy.

Mechanic, D. 1972. *Public Expectations and Health Care.* New York: Free Press.

Penchansky, R., and W. Thomas. 1981. "The Concept of Access: Definition and Relationship to Consumer Satisfaction." *Medical Care* 19: 127-40.

Racher, F., and A. Vollman. 2002. "Exploring the Dimensions of Access to Health Services: Implications for Nursing Research and Practice." *Research and Theory for Nursing Practice: An International Journal* 16, 2: 77-90.

Scott, J. 2000. "A Nursing Leadership Challenge: Managing the Chronically Ill in Rural Settings." *Nursing Administration Quarterly* 24: 21-32.

Shields, M., and S. Tremblay. 2002. "The Health of Canada's Communities." *Health Reports Supplement* I: 9-33. Statistics Canada Catalogue No. 82-003.

Thomas, J.W., and R. Penchansky. 1984. "Relating Satisfaction with Access to Utilization of Services." *Medical Care* 22, 6: 553-68.

Thurston, W.E., C.M. Scott, and A.R. Vollman. 2004. "Public Participation for Healthy Communities and Public Policy." In *Community as Partner: Theory and Practice,* Canadian ed., edited by A.R. Vollman, 124-56. Philadelphia: Lippincott.

World Health Organization (WHO). 1978. *Primary Health Care.* A joint report by the Director General of the WHO and the Executive Director of UNICEF presented at the International Conference on Primary Health Care, Alma Ata, USSR. Geneva: WHO.

Chapter 10   **Virtual Health-Care Communities: The Use of Web-Based and Mobile Intelligent Technologies for Risk Assessment and Health Management in Rural and Remote Communities**

A. Barranco-Mendoza and D. Persaud

Key Points

- Telehealth, e-health, and web-based clinical support systems are becoming more elaborate and inclusive across Canada regardless of rural or urban context.
- Information technology can provide professional support at a distance to many rural and remote nurses and other health practitioners who work alone or with little backup in their everyday practice.
- Web-based intelligent clinical decision support systems, such as DRAsTIK, and telehealth can assist both patients and health practitioners to manage collaboratively patients' health regardless of their place of residence, whether rural or urban, and their proximity to a health clinic.

The Internet has become a very useful tool for information exchange and continuing education (Dryburgh 2001) with the establishment of websites that provide health and medical knowledge on almost all known diseases and conditions that affect humans. The websites and, in some cases, downloadable software allow users to interact with others through a variety of means: emails, blogs, videoconferences, general and specialized forums for discussions, surveys, and interactive applications. The Internet user becomes part of a "virtual community" and interacts with health practitioners, other clients, or both. In some cases, clients get "real time" emotional support and information on a number of issues relevant to them. But in all cases, these websites are meant only to provide information and do not replace the advice of one's physician. The Internet is easily accessible in urban areas but might be limited in some rural and remote areas. Urban areas are equipped with high bandwidth data lines and more accessible hubs for Internet connection. However, in rural areas, wireless technology is becoming increasingly important as a means to overcome geographical limitations. As a result, there is growing Internet access to videoconferences, downloads of health data and images (teleradiology, telepathology, etc.), online intelligent risk assessment and decision support systems, and specialized health education websites; correspondingly, there has been a rise in the quality and availability of health support in those areas.

Although there are many web-based health risk assessment systems that utilize artificial intelligence, we focus on a system that has broader application and flexibility to assist in the early assessment of a person's risk of developing or having a condition such as autism, lung cancer, and type 2 diabetes mellitus (T2DM). The Disease Risk Assessment Temporal Intelligent Knowledge-Based (DRAsTIK) system (Barranco-Mendoza 2005; Barranco-Mendoza, Persaud, and Dahl 2004, 558-59) is being developed by the Trinity Western University (TWU) Health Informatics Research (HeIR) Group in collaboration with Infogenetica Bioinformatics, a Canadian non-profit bio-informatics R&D institute. DRAsTIK is currently being optimized for T2DM and can assist health-care providers to develop personalized prevention and monitoring strategies for high-risk populations, such as Aboriginals, many of whom live in rural or remote areas.

Health Care in Canada

Health care for all individuals in Canada falls under the auspices of Health Canada (Health Canada 2008a). This federal agency oversees the publicly funded Canadian health-care system (Medicare) and aims to provide universal coverage for necessary medical services. Services provided under Medicare are free of charge and are administered under the provincial and territorial governing bodies. Since Medicare is a national health insurance plan, it is funded by provincial and territorial governments with assistance from the federal government. Funding from the federal government to provincial and territorial governing bodies is contingent on the following criteria based on the Canada Health Act (1984): comprehensiveness, universality, portability, accessibility, and public administration (Health Canada 2008a). A challenge for health professionals has been to provide universal care and follow-up for Canadians living in urban and, more so, rural and remote communities. To deal with these issues, each province and territory has created legislated regional bodies, such as Shared Provincial Access Network for British Columbia (SPAN/BC), Alberta Health and Wellness Telehealth Program, and Telehealth Saskatchewan, to name a few (Health and the Information Highway Division, Health Canada, 2004), that are responsible for the proper management of health-related services. Unlike the other provinces and territories in Canada, Alberta has recently (as of 15 May 2008) assigned one provincial governance board, the Alberta Health Services Board (a superboard), to replace all regional and health authority boards. The purpose of this one provincial board is to provide more equitable and focused patient care (Healey and Pollock 2008). As of June 2011, Prince Edward Island has been the only other province to have a single health services board (Health PEI), which is responsible for the delivery and operations of health services on the island.

Because metropolitan areas have the latest and most accessible health services, it is expected that distance from Census Metropolitan Areas (CMAs) and Metropolitan Influenced Zones (MIZ) will influence the health of Canadians in rural and remote communities (Mendelson 2001). For a thorough explanation of the classification of "Rural and Small Town" communities (RST) into CMAs and MIZ, refer to Chapter 2 in this volume.

Health of Canadians in Rural Areas

Rural Canadians (Weak MIZ and No MIZ) have been noted to be less healthy than their counterparts in urban areas (Canadian Institute for Health Information [CIHI] 2006). For example, there are higher mortality rates and shorter life expectancies; in addition, chronic diseases (arthritis/rheumatism, high blood pressure, and diabetes) are significantly higher in rural populations than in urban populations (for further review, see Chapter 21, this volume). Using multivariate analytical methods, it was also revealed that socio-economic factors, place of residence, health behaviour, and attitude toward health contribute to weaker health prospects in rural communities (see Chapter 3).

Improvement of the health of rural Canadians, especially with regard to chronic diseases, comes under the administration of Health
Canada and the regional health bodies of the individual provinces and
territories, as stated earlier. Because rural communities can be some
distance apart and far from CMAs, various approaches (e.g., telehealth
and e-health) have been implemented to increase health services for
those in rural and remote areas.

Telehealth and E-Health Initiatives

An approach to providing health care to rural Canadians has been the
implementation of the Telehealth System (THS). In concise terms,
telehealth is the practice of medicine at a distance from the patient. The
THS has evolved from a simple telephone service between clients and
clinician into an elaborate, highly digital, information pathway involving the use of computers, videoconferences, and, in some cases, satellite
communications. Via telehealth, a patient can connect with a clinician
in an urban health centre through a secure network connection at a
local nursing station (LNS) in the rural or remote area. The LNS is
crucial since it is sometimes the only health facility in a rural or remote
community. An example of the use of the THS is the process by which
a patient grants access to his or her health records to health providers
stationed many kilometres away. These records are a composite of lab
tests, X-rays, CT or other imaging scans (digitalized), and past medical
diagnoses. Depending on the level of infrastructure of the telecom-
munication pathway, a client can be seen on a monitor in the clinician's
office and can interact by video-/audioconferencing. Telehealth also
provides patient follow-up care and ongoing health education for clinical practitioners in remote areas. However, successful implementation
of a telehealth system in rural communities is dependent on a number
of criteria, such as readiness of the environment, information technology and equipment availability, needs analysis, and the ability to recruit and retain qualified personnel (Jennett and Andruchuk 2001,
169-74; Jennett, Gagnon, and Brandstadt 2005, 279-85; Minore et al.
2005, 86-100).

Based on a number of crucial health conferences in Canada, such as
Vision 2020 (Léger 2000, 12-14) and Canada E-Health 2000: From
Vision to Action (Pascal 2001, 37-40), a number of important recommendations have been suggested for implementation of information
and communication technologies (ICTs) in the health-care system.

Participants at these conferences represented a broad spectrum of people from all areas of the health sector in Canada. The recommendations were for continued establishment and effective management, reliability, and security of electronic health records. Other key recommendations included strengthening the existing telehealth systems, improving client access to health information, and enhancing clinical decision support systems. The implementation of the above-mentioned recommendations resulted in a more efficient telehealth system, the Canadian Health Infoway (Infoway), in 2001. Infoway is a not-for-profit organization funded by the federal government that collaborates with provincial and territorial governments, health-care providers, and technology developers and providers. Its mission is to provide a conduit for using electronic health information systems and electronic health records (EHRs) across the country. An EHR is an electronic integrated version of a person's health records that can be viewed in a secure manner from all systems that are part of a secure network. Since its inception, Infoway has contributed to the development of standards in health care for e-health and the implementation of EHRs (Giokas 2005, 108).

E-health systems within Infoway and other web-based health information portals (a portal is a website that serves as an entry point to other relevant websites) present a solution to overcoming barriers created by geographical distance and the implementation of a universally accessible portal for delivering health care. The ultimate purpose of these e-health initiatives is to create more informed patients who are better able to assess the risks and benefits of different treatments for themselves (Henwood et al. 2003, 589-607). Table 10.1 summarizes some of the major websites that provide information to health-care workers and clients in Canada. Similar informative websites are available in the United States.[1] The websites shown in the table are only a few of the many sites available on the Internet. Some websites represented (e.g., Health Canada and the Canadian Health Network) are either government agencies or administered by the federal or a provincial government. Other websites (e.g., Health Line and WebMD) are broad and contain credible health-related information that is continuously reviewed by independent medical review boards for accuracy and timeliness. However, in general, one must be careful to verify the sources when accessing health-related websites since many of them are posted on the Internet by individuals without any medical or scientific training and can contain incomplete and/or erroneous information.

Table 10.1   A sample of web-based health information networks in Canada

Organization	Mission	URL address
Canadian Society of Telehealth	To provide a resource for improving health care by creating a forum for enhanced sharing of resources, advocacy, and communication. It claims to be the foremost telehealth organization in Canada.	www.cst-sct.org/
Health Canada	The federal department that is responsible for improving and maintaining the health of Canadians.	www.hc-sc.gc.ca/
Rural and Remote Canada Online	A broad range of services for rural communities: government of Canada programs and services and contacts to various rural organizations and associations.	www.rural-canada. ca/
Continuing Medical Education Directory	This Internet site provides a list of organizations and key contact members who are involved in continuing medical education in Canadian medical schools, medical associations, and industry.	www.mdcme.ca/
Canadian Health Network (Public Health Agency of Canada)	To promote and protect the health of Canadians through leadership, partnership, innovation, and action in public health.	www.phac-aspc. gc.ca/
Clinical Practice Guidelines and Protocols in BC - PDA Delivery	This site provides the guidelines and protocols that are developed by the Guidelines and Protocols Advisory Committee and makes them available to physicians in British Columbia on PDA format. The guidelines have been condensed and are viewable on both Windows Mobile (PocketPC) and Palm-type devices through synchronization with Microsoft Windows Operating System computers. The site is regularly updated with new guidelines for different diseases.	www.clinipearls.ca/ bcguidelines/
MyDoctorCa	1. Provides information about your family doctor (or any doctor) and the clinic s/he works at. 2. Has health and community links (i.e., identifies local groups in your communities with fundraising activities and group support). 3. Has online applications to monitor aspects of chronic disease (e.g., blood pressure tracking) and private email services so patients can contact their doctors directly. 4. Supported by the Canadian Medical Association. 5. Individual doctors may charge a block fee for the online service.	www.mydoctor.ca/

▶

◀ **Table 10.1**

Organization	Mission	URL address
Ontario Wait Times	1. To allow clients and doctors to search online in order to determine what are the wait times for a certain medical procedure at any hospital in Ontario. 2. It is possible based on the information you receive to request from your doctor a referral to another specialist or hospital with a shorter wait time.	www.health.gov. on.ca/en/public/ programs/ waittimes/

Government web portals are increasingly important to clients seeking information because they are more detailed compared with telehealth systems. Web portals contain information of a general nature, whereas telehealth systems contain information more specific to the client (e.g., a patient's data and health records). In a study performed in Ontario (which might reflect what is present in other provinces), the main uses of health information systems were to (1) look after someone else, (2) decide where to go to seek help or treatment, (3) decide which treatment to undertake, and (4) acquire information to discuss with physicians (Harris, Wathen, and Fear 2006).

On 1 April 2008, the Canadian Medical Association inaugurated www.mydoctor.ca. It is the first Canadian health portal or personal health record (PHR) that allows web-based risk assessment with physician communication and electronic medical record (EMR) implementation. The mydoctor.ca website can be accessed by any physician from any province or territory. Clients can assess their risk of hypertension, asthma, and obesity and selectively release information to their physicians, which will be automatically documented in an EMR. In other words, all client activities are stored and documented when the client is logged on to the website.

Critical to any e-health initiative is the development of clinical decision support and risk assessment information systems (discussed in the next section). They involve the use of medical health records, imaging data (X-ray, CT scans), and biochemical laboratory tests to help facilitate a more beneficial course of action or program for the efficient treatment of the patient using a more individualized approach (Burke and Weill 2005). These clinical decision support systems will be a significant part of the Canadian health infostructure. The term "health infostructure" is meant to convey the development of ICTs in Canadian health-care management (Health Canada 2008b).

Intelligent Technologies for Risk Assessment and Health Management

Risk assessment systems (RAS) are software-based tools that calculate the likelihood of a client developing a particular disease based on using computational and/or mathematical processes of varying complexity. Data input for algorithmic analysis is typically composed of representative genotypic (e.g., race) and environmental data (e.g., modifiable risk factors) to determine pathological output based on cohort studies. The intent, based on the risk outcome, is to inform a client of the likelihood of developing a particular disease in order to empower the client to take primary and secondary preventive action. Primary preventive actions are health measures taken to prevent the onset of a disease. Secondary preventive measures avert the onset of complications from an existing pathology. Web-based RAS are becoming increasingly popular due to their wide availability, accessibility, and low or no cost. This type of tool can become a valuable solution in rural and remote areas where specialized medical personnel are not readily available.

Intelligent risk assessment systems (IRAS) are RAS that utilize artificial intelligence methodologies in the algorithms used to perform the analysis. By an intelligent system, we refer to a system that perceives its environment and takes actions that maximize its chances of success. IRAS are different from standard RAS in that they can adapt to changes in the client's information and utilize the new information to refine the risk assessment. The more sophisticated IRAS are even able to learn from these changes (called machine learning) so that assessments of future clients will include the newly learned information for a better risk assessment.

Employers, government organizations, and health insurance firms might use RAS to calculate prime rates, promote wellness, and implement health promotion programs (Cardium Health 2005). RAS are useful for health education because they are cost effective to implement and highly accessible to the general population. They allow for client-individualized risk of disease, education, and monitoring. Most of the currently available web-based RAS are provided free of charge through niche web portals. Unfortunately, the use of RAS and the understanding of their impact on patient care and lifestyle remain in their infancy

(Brindle et al. 2006, 1752-59). One reason might be problems, such as user interface intuitiveness, experienced by users during portal use (Barranco-Mendoza and Grajales 2008; Grajales 2008).

Other critical areas that must be considered in the development of RAS are data interactivity and international standards. Large amounts of biological and medical data are becoming available, and, consequently, it is important to adhere to international standards so that this wealth of information can be usable by many applications.

Given that chronic diseases are the leading cause of worldwide death and a significant financial burden to both developed and developing countries (World Health Organization [WHO] 2005), a number of e-health initiatives around the world focus on these diseases. Table 10.2 shows some of the publicly available web-based RAS for chronic diseases. The majority are hosted outside Canada by reputable health-care organizations, most of them in the United States, have been tested by health professionals, and are available for anyone to use.

Legal and Ethical Aspects of Telehealth and Medical RAS

The use of telemedicine is growing, and with that growth come a number of ethical and legal implications. The following requirements have been recommended by attorneys for the prevention of malpractice regarding telemedicine: proper licensing for the province from which the medical service is being provided, maintenance of security and client confidentiality, determination of national and provincial reimbursements, responsibility of care (the legal obligation of an individual to adhere to a reasonable standard of care while performing any act that could harm others), product liability, and intellectual property rights (Johnson 2003, 101; Picot and Cradduck 2000; Pong and Hogenbirk 1999, 3-14; Stanberry 2006, 166-75). Such recommendations are also applicable to liability under tort law (i.e., negligence theory and product liability) for computer software for health risk assessment (Goodman and Miller 2006, 379-402).

The general concern of all Canadians is privacy and security of personal information. In Canada, two federal privacy laws protect citizens: the Privacy Act (1983), and the Personal Information Protection and Electronic Documents Act (2001). Personal information includes age, weight, ethnicity, blood type, and medical records. The Privacy Act therefore requires any business to seek your consent before it acquires

Table 10.2   Publicly available web-based RAS for chronic diseases

System name	Disease category	URL address
Comprehensive Stroke Program Risk Assessment	Cardiovascular	www.strokecenter.stanford. edu/test.html
Your Disease Risk: Heart Disease	Cardiovascular	www.yourdiseaserisk.wustl.edu/
Your Disease Risk: Stroke	Cardiovascular	www.yourdiseaserisk.wustl.edu/
Brain Australia: Stroke Risk Self Assessment Chart	Cardiovascular	www.brainaustralia.org.au/ stroke/stroke_risk_assessment _chart
C Health: Seniors' Health Stroke Assessment Quiz	Cardiovascular	www.chealth.canoe.ca/health_ tools. asp
Health Status Cardiac Risk Assessment	Cardiovascular	www.healthstatus.com/
AHA Heart Attack/Coronary Heart Disease Risk Assessment	Cardiovascular	www.heart.org/heartorg/
Your Disease Risk: Cancer	Cancer	www.yourdiseaserisk.wustl. edu/
National Cancer Institute Breast Cancer Risk Assessment Tool	Cancer	www.cancer.gov/bcrisktool/
Women's Cancer Network Cancer Risk Assessment Survey	Cancer	www. foundationforwomenscancer. org/
American Diabetes Association Diabetes Risk Test	Diabetes	www.diabetes.org/risk-test. jsp?WTLPromo=HOME_ risktestandvms= 211558071459
American Diabetes Association Diabetes PHD	Diabetes	www.diabetes.org
Your Disease Risk: Diabetes	Diabetes	www.yourdiseaserisk.wustl.edu
St. Luke's Diabetes Risk Calculator	Diabetes	www.sleh.com/
Beacon to Health: Risk Assessment and Prevention of Type 2 Diabetes	Diabetes	www.infogenetica.com/ beacontohealth
Valley Health Diabetes Self-Assessment	Diabetes	www.valleyhealth.com/
Health Status Diabetes Risk Assessment	Diabetes	www.healthstatus.com/

Source: Grajales (2008).

or discloses your personal information. The onus is on the organization to provide proven security measures that maintain the confidentiality of your personal information. Ethical issues in telehealth and electronic RAS are burgeoning. Common ethical priorities centre on the proper training and use of clinical software such that the system can work as designed in the effort to provide the best possible care for the client.

Artificial Intelligence in Medicine

Only recently have IRAS become more publicly accepted and widely available thanks to the Internet. However, the use of computers and artificial intelligence to assist in medical diagnosis dates back to the late 1950s (Altman 1999). In fact, one of the first areas that drew the attention of artificial intelligence (AI) researchers was that of medical diagnosis since it involves many common reasoning tasks. The seminal paper of Ledley and Lusted (1959) explained that medical reasoning, such as the process of diagnosing a disease based on the analysis of a patient's symptoms, involves well-recognized strategies of inference used in computational AI processes, such as Boolean logic (based on something being true or false; e.g., does the patient have a fever?), Bayesian probability (e.g., what is the probability of a patient having a certain disease based on the number of observed cases within a particular population?), and symbolic logic (the use of sentences that include logical operators such as "and," "or," "implies," "equals," and "not" to express logical statements; e.g., if a child's oral temperature is equal to thirty-eight degrees Celsius or higher, it implies that the child has a fever). Therefore, diagnostic reasoning can be formulated using these logical and computational techniques, and these concepts have influenced a large number of health risk assessment AI research projects over the past fifty years.

From the early days of expert systems, rules have been the essential means for expressing knowledge in a symbolic way. They offer simplicity, transparency, uniformity, and ease of inference, which make them very attractive to represent medical knowledge obtained from a human expert (see Figure 10.1). However, it quickly became evident that knowledge acquisition is the most complex part of the development of expert systems. Rules obtained from a human expert risk capturing the biases of one person on the subject. Even though they might appear as a coherent and modular set of knowledge, rules can reveal inconsistencies, gaps, and other problems.

Figure 10.1   Schema of an expert system of the early 1980s

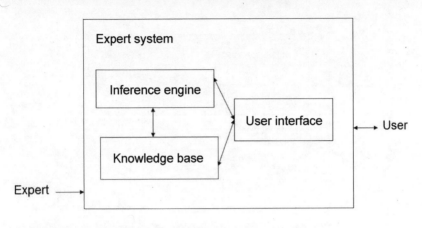

Source: Adapted from Lavrac, Keravnou, and Zupan (2000, 113-57).

These limitations, along with the high cost of acquiring the knowledge directly from the experts and the increasing availability of databases of sample cases, shifted the focus to learning the rules from such databases. The option of developing rules from databases was attractive since it is less prone to bias, more efficient, and cost effective. Human experts are still involved in the development of machine-learning systems, providing the sample cases and verifying the resulting rules. The advantage of the learning approach is that it ensures the resulting rules are hierarchically organized and consistent. The difficulty is that the sample dataset must be complete enough for the domain in question (without significant gaps in the knowledge); otherwise, the resulting rules will not provide adequate coverage and/or sufficient accuracy.

Research in the past decade has been characterized by efforts to bridge the gap between large amounts of data that have been captured but remain uninterpreted due to volume or complexity and understanding such data. Thus, the research emphasis now is on data analysis. Intelligent data analysis, such as knowledge discovery in databases, machine learning, data visualization, and so on, is the latest focus of health informatics research (Frawley, Piatetsky-Shapiro, and Matheus 1991).

The need for intelligent data analysis in medicine is evident in a number of ways, including support for the analyses of individual clients' raw data of specific knowledge-based problem-solving activities (e.g., diagnosis, prognosis, monitoring, treatment planning, etc.) and use of

Figure 10.2   Schema of a modern decision support system

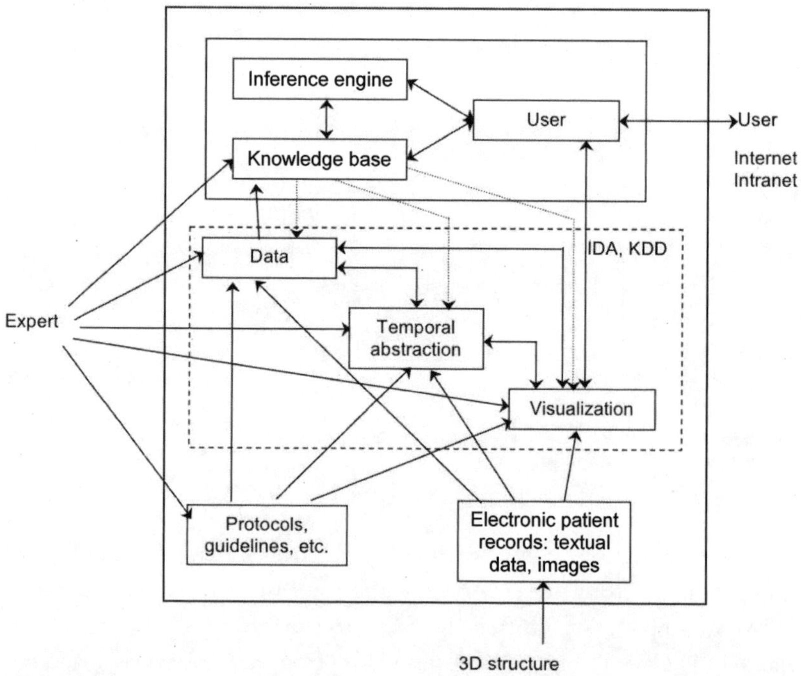

Source: Adapted from Lavrac, Keravnou, and Zupan (2000, 113-57).

data mining in the discovery of new medical knowledge that can be extracted from sample cases. Figure 10.2 represents a generic schema of a recent decision support system. In this schema, large volumes of data have to be processed, such as patient records comprising images and textual data, protocols, guidelines, and other important factors. The solid arrows denote the normal flow of information, and the dotted arrows show the flow of information in processes that involve loops and iterations between the different steps of the intelligent data analysis procedure.

Software Tools to Assist Diagnosis and Risk Assessment

Most of the work done on computer-assisted diagnosis (CAD) has focused on image analysis technologies. Many computer-aided image analysis systems use artificial neural networks to identify nodules in chest radiographs, CT scans, pap smears, and so forth Barranco-Mendoza et al. 1999, 25-40; Barranco-Mendoza et al. 1997; (Fausett 1994; Rumelhart and McClelland 1986).

Image analysis systems provide valuable information about the client's condition based solely on structural/textural information; however, in conditions such as lung and oral cancer at very early stages, the lesions are so small that structurally it is difficult to discern which are malignant and which are not. Therefore, it is important to consider symptoms in addition to the morphological features of the lesions to provide a more accurate early diagnosis.

As mentioned, most of the current research and development done on CAD systems has focused on image analysis. Yet a multi-axial analysis is required to obtain a more accurate diagnosis at the early stages of certain diseases such as cancer. By multi-axial analysis, we mean the involvement of distinct data types, such as bio-markers, gene loci, genomic, dietary, imaging, environmental, and socio-economic data, that by themselves and in combination affect the behaviour of a system.

As a case study that captures the ideas above, we will discuss our development of DRAsTIK. From the insights that we obtained from early work on image analysis for the early diagnosis of lung cancer (Barranco-Mendoza et al. 1999, 25-40; Barranco-Mendoza et al. 1997), we determined that it is absolutely necessary for complex conditions such as cancer to consider multi-axial patient data to perform a more accurate risk assessment. Therefore, the available client information, such as health history records, imaging, genetic, serum, and sputum cytology data, were incorporated into a multi-axial knowledge representation model, the Probabilistic Property-Based Model (PPBM). PPBM considers all these disease factors to estimate the likelihood that the client will develop a condition using an inference engine combined with Bayesian probability and temporal abstraction. This optimized Bayesian/Temporal module enables DRAsTIK to follow-up a client's progress over time and accurately adapts the risk assessment based on new and previous historical data (Barranco-Mendoza 2005; Barranco-Mendoza, Persaud, and Dahl 2004, 558-59).

PPBM can calculate probability even if only partial information is given and will recommend follow-up tests to be performed, the results of which will improve the accuracy of the assessment. Also, PPBM is sufficiently flexible to allow modification of the knowledge base as new scientific and medical information becomes available, such as newly discovered cancer bio-markers. The original knowledge base follows the accepted clinical practice guidelines for the condition, but the engine learns and identifies patterns in the client data that are presented to the expert health practitioner, who can validate them and enable their incorporation into the knowledge base to refine future assessments. This methodology is being further developed by the TWU HeIR Group to address risk assessment and prevention plans of T2DM. In collaboration with Infogenetica Bioinformatics, PPBM was used to develop DRAsTIK, an IRAS for chronic diseases for web and mobile devices that will integrate with standard EMR. A collaborative project with the University of British Columbia (UBC) Continuing Professional Development and Knowledge Translation group (CPD-KT) is being pursued to integrate DRAsTIK with CliniPEARLS, software for portable digital assistants (PDAs) (e.g., Palm and Windows mobile devices), developed by the CPD-KT in conjunction with the BC Ministry of Health's Guidelines and Protocols Advisory Committee, that facilitates quick reference of clinical practice guidelines (CPGs) at the point of care. (The software and guidelines can be downloaded free of charge for BC health practitioners with registration from http://www.clinipearls.ca/bcguidelines.)

The CliniPEARLS and DRAsTIK research groups are currently focusing on T2DM prevention and risk assessment among high-risk populations, Aboriginals – many of whom live in rural or remote communities – being one of the most at risk. T2DM is rapidly rising in incidence in both rural and urban communities. It is associated with high morbidity and mortality and imposes a significant economic burden on the Canadian health system. Evidence suggests that raising health consumers' knowledge of this disease and its associated risk factors can dramatically curb its incidence. Information technologies, such as IRAS, EMR, and PDA, have demonstrated efficacy in improving disease prevention and management through effective just-in-time knowledge translation and decision support to physicians and patients (Ho et al. 2004). We have been exploring the efficacy of combining DRAsTIK and CliniPEARLS, linking patient-specific health data with literature-based risk factors assessment strategies for T2DM, as health promotion and prevention tools for physicians and their patients to use in the primary prevention of T2DM. We have customized the system by using datasets that consider specific Canadian Aboriginal information on specific genetic markers, physiological characteristics, and social and lifestyle habits. These datasets will enable DRAsTIK to develop personalized electronic T2DM prevention plans sensitive to the particular physiological and sociological needs of Aboriginal users. Even though this phase is at an early stage, preliminary results look promising.

Future Directions

As we have seen, the advancement in communication infrastructure, the already widespread and expanding acceptance of mobile and web-based technologies, and the development of new and interactive health informatics systems are allowing Canadians in all kinds of communities – urban, rural, or remote – to have access to more and more accurate health information in a faster and more convenient way. Family physicians, nurse practitioners, and other primary health-care professionals now have tools at the point of care to enable them to provide more specialized diagnosis, treatment, and care that, in the case of rural and remote communities, would not have been easily available or were prohibitive in terms of cost.

Virtual health-care communities, online forums, and web-based RAS are enabling clients to become active participants in the maintenance of their own health. However, it is important that users of these technologies remain cautious of the accuracy of the information provided, for not all sources available on the Internet are reliable. Also, regardless of its accuracy, technology can never fully substitute for the professional advice, empathy, common sense, and care of a real-life health-care professional. These tools are meant to assist health providers to increase the accuracy and speed of their diagnoses at the point of care, regardless of their geographical location, expand their knowledge and training opportunities, and make communication with the patient and other health-care professionals more effective.

New technologies bring new legislations, processes, and procedures. The face of the Canadian health-care system is changing. The availability and functionality of these new technologies are increasing day by day. They will provide greater access to and flexibility in care for Canadians regardless of geographical location, and this is good news for rural and remote communities.

194   *Rural Health Services Delivery*

Acknowledgments

We would like to thank Francisco Grajales II, Varun Ramraj, Kendall Ho, and Infogenetica Bioinformatics for their continuing collaboration on some of the work presented here.

Note

1 Healthline (http://www.healthline.com); WebMD (http://www.webmd.com), Telehealth Information Exchange (http://tie.telemed.org); International Society for Telemedicine and eHealth (http://www.isft.net).

References

Altman, R.B. 1999. "AI in Medicine: The Spectrum of Challenges from Managed Care to Molecular Medicine." *AI Magazine* 20, 3: 67-77.

Barranco-Mendoza, A. 2005. "Stochastic and Heuristic Modeling for Analysis of the Growth of Pre-Invasive Lesions and for a Multidisciplinary Approach to Early Cancer Diagnosis." PhD diss., Simon Fraser University.

Barranco-Mendoza, A., C. Clem, A. Gupta, P. Fizzano, and M. Guillaud. 1999. "Predicting the Development of Pre-Invasive Lesions from Biopsies." *Archives of Control Sciences* 9: 25-40.

Barranco-Mendoza, A., C. Clem, A. Gupta, P. Fizzano, M. Guillaud, R. Aggarwala, and F. Beardwood. 1997. "Modelling Pre-Invasive Bronchial Epithelial Lesions." Paper presented at the First Pacific Institute for the Mathematical Sciences Industrial Problem Solving Workshop, Vancouver.

Barranco-Mendoza, A., and F. Grajales II. 2008. "Usability and Performance Analysis of Publicly Available Web-Based Chronic Disease Risk Assessment Systems." Manuscript, Trinity Western University.

Barranco-Mendoza, A., D.R. Persaud, and V. Dahl. 2004. "A Property-Based Model for Lung Cancer Diagnosis." Paper presented at Currents in Computational Molecular Biology, RECOMB 2004, San Diego, CA.

Brindle, P., A. Beswick, T. Fahey, and S. Ebrahim. 2006. "Accuracy and Impact of Risk Assessment in the Primary Prevention of Cardiovascular Disease: A Systematic Review." *British Medical Journal* 92, 12: 1752-59.

Burke, L., and B. Weill. 2005. *Information Technology for the Health Professions.* 2nd ed. New Jersey: Pearson Prentice Hall.

Canadian Institute for Health Information (CIHI). 2006. *How Healthy Are Rural Canadians? An Assessment of Their Health Status and Health Determinants.* Ottawa: CIHI.

Cardium Health. 2005. *Getting Real Value for Health Risk Assessments.* Cardium Health (now called Nurtur), Farmington, CT, http://www.cardiumhealth.com/.

Dryburgh, H. 2001. *Changing Our Ways: Why and How Canadians Use the Internet.* Ottawa: Housing, Family and Social Statistics Division, Statistics Canada. Catalogue No. 56F0006XIE.

Fausett, L.V. 1994. *Fundamentals of Neural Networks: Architectures, Algorithms, and Applications.* Upper Saddle River, NJ: Prentice Hall.

Frawley, W., G. Piatetsky-Shapiro, and C. Matheus. 1991. "Knowledge Discovery in Databases: An Overview." In *Knowledge Discovery in Databases,* edited by G. Piatetsky-Shapiro, 1-30. Menlo Park, CA: AAAI Press.

Giokas, D. 2005. "Canada Health Infoway: Towards a National Interoperable Electronic Health Record (EHR) Solution." *Studies in Health Technology and Informatics* 115: 108-40.

Goodman, K.W., and R.A. Miller. 2006. "Ethics and Health Informatics: Users, Standards, and Outcomes." In *Biomedical Informatics,* edited by E.H. Shortliffe and J.J. Cimino, 379-402. New York: Springer.

Grajales, F. II. 2008. "Internet-Based Self-Management of Chronic Disease: Usability and Performance Analysis of Publicly Available Risk Assessment Systems with Recommendations of Future System Design." Manuscript, Trinity Western University.

Harris, R.M., C.N. Wathen, and J.M. Fear. 2006. "Searching for Health Information in Rural Canada: Where Do Residents Look for Health Information and What Do They Do When They Find It?" *Information Research* 12, 1: paper 274, http://InformationR.net/.

Healey, R.R., and C. Pollock. 2008. *Between the Government and the Universities: The Alberta Heritage Foundation for Medical Research, 1980-2005.* Edmonton: University of Alberta Press.

Health Canada. 2008a. *About Health Canada.* Ottawa: Health Canada, http://www.hc-sc.gc.ca/.

–. 2008b. *Canada's Health Infostructure.* Ottawa: Health Canada, http://www.hc-sc.gc.ca/.

–. Health and the Information Highway Division. 2004. *Telemental Health in Canada: A Status Report.* Ottawa: Health Canada. Catalogue No. H21-236/2004E-HTML.

Henwood, F., S. Wyatt, A. Hart, and J. Smith. 2003. "Ignorance Is Bliss Sometimes: Constraints on the Emergence of the 'Informed Patient' in the Changing Landscapes of Health Information." *Sociology of Health and Illness* 25, 6: 589-607.

Ho, K., H.N. Lauscher, A. Best, G. Walsh, S. Jarvis-Selinger, M. Fedeles, and A. Chockalingam. 2004. "Dissecting Technology-Enabled Knowledge Translation: Essential Challenges, Unprecedented Opportunities." *Clinical and Investigative Medicine* 27: 70-78.

Jennett, P.A., and K. Andruchuk. 2001. "Telehealth: 'Real Life' Implementation Issues." *Computer Methods and Programs in Biomedicine* 64: 169-74.

Jennett, P.A., M.P. Gagnon, and H.K. Brandstadt. 2005. "Preparing for Success Readiness Models for Rural Telehealth." *Journal of Postgraduate Medicine* 4: 279-85.

Johnson, L.J. 2003. "Legal Risks of Telemedicine." *Medical Economics* 1: 101.

Lavrac, N., E. Keravnou, and B. Zupan. 2000. "Intelligent Data Analysis in Medicine." In *Encyclopedia of Computer Science and Technology,* vol. 42, edited by A. Kent and J.G. Williams, 113-57. New York: Dekker.

Ledley, R.S., and L.B. Lusted. 1959. "Reasoning Foundation of Medical Diagnosis: Symbolic Logic, Probability, and Value Theory Aid Our Understanding of How Physicians Reason." *Science* 130, 9: 9-12.

Léger, M. 2000. "Health Care of the Future: Vision 2020 Leads the Way – Part 1." *Healthcare Canada Information Management and Technology* 14, 2: 12-14.

Mendelson, R. 2001. *Geographic Structures as Census Variables: Using Geography to Analyse Social and Economic Processes.* Canada: Statistics Canada. Catalogue No. 92F0138MIE.

Minore, B., M. Boone, M. Katt, P. Kinch, S. Birch, and C. Mushquash. 2005. "The Effects of Nursing Turnover on Continuity of Care in Isolated First Nation Communities." *Canadian Journal of Nursing Research* 37: 86-100.

Pascal, W.J. 2001. "Canada E-Health 2000: From Vision to Action." *Healthcare Information Management and Communications Canada* 15, 1: 37-40.

Picot, J., and T. Cradduck. 2000. *The Telehealth Industry in Canada: Industry Profile and Capability Analysis.* Keston Group and Infotelmed Communications, Canada.

Pong, R.W., and J.C. Hogenbirk. 1999. "Licensing Physicians for Telehealth Practice: Issues and Policy Options." *Health Law Review* 8: 3-14.

Rumelhart, D.E., and J.L. McClelland. 1986. *Foundations.* Vol. 1 of *Parallel Distributed Processing,* edited by D.E. Rumelhart and J.L. McClelland. Cambridge, MA: MIT Press.

Stanberry, B. 2006. "Legal and Ethical Aspects of Telemedicine." *Journal of Telemedicine and Telecare* 12: 166-75.

World Health Organization (WHO). 2005. *Preventing Chronic Diseases: A Vital Investment: WHO Report.* Edited by Robert Beaglehole. Geneva: WHO Press.

Chapter 11   **Service Delivery Change in Three Prairie Communities**

D. Ramsey and K. Beesley

Key Points

- Understanding the health service implications of change, restructuring, and future development is crucial in Canadian rural communities.
- Health-care services are an important determinant of rural community well-being and, with community resilience, help to illustrate opportunities for and barriers to service enhancement.
- Evidence suggests that access to a family physician is critical because it is a frequently used service. Even though selected other health services are less frequently used, they are perceived to have declined in quality.
- Rural communities are concerned about not having health services at all. In the rural Prairies, this is a particular issue because so many communities are aging in place.

Economic restructuring in rural Canadian communities has led to dramatic changes in social, political, and economic life. Although rural areas have always been exposed to some degree of change, the past fifty years have demonstrated intensified and rapid restructuring as a result of mechanization, modernization, and downsizing, particularly in agriculture (Troughton 2005). Today the future of many rural areas across the country hinges on shifting demographics. Rural youth out-migration (Hamilton and Butler 2001), coupled with aging in place

(Joseph and Chalmers 1995; also see Chapter 23, this volume) and rural in-migration, especially of seniors, has contributed to rural change. These changing demographics have led to an increased focus on service provision (Halseth, Ryser, and Sullivan 2003). With approximately 80 percent of Canadians living in urban areas, the provision of services to the remaining 20 percent scattered over a large geographical area is difficult, particularly when this group is aging. It is undeniable that the rural Canadian population is aging. In fact, Statistics Canada data indicate that, from the time of the initial fertility decline in 1966 up to 2001, the population group aged nineteen and under declined by 8 percent, while the population group aged sixty-five and over more than doubled (Statistics Canada 2002). Rural communities, where almost 20 percent of all Canadian seniors live, are among the most affected by this "greying."

This chapter explores the issues of change, restructuring, and future development in rural communities in the Prairies. The research is based on two larger research projects interested in service delivery in rural Canada. The first is the New Rural Economy (NRE) Project based at Concordia University. This research has been examining service delivery issues in thirty-two rural communities across Canada since 1996 (Reimer 2006). The second is the Determinants of Rural Health Project based at Brandon University (Annis, Beattie, and Racher 2004). As illustrated in the title, the purpose of the project was to identify what determines health in rural communities. Follow-up research examined implications for the provision of services deemed important to these communities (Ramsey and Beesley 2006, 2007). Both the NRE and the Determinants of Rural Health utilized a variety of methods to identify service delivery issues and how best to address them. The research instruments implemented in the three community surveys reported in this chapter were drawn from this larger research. The intent of the research was to assess changes in level of service and to identify how resilient communities were in addressing changes, including changes in service provision.

The results presented here are based on household surveys conducted in three communities: Benito and Manitou, Manitoba, and Carnduff, Saskatchewan. Each community has strengths and weaknesses, and each provides examples of efforts to maintain, if not enhance, services. The latter is viewed as resiliency. Resiliency in biological systems refers to the ability to both withstand and respond to change. In human communities, such resiliency can be measured in its capital and capacity.

We begin the chapter with a brief overview of the literature that pulls together approaches to assessing rural health and well-being (e.g., including access to health-care services), understanding capital in communities as a measure of response to change (e.g., campaign to keep a hospital open), and considering community resiliency as one perspective from which to examine a community's ability to recover from certain elements of change (e.g., closure of a hospital). We then analyze the results of the household surveys. Although we focus on health-care service issues in the communities, we describe other services and issues to illustrate the relative importance of health-care issues compared with all other issues. In the conclusion, we offer recent examples of initiatives in other prairie communities to address issues of health-care services as possible solutions for other communities.

Rural Well-Being and Resiliency

With regard to rural studies, health and well-being can be viewed as both measures and determinants (Ramsey and Beesley 2006). The Manitoba Department of Health (2004, 5), for example, identified eighty-five indicators of health based on three general categories:

1 *Healthy Living:* self-reported health, life expectancy, infant mortality, low birth weight, chronic diseases, and health promotion and disease prevention.
2 *Access to Health-Care Services:* health information or advice, primary health care, family physician, immediate care, routine care, ambulatory care sensitive conditions, wait times for elective diagnostic services, and prescription drug expenditures.
3 *Patient Satisfaction and Quality of Care Received:* telehealth services, community-based care, physician care, and hospital care.

A number of frameworks for determinants of health can be identified, including social and economic dimensions of well-being (Health and Welfare Canada 1992) and broader frameworks such as that developed by Hamilton and Bhatti (1996), which includes income and social status, social support networks, education, working conditions, physical environments, biology and genetics, personal health practices and coping skills, healthy child development, and health services. Hancock, Labonte, and Edwards (1999) identified six general determinants of health for community-level measurement, including sustainable ecosystems, environmental viability, livability of built environments, community conviviality, social equity, and economic adequacy. Also at the community level, Halseth and Williams (1999) addressed issues of community participation and empowerment in relation to health-care service provision and related decision-making processes.

In southwestern Manitoba, previous research illustrated the importance of rural health-care services as a determinant of rural community well-being (Annis 2005). Specifically, health-care centre managers in the region indicated that access to services in rural communities is crucial not only to rural community health and well-being but also to community survival (Ramsey and Beesley 2006, 2007). Maintaining such services depends on the capital and capacity that exist within the community. Known colloquially as the "three Cs," social capacity, capital, and cohesion have been adopted as both concepts and attributes for assessing rural changes and conditions (Gauthier and Weiss 2005; Ramsey and Beesley 2006; Reimer 2006). Whereas social capital can be viewed as the stock that a community or institution has to address change, capacity refers to the ability of a community or institution to access and utilize capital. Cohesion, in turn, relates to how well community members and institutions work together to utilize capital. In recent years, social capital has been adopted as a concept and attribute in the area of health studies in a number of ways, including an attribute of health (Pollack and von dem Knesebeck 2004), a determinant of health (Health Canada 2006), and a network (Rose 2000). This chapter recognizes that capital includes physical (e.g., bricks and mortar), human (e.g., health-care professionals), social (e.g., relations), financial (e.g., tax base), and environmental (e.g., natural resources) dimensions and that they influence health and well-being. The chapter takes capital to be an indicator of what communities and regions have in place to help them address particular issues (Gauthier and Diaz 2005) by focusing on physical and human capital.

Communities change, including their conditions. One approach to assessing change is to try to understand better a community's resiliency (Adger 2000; Kulig 1999; Olsson 2003; Peterson 2000). Kulig, Edge, and Joyce (2008, 76) state that community resiliency "can be viewed as both a theoretical framework and social process that explains community responses to external forces, such as economic downturns, natural disasters, or other threats to sustainability." This chapter adopts the definition put forth by Kulig (1999, 223), "the ability to bounce back from adversity," to which we can add that community resiliency is "the ability of a community to not only deal with adversity but, in doing so, to reach a higher level of functioning" (Brown and Kulig 1996, 97). Kulig (1999, 223) suggests that "this definition emphasizes a community engagement process that includes both proactive and reactive responses." Resiliency, in essence, is the ability to withstand change, and this ability is based in part on the health of the community, which includes its capital. Kulig (1999, 223-24) further argues that within this context there are useful mechanisms through which "community members can articulate how their community is functioning ... [and] suggest opportunities to work together and to further build the resiliency of their community." This chapter illustrates how communities have identified such opportunities and barriers through service maintenance and enhancement.

Study Area and Methodology

An important dimension of the research design was to facilitate the analysis of change linked to community resiliency. We asked respondents to address, in an open-ended fashion, their feelings about changes in selected community services over a five-year period. Clearly, a satisfactory response to such change would be a marker of resiliency. A number of factors determined community selection for the analysis. First, given recent restructuring in the grain sector in the Prairies, we selected communities where agriculture formed part of the community and its surrounding region's economy. Second, we sought a range of locations in the Prairies, including degrees of isolation from larger centres (see Figure 11.1). Benito represents an agricultural community at the northern fringe of grain production and is located on the border between Manitoba and Saskatchewan. Carnduff is located in the southeast corner of Saskatchewan. Manitou is located in south-central Manitoba. Although all three communities have seen a decline in population since 1996, Benito has been the hardest hit, losing 20 percent of its population in a ten-year period (see Table 11.1). The unemployment rate in Benito has risen the highest of the three communities, from 6.2 percent in 1996 to 14.3 percent in 2006. This compares to Manitoba unemployment rates of 7.9 percent and 5.5 percent respectively. All three communities fall within the Statistics Canada definition of "Rural and Small Town," as defined in Chapter 1 in this volume.

Figure 11.1 Map showing locations of study areas

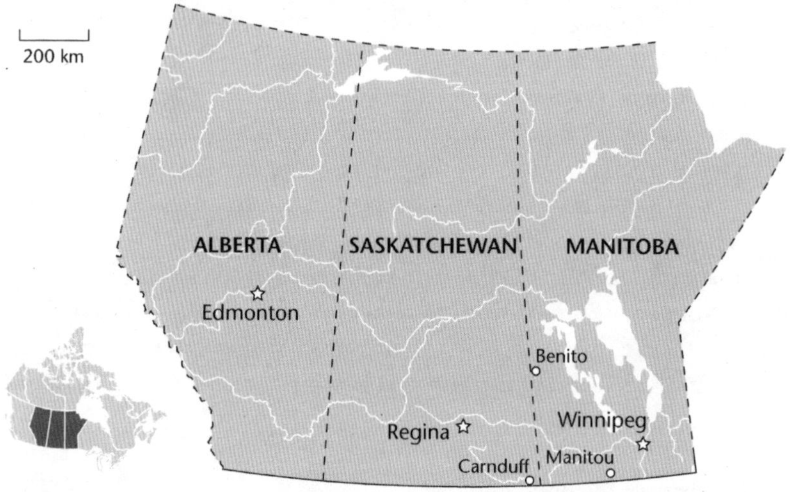

The research began with a household survey in Benito in 2003 (Walsh and Ramsey 2003). The instrument was developed based on a detailed household survey of twenty communities in 2002 ($n = 1,995$) as part of an initiative of the NRE Project at Concordia University. A shortened instrument focusing on core services was developed and pilot tested for Benito. Benito is one of thirty-two communities included in the NRE. However, it was not included in the 2002 NRE. This survey was an attempt to provide a greater prairie comparative within the NRE research.

A knock-and-drop technique was employed to deliver a question-naire to all residents of Benito in early August 2003. With this technique, researchers attempt to make personal contact with respondents, giving them the opportunity to describe the research and their role in it (Steele et al. 2001; Walsh and Ramsey 2003). Reminder letters were sent to all households in late August. In parts of rural Canada, the zero in the second digit of the six-digit postal code denotes Rural and Small Town. Furthermore, all households in such a community or region have the same postal code. In Benito, Canada Post delivered the reminder cards to all households. A 33 percent ($n = 63$) response rate was achieved (Walsh and Ramsey 2003). Based on the results of the Benito survey, comparisons with other communities were considered useful to

Table 11.1   Demographic structure of selected communities, 1996-2006

Measure	Community	1996	2001	2006	Change, 1996-2006
Population	Benito	460	415	370	-90 (-19.6%)
	Carnduff	1,069	1,017	1,012	-57 (-5.3%)
	Manitou	781	775	718	-63 (-8.1%)
Unemployment rate (%)	Benito	6.2	11.1	14.3	+8.1
	Carnduff	6.0	4.3	1.8	-4.3
	Manitou	8.1	0.0	0.0	-8.1
Total experienced workforce	Benito	160	135	175	+10
	Carnduff	495	460	560	+65
	Manitou	370	390	410	+40

Source: Statistics Canada, Community Profiles, 2001, 2006.

understand better the larger context of change and resiliency. A modified instrument, with a length of two double-sided pages that focused on service delivery and change, was mailed to all residences of Manitou and Carnduff in December 2004. All households in each community were sent a questionnaire, which included an addressed and stamped envelope for return. Following reminder letters sent out in early January 2005, a 28 percent ($n = 99$) response rate was achieved in Manitou and an 18 percent ($n = 65$) response rate in Carnduff.

A major limitation of the research was that the overall response rates were low, ultimately impacting the representativeness of the findings to the larger communities (Hikmet and Chen 2003). Interestingly, the researchers had been working in Benito for one year prior to conducting the household survey. In fact, community leaders expressed disappointment at not being part of the larger NRE survey. An announcement was made in the regional newspaper indicating times when the researchers would be in the community to assist with any questions. Only two residents attended these sessions. The Carnduff and Manitou surveys were conducted with no prior contact or any advertising or community visit. The respondents, overall, approximated the gender breakdown of each community but over-represented seniors. These respondents, with a strong vested interest in the health-care system, are important commentators in any health-related research in Rural and Small Town Canada (Beesley et al. 1996).

Despite employing the Total Design Method established by Dillman (1978) and Salant and Dillman (1994) for each community, response rates were low. Because of the low rates, the results are not considered representative of each community. We are confident, though, that given the scale of the services (e.g., hospitals, schools, policing, business services) the responses are a true indication of levels of capital within the community. The positive and negative impressions of development and service provision provide indications of resiliency. Furthermore, though a small percentage of respondents provided detailed open-ended comments, those who did clarified the details surrounding the issues related to service delivery and economic development in their respective communities. The capital and resiliency witnessed in the communities illustrate, at a minimum, maintenance if not enhancement of rural community well-being.

Service Delivery Change in the Three Communities

This section provides a contextual comparison between health and other services. Key points from the analysis include improved school access in Carnduff (70.8 percent), improved library access in Carnduff (84.6 percent) and Manitou, worsened RCMP service in Manitou (56.6 percent), and improved recreational facilities in Manitou (57.6 percent) (see Table 11.2). Although libraries were omitted as a service in the Benito survey, their importance as an improvement was noted in other sections of the questionnaire. Interestingly, for many services in each community, a large percentage of respondents had no opinion or thought that services had not changed. Given the aging of rural communities, many respondents had little or no contact with some community facilities, such as schools and recreation centres. Yet it was possible to assess service change in the section that asked respondents to identify the top three positive and negative changes in their respective communities over the past five years.

Respondents were asked to provide details about access to four specific aspects of health services: family physician, ambulance, emergency room, and physiotherapy. Interestingly, very few respondents thought that these services had improved (see Table 11.2). In each of the three communities, more people thought that accessing a family physician was more difficult than those who thought that it was easier than in the previous five years. Although a lack of physicians is an issue across Canada (CIHI 2002), urban residents have the option of visiting

Table 11.2   Perceptions of change over a five-year period (percentages), 2000-5[1]

Service	Community	Perceptions of change in quality of services			
		Better	Same	Worse	Neutral/ no response
Schools	Benito	6.3	15.9	28.8	49.2
	Carnduff	70.8	16.9	1.5	10.8
	Manitou	8.1	47.8	15.2	29.9
Libraries	Benito[2]	–	–	–	–
	Carnduff	84.6	6.2	3.1	6.2
	Manitou	34.3	50.5	0.0	15.2
RCMP	Benito	1.6	61.9	17.5	19.0
	Carnduff	10.8	72.3	6.2	10.8
	Manitou	4.0	26.3	56.6	13.1
Recreation	Benito	7.9	68.3	3.2	20.6
	Carnduff	38.5	52.3	0.0	8.2
	Manitou	57.6	26.3	4.0	11.1

Health service	Community	Perceptions of change in access to health-care services			
		Easier	Same	Harder	Neutral/ no response
Doctor	Benito	1.6	23.8	66.7	7.9
	Carnduff	1.5	18.5	70.8	9.2
	Manitou	11.1	36.4	46.5	6.1
Ambulance	Benito	1.6	19.0	1.6	78.2
	Carnduff	3.1	0.0	10.8	86.2
	Manitou	5.1	3.0	10.1	81.8
Emergency	Benito	1.6	17.5	17.5	63.5
	Carnduff	1.5	9.2	20.0	69.2
	Manitou	8.1	13.1	13.1	65.7
Physiotherapy	Benito	0.0	14.3	9.5	76.2
	Carnduff	3.1	4.6	6.2	86.2
	Manitou	6.1	3.0	6.1	84.8

Note: Percentages may not add up to 100 due to rounding.
1 The Benito survey covers the years 1998-2003.
2 Libraries were not included as a service in the Benito survey.
Source: Authors' surveys.

walk-in clinics or hospitals. A community unable to attract even one physician presents safety concerns for residents, especially older residents. Basic health-care service provision is of particular concern in remote regions of the Prairies. This issue is described in detail in Chapter 9 in this volume.

Two-thirds (66.7 percent) of respondents in Benito and 70.8 percent of those in Carnduff thought that access to a physician was harder. The percentage was much lower (46.5 percent) in Manitou. Perceptions of access to ambulance, emergency, and physiotherapy services were markedly different. More than three-quarters of respondents from each community did not respond or were neutral on the topic. Two reasons can be identified for such a high percentage. First, none of the communities has ambulance, emergency, or physiotherapy facilities. However, respondents were given the opportunity to indicate whether the service was available within a thirty-minute drive or was farther away. Second, though over 80 percent in each community visited a physician, less than 10 percent used an ambulance, about 30 percent used emergency services, and 12 percent used physiotherapy services. A key barrier to service use is the physical distance between user and service, not unlike the case described in Chapter 16 in this volume.

Benito

Of the four service categories, that of family physician garnered the greatest rate of question completion, which supports the belief that a family physician is a needed and used service and that the absence of one is of concern to community residents. Of the sixty-three respondents who completed the family physician access question, only one respondent indicated that access had improved. Although some respondents can easily make the half-hour (twenty-seven-kilometre) trip north to Swan River to see a family physician, many elderly and lower-income residents find such travel more difficult. Although the high degree of "Neutral" or "No Response" responses to the other services is related to not accessing them, those who had fewer respondents thought that access to ambulance, emergency room, or physiotherapy services was easier.

Fifty-nine respondents also provided comments in response to the question "what are the most important things you feel Benito should attempt to achieve over the next few years?" The need to maintain and improve businesses and the ability to obtain a physician were the dominant comments. Almost half of the comments (47.5 percent) by respondents specifically mentioned the lack of a physician. Most of the comments were simple statements. However, a number of respondents provided more detailed comments, particularly related to issues facing seniors. For example, one respondent noted that "[we need to] have a doctor in Benito. It's mostly seniors living here, some don't drive. As it is now, you have to go to Swan River or Kamsack to see a doctor. Even for a prescription, you have to hire someone to take you."

Swan River is a larger rural service community twenty-five minutes north of Benito, and Kamsack to the west in Saskatchewan (population of 1,713 in 2006) takes slightly longer to reach and is subject to the Saskatchewan health-care system. Another respondent lamented that it appears that officials in Swan River are "calling the shots" in deciding for Benito whether it ought to have a resident physician. This comment was reinforced by this respondent at the end of the questionnaire in providing "any other comments": "Why should Swan River have eight doctors sitting there and not one to come to Benito for even two days per week? It's disgusting. We're a village of mostly seniors and find it very hard to get to Swan River all the time."

In total, twenty-eight respondents also provided viewpoints in the "any other comments" section. The space for comments was small, so most responses were only a few words, including "need a doctor," "no doctor on call," "need a doctor on duty," and "have a local hospital facility with no doctor." Another respondent commented that, though the hospital includes a personal care facility and seniors' housing, it lacks the services of a physician.

The issues in Benito are not unique to parts of rural Canada. However, the community has both physical capital and human capacity to respond to such adversity. In fact, the community owns a house for a physician to live in and has used it in international recruitment initiatives. The community thus far has been unsuccessful. The health-care and long-term-care home are located in the same complex and are staffed by a registered nurse. There are still concerns about the lack of a physician in the community. As noted by one resident, "with no doctor, no doubt our drugstore will close, that leaves us with just our grocery stores. Elevators all closed, you're looking at another little dead town in a few years."

Carnduff

In Carnduff, 117 initiatives were raised regarding what the community needs to do in the next few years. The dominant issues were related to maintaining and upgrading community services. Unlike in Benito, in Carnduff fewer respondents mentioned issues related to health-care services. Most comments related to business development and recreational facilities: "Carnduff has heavily capitalized on education and recreation. Now it needs to encourage each individual business to update and expand ... to attract people to this centre." Respondents also noted existing efforts in the community, such as construction of the new school (mentioned by most respondents), establishment of new businesses and services, and community spirit and pride, yet they mourned the loss of the grain elevators. Division over the importance of the original elevators in communities was noted. Although not mutually exclusive, ten respondents thought that construction of the new inland grain terminal was positive, compared with sixteen who mourned demolition of the small elevators. With respect to health care, nine respondents identified the need for a new or improved seniors' home, seven identified the need for a new or improved health-care facility (e.g., hospital), and five identified the need for a new physician.

Almost 30 percent of respondents (nineteen out of sixty-five) made entries in the "any other comments" section. The issues ranged from concerns about trains blowing horns through town at two in the morning to paying coaches in hockey and baseball and from the community being a nice place to live to Carnduff not needing any more recreational facilities. Only three provided comments related to health-care services. One respondent simply stated that the "doctor in town should retire, and a new one should come in." Another expressed concern through a personal story: "It is frustrating to have to go to Oxbow for hospital and doctor. My husband has a serious illness, and we have to go to Regina at least once a month – very costly, and [it] takes time from work for appointments." The third respondent, though not specifically mentioning health-care services, suggested that sharing services across communities is a necessary response to declining populations: "I believe that we need to reduce local municipal administration and council and amalgamate those services with other towns the same size and share expenses and costs in order to make our community able to operate without increasing taxes. Small communities and senior populations can no longer afford increasing costs." Other respondents noted similar points with regard to business development and rural revitalization more generally.

For Carnduff, the most important issues of the day were articulated in the question that asked what the positive and negative changes in the community had been in the past five years. A total of 154 positive changes were identified, an average of 2.6 per respondent. Of these respondents, 51 (33.1 percent) identified construction of the new K-12 school as a positive change. This translates to 85 percent of respondents (51 of 60). Other positive changes included new businesses (21), the new inland grain terminal (10), a new library (9), new baseball diamonds (9), and expansion of oil-related service companies. No positive changes were identified with regard to health care or seniors' services. In contrast, only 78 percent negative changes were identified, among them loss of the elevator and its tax base (16), loss of the local pregnant mares' urine (PMU)[1] business (10), impacts of bovine spongiform encephalopathy (BSE)[2] (10), and loss of businesses/dealerships (7). Only 3 respondents identified negative changes related to health care – the need to replace a soon-to-be-retiring physician.

The responses to the survey for Carnduff were very different compared with those for Benito. Perhaps this is not surprising. Even though Benito has a much smaller population, it does have a health centre and facilities for a physician, including a home. Carnduff does not have such facilities and has long relied on services in adjacent communities. Having a local physician, however, was deemed to be important by some. Also, a number of recent developments (e.g., new school, new recreational facilities, new inland grain terminal, loss of old elevators, and BSE crisis) could have affected the results.

Manitou

Responses in Manitou were similar to those in Carnduff in terms of what the community should strive to do in the next few years. Of the 178 comments made, 61 (34.2 percent) related to providing health-care services. Close to half of them (28) related to completing the wellness centre. Other issues included restoring (21) or maintaining (7) health-care services and recruiting registered nurses (2). Two respondents were against placing any more resources in the wellness centre. One respondent made the general point that "we need to provide services such as hospitals, child care, education and recreation to keep families from moving to larger centers." Other issues identified included improving streets and walkways (12) and the need to create more businesses (11). Resiliency was further noted in the identification of new services and tourism development in the community. As noted by one respondent, however, "the test will be balancing these developments with the loss of core services (hospital, elevator, business, etc.) and declining school enrolments." Yet another respondent stated that Manitou "should become more of a draw to young people to 'live' in rather than one for the old people to 'die' in."

As in Benito, in Manitou health-care services were prominent in the "any other comments" section of the questionnaire. Thirty-five (55.6 percent) of the sixty-three total respondents provided comments. Nine comments related in some way to the wellness centre and other health-care services. The wellness centre proposal includes recreational and therapy pools, a new community hall, a day-care centre, and swimming, fitness, physiotherapy, and other recreational services. To date, only the outdoor swimming pool has been completed. Three respondents stated that no further resources should be put into the new wellness centre – each mentioning wasted tax dollars.

> *I am very concerned in regard to the new proposed wellness centre. We have one person on payroll for the last few years trying to allocate funds for this project – what a waste. If we should get this new facility, how are we going to keep it going? Everyone is short of cash, our population is mostly older seniors. We should have a town vote where everyone can vote and decide on this issue.*

Others related concerns about access to a physician. One respondent wrote, "please keep our doctors in town." Similarly, another indicated that a "lack of continuous doctor service causes people to go to Swan Lake or Morden. The possibility of four levels of senior housing is here if the town would concentrate on it. There will always be retirees, and the houses in town are getting older and need replacement by young people." Another suggested the need to "promote doctors so [that the] hospital can stay and more people [can access] a doctor."

Other issues ranged from gun control to government control and loss of personal freedom. Other respondents pointed to the general need to provide jobs to keep and attract young people to the community. For example, "people are becoming more interested in living in small rural communities, but we need to give them services. Marketing the community on these assets may be necessary." Although the survey results seem to indicate divisions in the community regarding the new wellness centre, others see such services as assets, or social capital, on which the town needs to act.

Interestingly, issues identified in the positive and negative changes section of the questionnaire were not raised in any of the other sections.

Positive changes included the new swimming pool, a new dance studio, artificial ice for the rinks, the opening of a new Internet pharmacy business, the new tourism facility, an upgraded sewer system, access to high-speed Internet, and improved golf courses. Negative issues included declining school enrolments, demolition of the grain elevator, loss of the local restaurant, and declines in emergency services due to the shortage of registered nurses. One respondent identified plans for the new wellness centre as a negative change. Although Manitou appears to have shown resiliency in the face of change, it also appears to face a number of important issues, including community division.

Discussion

This chapter is embedded in two linked scholarly areas, rural well-being and resiliency, drawing largely on the work of Kulig (1999) and Kulig, Edge, and Joyce (2008) in identifying community resiliency as a process for understanding how communities respond to change, including change in well-being. The chapter further argues that building capital contributes to the resiliency of rural communities. In Carnduff, for example, resiliency was noted in the identification of new services and tourism development in the community. Similar efforts were identified in Manitou. In Benito, continued efforts by community leaders to attract a physician to their community were identified as examples of resiliency aimed at improving community well-being. Health care is but one, albeit large, component of the strategy to facilitate rural community well-being at both the individual and the collective scales. We need more work, research, and action designed to make our rural communities in the Prairies (and beyond) desirable places to live, work, and play, including ensuring appropriate levels of care.

Conclusion

Health-care service provision in Canada has been a dominant issue for a number of years. While urban centres are concerned with waiting lists for particular services, rural communities are concerned about not having services at all. Similarly, urban centres must often address issues related to school safety and increasingly large class sizes, whereas many rural communities are faced with the task of keeping their schools open. The core rural business of the southern rural Prairies is agriculture. Shifts in economic structure have often meant the loss of the local grain elevator. The closure of hospitals, schools, and elevators is most often followed by the closure of other services and businesses. The lack of services results in a loss of population, the final result being the demise of the community. These issues and fears are common in Benito, Carnduff, and Manitou.

Under circumstances such as those described above, a sense of well-being and self-reported health might be entirely satisfactory until some threshold is met, such as health problems that require attention from health-care professionals who are not available. When such a threshold is met, the sense of well-being can be expected to decline, pressure to relocate to where needed services are available can be expected to increase, and the future of the rural community can be in trouble. At the same time, when demand for health services increases, one reasonable response is to provide the required services. Some might argue, in relatively simplistic terms, that rural communities live and die, and those in the throes of death should be allowed to pass on. Others might suggest that rural communities are worth saving, even if many of their senior citizens are leaving, one way or another. In the mental health service context, this chapter offers some insights into rural communities and includes a call to action to address community concerns.

As a final note, there are examples of communities across southern Manitoba that are building capacity by sharing capital to provide health-care services. The most recent example involves the communities of Neepawa (thirty-eight-bed hospital) and Minnedosa (twenty-seven-bed hospital), located northeast of Brandon in southwestern Manitoba. The proposal is to build a large hospital between the two communities, with the existing facilities being retrofitted into seniors' homes (Assiniboine Regional Health Authority 2008). Other smaller communities with health-care facilities, however, think that such a development would result in the closure of their facilities. Dave Dauphinais, mayor of the town of Erickson, is one example. He thinks that their nine-bed hospital would not be kept open. He believes that the proposed site, sixty kilometres from Erickson, is too far for residents to travel: "Our people want and deserve an adequate level of health care, and I'm not going to give up. I'm going to keep at it until somebody listens" (CBC 2007). The struggles continue in the Prairies. In responding to restructuring, only one thing seems to be clear: some communities will gain services; others will not.

Notes

1 The estrogen content of PMU has a market in treating women in menopause through estrogen replacement therapy. The industry is not without controversy over the treatment of animals and health concerns that PMU could pose for women (Parisien 2008). The issue raised by respondents related to the loss of contracts by prairie farmers in Canada in October 2003.
2 BSE is a disease that attacks the brain and central nervous system of a range of mammals, including cattle. Its discovery on an Alberta farm in May 2003 resulted in the border closing for trade with the United States. Prices dropped immediately. The border was closed until July 2005.

References

Adger, W.N. 2000. "Social and Ecological Resilience: Are They Related?" *Progress in Human Geography* 24, 3: 347-64.
Annis, R.C. 2005. "Determinants of Health of Rural Populations and Communities Research Project: Final Report 1999-2005." Report for Social Sciences and Humanities Research Council Grant No. 828-1999-1029.
Annis, R., F. Racher, and M. Beattie. 2004. *Rural Community Health and Well-Being: A Guide to Action.* Brandon: Rural Development Institute, Brandon University.
Assiniboine Regional Health Authority. 2008. Minutes of the Assiniboine Regional Health Authority, 19 March, Shoal Lake, MB.
Beesley, K.B., R.T. Bowles, P.J. Macintosh, and C. Johnston. 1996. "Retirees Engaging Community: Seniors and Their Lives in Bobcaygeon, Ontario." In *The Challenges of Managing Change: A Towns and Villages Perspective,* edited by C. Mitchell and F.A. Dahms, 217-42. Waterloo: University of Waterloo.
Brown, D., and J. Kulig. 1996. "The Concept of Resiliency: Theoretical Perspectives from Community Research." *Health and Canadian Society* 41, 1: 29-50.
Canadian Broadcasting Corporation (CBC). 2007, 24 August. "New Hospital Would Kill Erickson Facility, Mayor Says." Ottawa: CBC, http://www.cbc.ca/news/.
Canadian Institute for Health Information (CIHI). 2002. "New Canadian Institute for Health Information (CIHI) Report Sheds Light on Physician Shortage Perception." Ottawa: CIHI, http://secure.cihi.ca/.
Dillman, D. 1978. *Mail and Telephone Surveys: The Total Design Method.* New York: John Wiley and Sons.
Gauthier, D.A., and P. Diaz. 2005. "Rural Adaptation and Social Cohesion for Sustainable Development of the Prairies." *Prairie Forum* 30, 2: iii.
Gauthier, D.A., and S. Weiss. 2005. "Assessing Performance: Indicators, Social Cohesion, and Community Sustainability." *Prairie Forum* 30, 2: 313-28.
Halseth, G., L. Ryser, and L. Sullivan. 2003. "Service Provision as Part of Resource Town Transition Planning: A Case from Northern British Columbia." In *Opportunities and Actions in the New Rural Economy,* edited by D. Bruce and G. Lister, 29-56. Sackville, NB: Rural and Small Town Programme, Mount Allison University.
Halseth, G., and A. Williams. 1999. "Guthrie House: A Rural Community Organizing for Wellness." *Health and Place* 5, 1: 27-44.
Hamilton, N., and T. Bhatti. 1996. *Population Health Promotion: An Integrated Model of Population Health and Health Promotion.* Ottawa: Health Promotion Development Division.

Hamilton, L.C., and M.L. Butler. 2001. "Outdoor Adaptations: Social Indicators through Newfoundland's Cod Crisis." *Research in Human Ecology* 8, 2: 1-11.

Hancock, T., R. Labonte, and R. Edwards. 1999. *Indicators that Count! Measuring Population Health at the Community Level.* Ottawa: Health Canada.

Health Canada. 2006. *Health Policy Research.* Ottawa: Minister of Public Works and Government Services Canada.

Health and Welfare Canada. 1992. *User's Guide to 40 Community Health Indicators.* Ottawa: Ministry of Supply and Services Canada.

Hikmet, N., and S. Chen. 2003. "An Investigation into Low Mail Survey Response Rates of Information Technology Users in Health Care Organizations." *International Journal of Medical Informatics* 72, 3: 29-34.

Joseph, A.E., and A.I. Chalmers. 1995. "Growing Old in Place: A View from Rural New Zealand." *Health and Place* 1, 2: 79-90.

Kulig, J.C. 1999. "Sensing Collectivity and Building Skills: Rural Communities and Community Resiliency." In *Health in Rural Settings: Context for Action,* edited by W. Ramp et al., 223-44. Lethbridge: University of Lethbridge.

Kulig, J.C., D.S. Edge, and B. Joyce. 2008. "Understanding Community Resiliency in Rural Communities through Multimethod Research." *Journal of Rural and Community Development* 3, 3: 77-94.

Manitoba Department of Health. 2004. *Manitoba's Comparable Health Indicator Report: November 2004.* Winnipeg: Government of Manitoba.

Olsson, P. 2003. "Building Capacity for Resilience in Social-Ecological Systems." PhD diss., Department of Systems Ecology, Stockholm University.

Parisien, C. 2008. "Producing Pharmaceuticals." *Manitoba Farmers' Voice* (summer): 21-22.

Peterson, G. 2000. "Political Ecology and Ecological Resilience: An Integration of Human and Ecological Dimensions." *Ecological Economics* 35: 323-36.

Pollack, C.E., and O. von dem Knesebeck. 2004. "Social Capital and Health among the Aged: Comparisons between the United States and Germany." *Health and Place* 10, 4: 383-91.

Ramsey, D., and K. Beesley. 2006. "Rural Community Wellbeing: The Perspectives of Health Care Managers in Southwestern Manitoba, Canada." *Journal of Rural and Community Development* 2: 86-107.

–. 2007. "'Perimeteritis' and Rural Health in Manitoba, Canada: Perspectives from Rural Health Care Managers." *Rural and Remote Health* 7: 1-11.

Reimer, W. 2006. "The Rural Context of Community Development in Canada." *Journal of Rural and Community Development* 1, 2: 155-75.

Rose, R. 2000. "How Much Does Social Capital Add to Individual Health? A Survey Study of Russians." *Social Science and Medicine* 51, 9: 1421-35.

Salant, P., and D. Dillman. 1994. *How to Conduct Your Own Survey.* New York: John Wiley.

Statistics Canada. 2001. *Community Profiles, 2001.* Ottawa: Statistics Canada, http://www.statcan.ca/.

–. 2002. *Census of Population, 2001.* Ottawa: Supply and Services Canada.

–. 2006. *Community Profiles, 2006.* Ottawa: Statistics Canada, http://www.statcan.ca/.

Steele, J., L. Bourke, A.E. Luloff, P. Liao, G. Theodori, and R. Krannich. 2001. "The Drop-Off/Pick-Up Method for Household Survey Research." *Journal of the Community Development Society* 32, 2: 238-50.

Troughton, M. 2005. "Fordism Rampant: The Model and Reality, as Applied to Production, Processing, and Distribution in the North American Agro-Food

System." In *Contrasting Ruralities: Changing Rural Economies, Societies, and Landscapes,* edited by S. Essex et al., 13-27. Wallingford, UK: CABI.

Walsh, D., and D. Ramsey. 2003. "'If It Came in the Mail, I Wouldn't Even Have Opened It'! New Approaches to Survey Techniques." *Prairie Perspectives* 6: 191-207.

Part 4: Rural Health Policy and Research

Chapter 12   **Integrating Policy, Research,
and Community Development:
A Case Study of Developing
Rural Palliative Care**

M.L. Kelley, W. Sletmoen, A.M. Williams,
S. Nadin, and T. Puiras

Key Points

- The need for palliative care is increasing in rural areas; however,
  rural people have less access to palliative care services than their urban
  counterparts.
- An integrated capacity development approach using policy, research,
  and community development can improve access and quality of rural
  palliative care.
- The four-phase capacity development model, Developing Rural Palliative Care, can be used as a theory of change to guide policy and
  practice in rural health.

People who are terminally ill express a desire to end their lives in their
home communities, where they can be surrounded by family and
friends. They do not want to travel long distances to urban centres to
receive palliative care (Hawker et al. 2006; Romanow 2002). However,
rural Canadians have limited access to palliative care (Cinnamon,
Schuurman, and Crooks 2008; Senate Committee on Social Affairs,
Science and Technology 2000). Strategies to develop palliative care
programs in rural communities are therefore needed.

This chapter offers a case study of developing palliative care in
northwestern Ontario using an integrated approach that includes three
components: (1) a provincial end-of-life care strategy that provides a

policy framework for rural health system change; (2) participatory action *research* (PAR) that applies and evaluates a model for planning, implementing, and evaluating palliative care programs; and (3) *community development* strategies to implement the model into practice. The case study, based on three years of experience by the authors developing palliative care in sixteen rural communities (see Chapter 1, this volume, for the definition of "Rural and Small Town"), is applicable to developing palliative care programs in rural communities throughout Canada and elsewhere.

Rural Health Services

The rural population is aging, with a high prevalence of chronic and terminal disease (Bollman and Clemenson 2008). For example, this volume presents the unique challenges faced by older adults with dementia and social isolation (see Chapters 24 and 25), people coping with HIV/AIDS (Chapter 16), and those with mental health issues (Chapter 13). Although approximately 30 percent of the Canadian population lives in rural areas, they have less access to health-care services than their urban counterparts (Ministerial Advisory Council on Rural Health 2002). Issues of rural health status and health services utilization are further examined in Section 1 of this volume.

The major issues of providing health services in rural communities are access to and quality of care (Ministerial Advisory Council on Rural Health 2002; Romanow 2002). These problems are mostly due to lack of resources, in particular health-care professionals and hospitals (Chapter 5, this volume; O'Toole et al. 2008; Pong 2008; Strasser 2003). Consequently, rural residents might need to travel significant distances to receive health services (Cloutier-Fisher and Joseph 2000; Grafton, Troughton, and Rourke 2004).

Rural health-care professionals have a broad scope of practice, simultaneously providing comprehensive general care, specific interventions, and community-based health promotion interventions (Hays, Evans, and Veitch 2005; Molinari and Monserud 2008). Rural providers thus need to be highly skilled generalists, rather than specialists, and practise in ways that are innovative and flexible (Hays, Evans, and Veitch 2005). Teamwork is a common feature of rural practice (Strasser 1999), motivated by the need to work together to get the job done (Kelley 2007) and a strong sense of team belonging (Sedgwick and Yonge 2008).

Rural health-care professionals who are also community members respect community norms, values, and existing social networks (Martinez-Brawley 2000).

Community Capacity Development

Given the geographical isolation and limited resources of many rural communities, capacity development has become an accepted approach to developing rural health services (Alfonso et al. 2008; Chapter 7, this volume; Craig 2007). Capacities are the collective capabilities found within and among people, organizations, community networks, and society in general (Norton et al. 2002). Essentially, capacity development involves building on what already exists.

From this perspective, communities are seen to have the capacity to tackle their problems through collective problem solving. Development is seen as an innate and natural process found in communities. Raeburn et al. (2006) reviewed the health promotion literature on community capacity building and identified three common features: the concepts of capacity and empowerment; the use of bottom-up, community-determined agendas and actions; and processes for developing competence. The need for a long-term investment in the community has also been identified (Bolger 2000).

It is less well documented how to actually practise capacity development. The method of promoting change is to enhance local capacity and not to impose solutions from outside (Morgan 1998). However, capacity developers lack comprehensive theories of change[1] to assist them in understanding the process of development and to guide the nature and timing of their community interventions (Alfonso et al. 2008). This lack has limited the ability to evaluate processes and outcomes of capacity development (Minkler and Wallerstein 2002). The PAR described in this case study evaluates a community capacity development model for use as a theory of change.

Rural Palliative Care Services

Palliative care is for patients with life-limiting, chronic, or terminal illness, when the focus of care is on relieving or preventing suffering and maximizing quality of life. The goal is not curing the illness but providing comfort to the dying individual and his or her family and friends. It incorporates the physical, social, psychological, and spiritual domains of care (Ferris et al. 2002).

Although palliative care is not specific to any illness or group, most of the literature has focused on caring for adults with cancer (Byock 2000) and HIV/AIDS (Grothe and Brody 1995). Since the population is aging, there is an increasing focus on death in older years (Davis and Higginson 2004) and palliative care for persons dying from non-malignant diseases (Murtagh, Preston, and Higginson 2004). Specialized palliative care programs are primarily urban based (Bosanquet and Salisbury 1999; Skilbeck and Payne 2005).

Rural approaches to providing palliative care are beginning to develop (Government of Nova Scotia 2001; Robinson et al. 2009; Wilson et al. 2006). Most dying rural people are cared for by generalist practitioners (physicians, nurses, social workers) in local hospitals, long-term-care facilities, and homecare programs, usually without the benefit of formal palliative care teams and programs (Seamark and Seamark 2004). Care can be enhanced by trained hospice volunteers (McKee, Kelley, and Guirguis-Younger 2007) or a designated palliative care bed in the local hospital (Sach 1997).

Development of rural palliative care programs has been hampered by lack of palliative care education and training for rural health-care providers (Chapter 7, this volume; Kortes-Miller et al. 2007; McConigley, Kristjanson, and Morgan 2000). Models to guide the development of rural programs have also been lacking (Robinson et al. 2009; Wilson et al. 2006). Given past successes in developing rural health services using a capacity development approach, a capacity development model was applied in this case study.

PAR as a Strategy of Inquiry

Community-based participatory action research is appropriate for developing rural health programs (Flicker and Savan 2006; Lyons and Gardner 2001). PAR is distinguished from other types by its goal and methodology. Collaboration, education, and action are the three key elements of PAR. It seeks to produce new knowledge by systematic inquiry, with the collaboration of those affected by an issue, for the purposes of education and taking action or effecting social change (Kemmis and McTaggart 2005). Methodologically, the subjects of the research (not the researcher) control all aspects of the research process (Cashman et al. 2008).

In PAR, knowledge is co-created by the researcher and subjects through a reflective spiral of activity: planning a change, acting and observing the processes and consequences of the change, reflecting on these processes and consequences, and then repeating the cycle of planning, acting and observing, and reflecting (Kemmis and McTaggart 2005; Ramsden 2003). The research plan is constantly evolving based on current experience (Minkler et al. 2008). Thus, unlike other methodologies, knowledge is embedded in the process rather than viewed as an outcome of the research. It is the evolutionary process of change (planning, acting/observing, and reflecting) that is documented by the researcher.

The research process begins with a social problem (e.g., lack of palliative care for dying people in a rural community) that calls for a collective solution. The researcher participates in solving the problem and uses the research process as a means to mobilize social change (Kemmis and McTaggart 2005; Ramsden and Cave 2002). The PAR process often begins with the introduction of a conceptual framework, a theory of change, or findings of previous research as a basis for reflecting, planning, and implementing the PAR (Kemmis and McTaggart 2005).

PAR can use any method for data collection and includes both qualitative and quantitative data. Common methods of data collection are conducting interviews, keeping personal journals and field notes, collecting questionnaires and narratives, and reviewing documents (Flicker and Savan 2006). The research outcome is often a case study report that documents the process of solving the problem and the relationships among people and events that operate as facilitators and barriers to the change process (Kemmis and McTaggart 2005). Participatory action researchers judge the validity of their research by the accomplishment of its goal and not in relation to its methods. Validity of the research process is maintained by the strong commitment of participants who must live with the outcome of their work (Minkler et al. 2008). Investment in the outcome of the research provides a strong incentive for participants to continue to make the best decisions to achieve their goal (see Chapter 9, this volume, for another example of PAR).

Given that the goal of PAR is to empower participants and implement social change, it is a logical methodological choice for research that aims to engage communities in solving problems of rural health. In the PAR project in northwestern Ontario, the "problem" to be solved was how to develop palliative care services in rural communities when health services are limited to basic homecare (case management, nursing, and personal care) and small hospitals or health centres that focus on primary care, emergency care, and long-term care. The number of "expected" deaths per year is also quite low.

Integrating Policy, Research, and Community Development: A Case Study

Northwestern Ontario covers an area that represents approximately 60 percent of Ontario's landmass (see Figure 7.1 for a map of northwestern Ontario), extending from White River in the east to the Manitoba border in the west, to James Bay and Hudson Bay in the north, and to the US border in the south (North West Local Health Integration Network [NWLHIN] 2005). It is composed of the districts of Kenora, Rainy River, and Thunder Bay. The distance between eastern and western boundaries is slightly over 1,000 kilometres, with a population density of 0.5 persons per square kilometre. Despite its large geographical size, the population of northwestern Ontario (234,770) accounts for only 2.06 percent of the total population of Ontario (NWLHIN 2005). There are only two cities in northwestern Ontario with populations of over 10,000 people – Thunder Bay (109,016) and Kenora (15,838) – and it is estimated that 35.2 percent of the population lives in rural areas (Northwestern Health Unit 2007) comprised of numerous rural, remote, and First Nations communities.[2]

The economy of northwestern Ontario has traditionally been based upon resource sectors such as forestry and mining. However, significant layoffs in the forestry industry have impacted the region in the past few years, leading to unemployment and forcing people to leave their home communities to seek employment elsewhere (Northwestern Ontario Municipal Association [NOMA] 2007). This downturn in economic growth, coupled with geographical isolation and low population density, has made the planning and delivery of health services in northwestern Ontario challenging. There has been a chronic shortage of family physicians throughout the region, and many residents are required to travel long distances to receive health care. Poor weather and road conditions further complicate the population's access to much-needed health services (NWLHIN 2005). The challenges encountered in northwestern Ontario in trying to provide quality care to residents are representative of the challenges faced by many rural communities across Canada.

The Health Policy Challenge: Implementing the Ontario End-of-Life Care Strategy in a Rural Context

In July 2000, the Ontario Ministry of Health and Long Term Care announced funding to support a comprehensive, provincial, End-of-Life (EOL) Care Strategy that mandated the establishment of regional EOL Care Networks as well as local, interdisciplinary, and integrated service delivery. The desired outcome of the four-year strategy was to enhance homecare and respite services and reduce hospitalization and caregiver burnout (Seow, King, and Vaitonis 2008). Community Care Access Centres (CCACs), organizations that provide one-stop access to government-funded home and community services,[3] were charged with implementing the new policy within their catchment areas.

In northwestern Ontario, implementation fell to the North West CCAC, which provided services to the districts of Kenora-Rainy River and Thunder Bay. As the largest and most northern CCAC in the province, the North West CCAC faced challenges in providing services not faced in other areas of the province. Table 12.1 provides profiles of the communities serviced. Populations of all but two communities are fewer than 9,000 people, and most community populations are declining. The median age of residents is generally higher than the provincial average. Although the number of deaths per year can be as low as six, the aging population suggests that palliative care will be an increasing community need. Given this context, a unique "rural" approach to implementing the EOL Care Strategy was required.

The initial task for the CCAC was to develop an implementation plan that would achieve the goals of the provincial EOL Care Strategy while at the same time recognizing the unique strengths and attributes of the rural communities in the region. In 2005, under the direction of Puiras, this regional plan was developed. The core element of the plan was rural community capacity development, specifically the development of local, multidisciplinary, palliative care teams in each community that would be supported by educational programs, clinical consultations, and co-ordinated access to services at the regional level. The Northwestern Ontario EOL Care Network was established to oversee and support development of the community palliative care programs.

Table 12.1   Rural community demographics

Community	Population (2001)	Population (2006)	Median age (2006)	Number of deaths (2005)
Atikokan	3,632	3,293	43.0	25
Dryden	8,198	8,195	41.8	99
Emo	1,331	1,305	39.9	9
Fort Frances	8,315	8,103	42.3	119
Greenstone	5,662	4,906	39.8	25
Kenora	15,838	15,177	42.4	198
Manitouwadge	2,949	2,300	42.8	6
Marathon	4,416	3,863	39.8	22
Nipigon*	1,964	1,752	43.6	31
Red Rock*	1,233	1,063	43.8	n/a
Rainy River	981	909	47.8	21
Red Lake*	4,233	4,526	37.9	27
Ear Falls*	1,150	1,153	39.1	n/a
Sioux Lookout	5,336	5,183	35.1	52
Terrace Bay*	1,950	1,625	45.6	18
Schreiber*	1,448	901	42.9	n/a
City of Thunder Bay†	*109,016*	*109,140*	*41.7*	*1,195*
Ontario	*11,410,046*	*12,160,282*	*39.0*	*85,808*
Canada	*30,007,094*	*31,612,897*	*39.5*	*n/a*

* These rural communities are close together and share health services so were treated as one site.

† The only urban community in northwestern Ontario is also the regional health service referral centre.

Sources: The data in columns 2-4 are from Statistics Canada (2008). The data in column 5 are from Habjan, Diamond, and Kelley (2008).

The Research Goal: Implementing and Evaluating the Developing Rural Palliative Care Model

An extensive review of the rural health and rural palliative care literature in 2003 revealed no community capacity development model to guide rural communities through the process of creating palliative care programs. Thus, Kelley (2007) collected data from sixty-six rural palliative care providers and created a model called Developing Rural Palliative Care (DRPC). Through subsequent research, the DRPC model has been validated (Kelley and Williams 2008) and is currently being used in intervention research by Kelley and Williams. The PAR reported in this chapter forms one component of this research.

Located at Lakehead University in northwestern Ontario, Kelley is a founding member of the Northwestern Ontario EOL Care Network's steering committee. In 2005, the DRPC model was presented to the steering committee, which adopted it as their guide for regional palliative care development. This presented a unique opportunity for the researchers to evaluate the model's utility to plan and implement a multi-year, region-wide capacity development initiative.

The DRPC model is essentially a theory of change that depicts a bottom-up community development approach. It draws on community capacity development as its theoretical perspective and incorporates the rural attributes of teamwork, generalist practice, and limited infrastructure. The model addresses how rural providers manage challenges such as lack of resources, resistance to palliative care, and bureaucracy. Enabling factors identified in the model are being community focused, educating providers, working together, fostering local leadership, and taking pride in accomplishments (Kelley 2007). Because the DRPC model is a theory of change within a local context, it can be applied in any rural community.

The model outlines a rural community's process of developing palliative care in four sequential phases: (1) having antecedent community conditions; (2) experiencing a catalyst; (3) creating a local palliative care team; and (4) growing the palliative care program. Each phase of the model incorporates broad themes and specific strategies to guide community members. Ultimately, the model can create a local palliative care program that provides clinical care, education, and advocacy and is supported by strong links both within the community and with outside expert resources. Further details of the model are published elsewhere (Kelley 2007). The DRPC model, depicted as a growing tree, is shown in Figure 12.1.

An important feature of the model is its sequential nature: that is, each phase builds upon the capacities developed during the previous one. In implementing the EOL Care Strategy, use of the model highlighted the importance of strengthening each community's antecedent conditions prior to creating local palliative care teams. The antecedent conditions are collaborative practice, sufficient infrastructure, a vision for change, and a sense of community empowerment. To assess local antecedent conditions and begin the PAR, ten questions were created by Kelley and used by the EOL Care coordinator to engage community stakeholders in self-reflection on their readiness to develop a palliative care program. Three examples of these questions follow. What is the

Figure 12.1   DRPC model, depicted as a growing tree

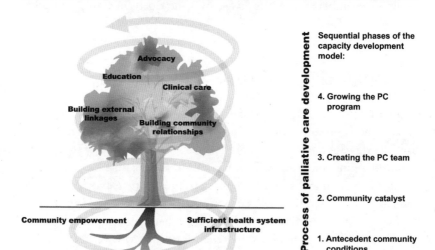

quality of dying in your community now? What is your vision for change? What are the strengths/challenges for palliative care in your community? This discussion was the catalyst for change (phase 2 of the DRPC model) in the local communities. Likewise, use of the model emphasized that investing the time to establish a strong local team (phase 3 of the DRPC model) of committed stakeholders in each community was important prior to delivering palliative care services.

An overview of the PAR process is presented in Figure 12.2. The purpose of the research is to apply and evaluate the DRPC model as a tool for planning, implementing, and evaluating community capacity development for palliative care. The model was introduced in each community as the theory of change to guide the process of development.

After two and a half years of implementation, the model has proven to be a useful tool to guide the process of community development and evaluate regional progress. Each community has been assessed according to the four phases of the model, and the tasks that need to be accomplished within each phase have been identified. As of May 2008, the EOL care coordinator is undertaking community development with thirteen rural communities. Of them, eight now have the antecedent

Figure 12.2 Overview of the PAR process

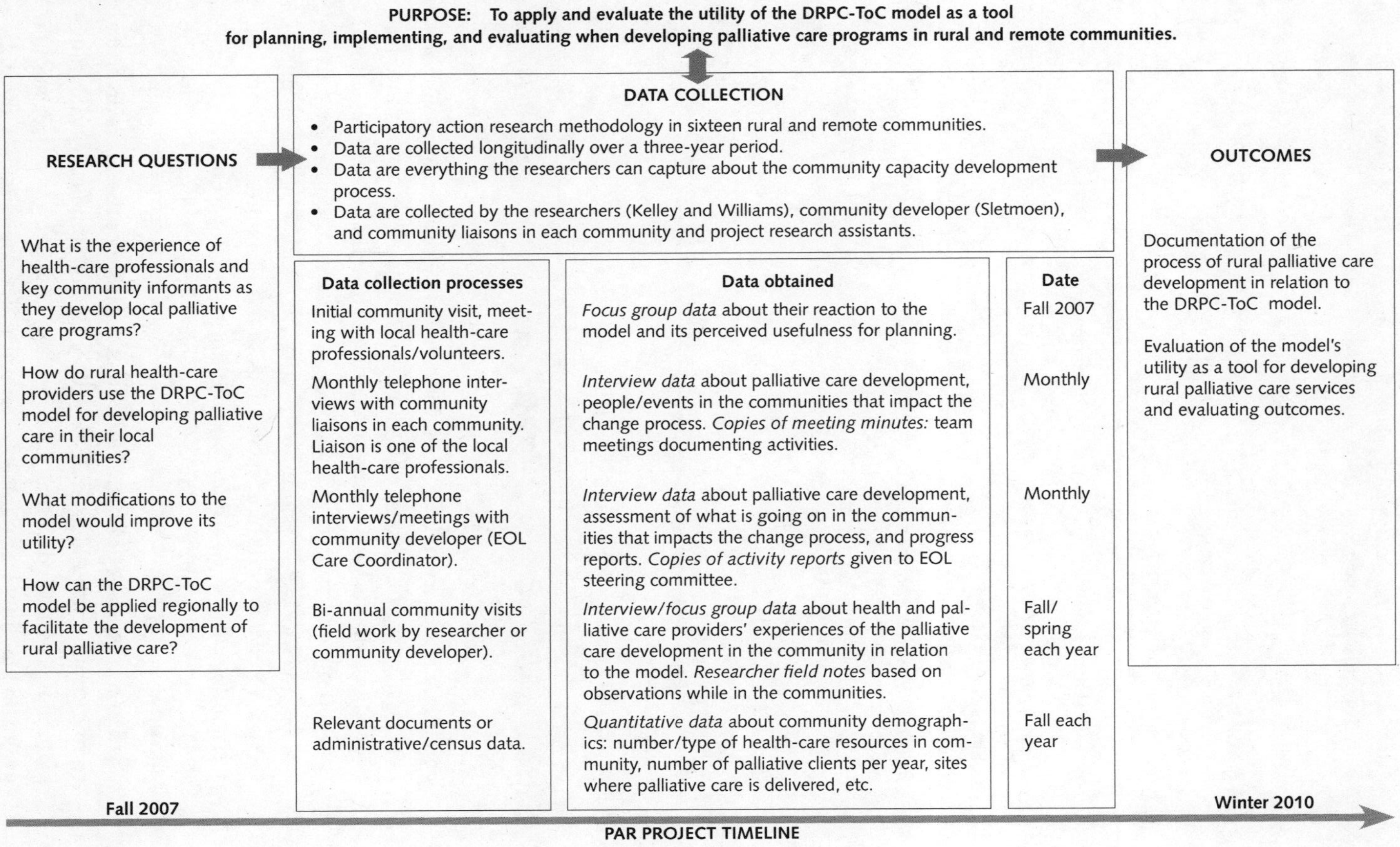

PURPOSE: To apply and evaluate the utility of the DRPC-ToC model as a tool for planning, implementing, and evaluating when developing palliative care programs in rural and remote communities.

RESEARCH QUESTIONS

What is the experience of health-care professionals and key community informants as they develop local palliative care programs?

How do rural health-care providers use the DRPC-ToC model for developing palliative care in their local communities?

What modifications to the model would improve its utility?

How can the DRPC-ToC model be applied regionally to facilitate the development of rural palliative care?

DATA COLLECTION

- Participatory action research methodology in sixteen rural and remote communities.
- Data are collected longitudinally over a three-year period.
- Data are everything the researchers can capture about the community capacity development process.
- Data are collected by the researchers (Kelley and Williams), community developer (Sletmoen), and community liaisons in each community and project research assistants.

Data collection processes	Data obtained	Date
Initial community visit, meeting with local health-care professionals/volunteers.	*Focus group data* about their reaction to the model and its perceived usefulness for planning.	Fall 2007
Monthly telephone interviews with community liaisons in each community. Liaison is one of the local health-care professionals.	*Interview data* about palliative care development, people/events in the communities that impact the change process. *Copies of meeting minutes:* team meetings documenting activities.	Monthly
Monthly telephone interviews/meetings with community developer (EOL Care Coordinator).	*Interview data* about palliative care development, assessment of what is going on in the communities that impacts the change process, and progress reports. *Copies of activity reports* given to EOL steering committee.	Monthly
Bi-annual community visits (field work by researcher or community developer).	*Interview/focus group data* about health and palliative care providers' experiences of the palliative care development in the community in relation to the model. *Researcher field notes* based on observations while in the communities.	Fall/ spring each year
Relevant documents or administrative/census data.	*Quantitative data* about community demographics: number/type of health-care resources in community, number of palliative clients per year, sites where palliative care is delivered, etc.	Fall each year

OUTCOMES

Documentation of the process of rural palliative care development in relation to the DRPC-ToC model.

Evaluation of the model's utility as a tool for developing rural palliative care services and evaluating outcomes.

PAR PROJECT TIMELINE

Fall 2007 → Winter 2010

Table 12.2   Using the growing rural palliative care model to track community palliative care development

Phase	Community 1	Community 2	Community 3
PHASE 1: Antecedent conditions			
Collaborative general practice	✓	✓	✓
Vision for change		✓	✓
Sufficient health-care infrastructure	✓	✓	✓
Sense of empowerment		✓	✓
PHASE 2: Catalyst	Beginning	✓	✓
PHASE 3: Creating the team			
Dedicated providers	✓	✓	✓
Right people involved		Not complete	✓
Leader		Informal	✓
PHASE 4: Growing the program			
Strengthening the team			
Engaging the community			A and B
Sustaining palliative care		A	A

KEY FOR PHASE 4
Engaging the community:
A   Changing clinical practices: developing/implementing tools for care, care planning, family education and support.
B   Educating and supporting community providers.
C   Building community relationships to improve service delivery.

Sustaining palliative care:
A   Volunteering time.
B   Getting palliative care staff and resources.
C   Developing policies and procedures.

conditions necessary to build their local palliative care teams. Four communities have progressed to develop local teams. One community has begun its palliative care program, which includes providing clinical care and offering palliative care education to other health-care providers. Progress in five communities is currently stalled by lack of one or more antecedent conditions, such as lack of infrastructure, collaboration, a vision for change, or a sense of community empowerment.

Using three examples, Table 12.2 depicts how the model is used by the EOL care coordinator to evaluate each community's progress in relation to the phases of the model. It also illustrates the great diversity among communities. The EOL care coordinator completes evaluations biannually based on data that she collects in each community. Ongoing evaluation is important since community development is a dynamic process. Changes in each community are tracked over time. The progress of palliative care development at the regional level is also tracked by aggregating individual community progress.

The Community Development Goal: Developing Local Palliative Care Programs in Rural Communities

The North West CCAC hired an EOL care coordinator, Wilma Sletmoen, to act as rural community developer. Her role was to support the establishment of local palliative care programs using existing resources: that is, the local community services and health-care providers who were already caring for dying people within their generalist practices. Her goal was to engage local community members committed to working together to provide comprehensive, compassionate, and seamless palliative care to the individuals and families in their communities. The community developer recognized the challenges of rural generalist practice, the sense of uniqueness and autonomy of each community, and the distrust of outsiders that local people can have. The principles of capacity development and PAR are evident as Sletmoen describes her approach: "There is a need to respect the resources and strengths which already exist – small communities have a tremendous amount of ingenuity and the ability to work out ways of accomplishing things that do not wait on the wheels of bureaucracy to turn or policies and procedures to be developed."

Consistent with the principles of PAR, Sletmoen became an active collaborator in the research. She incorporated the DRPC model into her practice and assisted the researchers in documenting the ongoing experience of the rural communities as they developed their local palliative care programs. She also provided valuable insight and information through regular interviews held face to face or by telephone. Interviews were audiotaped and transcribed for analysis.

As a user of the model, the community developer also provided constructive critiques of its utility and enhanced the researchers' understanding of contextual factors affecting local palliative care development. For example, she identified that two levels of "team" have been created by the communities. One is the community team that meets several times a year to facilitate palliative care program development and provide a forum for communication and community problem solving. This team could have twenty members. The second is the clinical team of two or three health-care professionals that develops when needed to care for a dying person and his or her family. A contextual issue that emerged is that the local palliative care teams are community based, but many of the agencies that employ the members have a regional structure and region-wide policies and procedures. This creates the challenge of balancing community autonomy and meeting individual community needs with the requirement to maintain consistency in policy and procedure in regionally based agencies.

Through her practice, the community developer further enhanced the model by identifying specific tasks that need to be accomplished at each phase of development. For example, she created a work plan outlining activities associated with entering the community and "becoming a catalyst" for change (phase 2 of the DRPC model). The plan included visiting communities and meeting individually with a wide range of community members to explain the EOL Care Strategy, seek their personal commitment, and listen to their issues/challenges regarding palliative care. In phase 3, "creating the team," the community developer identified the need for a "toolkit" to assist the local community with team development. Working with the community, she successfully applied for funds to develop this practical resource that will now be used by other communities as they go about forming their own teams and growing their own programs. The community developer thus enhanced the DRPC model with practical strategies.

The EOL care coordinator perceived many benefits from using the DRPC model and participating in the research. The model guided her planning for regional community development. It offered a number of benefits, including a theoretical foundation to support her practice experience and wisdom; greater consistency (though not necessarily conformity) in her practice; a tool to help assess which communities would benefit from which intervention at what time; and a means for evaluating progress in her work. Furthermore, the model provided a common language (e.g., phases) to discuss the experiences of different communities with others.

Community members have repeatedly reported benefits from using the model. It helps them to reflect on and better understand their own experiences and envision future tasks. It provides them with a sense of reassurance that the process they are embarking on is purposeful and shared. Individuals have remarked that it is very helpful to see the process of building the team and program, as framed by the model. They also like to use the model to self-evaluate their progress.

The challenges of community development work are consistent with those of capacity development in general and PAR in particular. Each community determines its own destiny, rate of progress, and priorities; these principles are inherent in the model. Communities develop palliative care at different rates. This variability creates an interesting tension for the EOL care coordinator, who facilitates community development but ultimately cannot control the outcome; each community is responsible for the outcome of the program. Accepting this community control can relieve the community developer of feeling responsible for developing the program but requires that the person is able to relinquish control and trust the community.

Bridging Silos: The Value of Integrating Policy, Research, and Practice

Given the challenges faced by rural communities in delivering health services, implementing the EOL Care Strategy and the related expectation to provide more palliative care at the community level had to be respectful of local realities. Although additional funding was made available through the CCAC to provide palliative homecare services, all other palliative care services needed to be provided within existing resources. Furthermore, the large psycho-social and spiritual components and the importance of providing support to family caregivers required a whole-community team approach. In short, it was a lot of work that involved many people. Communities could easily have resisted. However, by taking an approach that integrated policy implementation with the DRPC model and PAR, supported by local community development, the EOL Care Strategy has been successful in northwestern Ontario.

The integrated approach was most appreciated on the ground in the rural communities. Using the capacity development approach avoided imposing externally devised palliative care programs on communities. Rather, implementing the EOL Care Strategy was accompanied both by concrete help from the community developer and research to guide communities' local processes of developing rural palliative care. Community members have acknowledged the value of having the DRPC model as a theory of change to guide local experience. Through this work, rural health-care providers have been supported to manage their changes and challenges using the enabling factors identified in the model: being community focused, educating providers, working together, empowering local leadership, and valuing local accomplishments (Kelley 2007).

In northwestern Ontario, the roles of policy, research, and community development were complementary and synergistic for developing rural palliative care services. Without all three components, developing these services would have been more difficult. Initially, policy provided a clear goal and mandate for the work. The research provided the DRPC model as a theory of change to guide and evaluate the processes and outcomes of the policy implementation. The PAR cycle of planning, acting, observing, and reflecting guided the process. The community developer incorporated both the policy and the research into her day-to-day practice, demonstrated the "practice" of capacity development, and provided valuable data for evaluating the DRPC model. Overall, our experience has demonstrated that the model is plausible, doable, and testable as a theory of change for developing rural palliative care.

Recommendations

The need for palliative care services is growing throughout Canada, including rural communities. By undertaking this integrated approach to rural palliative care development in northwestern Ontario, several outcomes are being achieved. The policy goal of the Ontario Ministry of Health and Long Term Care to increase community-based palliative care services is being met. The CCAC community developer and Northwestern Ontario End-of-Life Care Network are successfully creating local palliative care teams in rural communities, resulting in better access to and quality of palliative care services for rural people. The researchers are validating the applicability of the DRPC model as a theory of change to guide and evaluate palliative care service development while refining its use for policy and practice.

This integrated process undertaken in northwestern Ontario could be replicated elsewhere in Canada where there is a policy goal to develop rural palliative care services because the DRPC model outlines a process of change applied within a local context. It incorporates geographical space by building on antecedent community conditions and adapts to place by emphasizing local community control. Policy makers anywhere can be guided by the model's emphasis on understanding antecedent community conditions and using an incremental, bottom-up capacity development process to develop rural health services.

In the future, the four-phase model could be evaluated for its applicability to establishing programs other than palliative care. The feasibility of doing so is suggested by the findings of other authors that are consistent with our work. Chapter 13 in this volume emphasizes that services must be designed to meet the specific needs of the community, and both that chapter and Chapter 16 recommend the establishment of collaborative teams as a foundation to develop rural programs for mental health and HIV/AIDS. Our experience in northwestern Ontario suggests that the integrated, capacity development approach described in this case study can achieve sustainable change in rural health services.

Acknowledgments

The research presented here was funded by the Canadian Institute of Health Research through the Interdisciplinary Capacity Enhancement Grant Timely Access and Seamless Transitions in Rural Palliative and End-of-Life Care in Canada. The community development work described was funded by the Northwestern Ontario Community Care Access Centre. The authors thank the Northwestern Ontario End-of-Life Care Network for their ongoing support of this initiative.

Notes

1 Creating and implementing theories of change (ToC) have comprised a popular approach for evaluators of complex social programs and interventions. ToC summarize the links among contexts, planned activities, and predicted outcomes of an intervention. A good ToC is plausible, doable, and testable (Fulbright-Anderson, Kubisch, and Connell 1998; MacKenzie and Blamey 2005; Mason and Barnes 2007).
2 The population density of northwestern Ontario is 0.5 persons per square kilometre versus 12.5 persons per square kilometre for Ontario as a whole (NWLHIN 2005).
3 The CCACs help people to remain living independently at home by arranging support services while also assisting people with applying for admission to long-term-care facilities when required. Their mandate includes information and referral, home and community health and supportive services, and placement in long-term-care homes.

References

Alfonso, M., J. Nickelson, D. Hogebroom, J. French, C. Bryant, R.J. McDermott, and J.A. Baldwin. 2008. "Assessing Local Capacity for Health Intervention." *Evaluation and Progam Planning* 31, 2: 145-59.
Bolger, J. 2000. *Capacity Development: Why, What, and How.* Capacity Development, Occasional Series, CIDA, Policy Branch. Gatineau, QC: CIDA.
Bollman, R., and H. Clemenson. 2008. "Structure and Change in Canada's Rural Demography: An Update to 2006." *Rural and Small Town Canada Analysis Bulletin* 7, 7: 1-29. Statistics Canada Catalogue No. 21-006-X. http://www.statcan.gc.ca/.
Bosanquet, N., and C. Salisbury. 1999. *Providing a Palliative Care Service: Towards an Evidence Base.* Oxford: Oxford University Press.

Byock, I. 2000. "Completing the Continuum of Cancer Care: Integrating Life-Prolongation and Palliation." *CA: A Cancer Journal for Clinicians* 50, 2: 123-32.

Cashman, S.B., S. Adeky, A.J. Allen, J. Corburn, B.A. Israel, J. Montano, et al. 2008. "The Power and the Promise: Working with Communities to Analyze Data, Interpret Findings, and Get to Outcomes." *American Journal of Public Health* 98, 8: 1407-17.

Cinnamon, J., N. Schuurman, and V.A. Crooks. 2008. "A Method to Determine Spatial Access to Specialized Palliative Care Services Using GIS." *BMC Health Services Research* 8: 140, http://www.biomedcentral.com/.

Cloutier-Fisher, D., and A.E. Joseph. 2000. "Long-Term Care Restructuring in Rural Ontario: Retrieving Community Service User and Provider Narratives." *Social Science and Medicine* 50: 1037-45.

Craig, G. 2007. "Community Capacity Building: Something Old, Something New?" *Critical Social Policy* 27, 3: 335-59.

Davis, E., and I. Higginson, eds. 2004. *Better Palliative Care for Older People.* Copenhagen: WHO, Regional Office for Europe.

Ferris, F., H. Balfour, L. Bowen, J. Farley, M. Hardwick, C. Lamontagne, M. Lundy, A. Syme, and P. West. 2002. *A Model to Guide Hospice Palliative Care.* Ottawa: Canadian Hospice Palliative Care Association.

Flicker, S., and B. Savan. 2006. *A Snapshot of CBR in Canada.* Toronto: Wellesley Institute, http://www.wellesleyinstitute.com/.

Fulbright-Anderson, A., A.C. Kubisch, and J.P. Connell, eds. 1998. *New Approaches to Evaluating Community Initiatives: Theory, Measurement, and Analysis.* Washington, DC: Aspen Institute.

Government of Nova Scotia. 2001. *A Rural Palliative Home Care Model: The Development and Evaluation of an Integrated Palliative Care Program in Nova Scotia and Prince Edward Island: A Federal Health Transition Fund Project Report.* Truro, NS: Communications Nova Scotia.

Grafton, D., M. Troughton, and J. Rourke. 2004. "Rural Community and Health Care Interdependence: An Historical, Geographic Study." *Canadian Journal of Rural Medicine* 9, 5: 156-63.

Grothe, T.M., and R.V. Brody. 1995. "Palliative Care for HIV Disease." *Journal of Palliative Care* 11, 2: 48-49.

Habjan, S., L. Diamond, and M.L. Kelley. 2008. *Northwestern Ontario Palliative Care Needs Assessment.* Thunder Bay: Centre for Education and Research on Aging and Health (CERAH), Lakehead University, http://www.cerah.lakeheadu.ca/.

Hawker, S., C. Kerr, S. Payne, D. Seamark, C. Davis, H. Roberts, et al. 2006. "End-of-Life Care in Community Hospitals: The Perceptions of Bereaved Family Members." *Palliative Medicine* 20, 5: 541-47.

Hays, R.B., R.J. Evans, and C. Veitch. 2005. "The Quality of Procedural Rural Medical Practice in Australia." *Rural and Remote Health* 5: 474, http://www.rrh.org.au/.

Kelley, M.L. 2007. "Developing Rural Communities' Capacity for Palliative Care: A Conceptual Model." *Journal of Palliative Care* 23, 3: 143-53.

Kelley, M.L., and A. Williams. 2008. "Developing Rural Palliative Care: Validating a Conceptual Model." Paper presented at the Interdisciplinary Capacity Enhancement (ICE) Team Conference, Edmonton, 7-9 May.

Kemmis, S., and R. McTaggart. 2005. "Participatory Action Research." In *Handbook of Qualitative Research: Third Edition,* edited by N.K. Denzin and Y.S. Lincoln, 559-603. Thousand Oaks, CA: Sage.

Kortes-Miller, K., S. Habjan, M.L. Kelley, and M. Fortier. 2007. "Development of Palliative Care Education Program in Rural Long-Term Care Facilities." *Journal of Palliative Care* 23, 3: 154-62.

Lyons, R., and P. Gardner. 2001. *Strategic Initiative in Rural and Northern Health Research: Canadian Institute of Health Research.* Ottawa: Canadian Institute of Health Research.

MacKenzie, M., and A. Blamey. 2005. "The Practice and the Theory: Lessons from the Application of a Theories of Change Approach." *Evaluation* 11, 2: 151-68.

Martinez-Brawley, E.E. 2000. *Close to Home: Human Services and the Small Community.* Washington, DC: NASW Press.

Mason, P., and M. Barnes. 2007. "Constructing Theories of Change: Methods and Sources." *Evaluation* 13, 2: 151-70.

McConigley, R., L. Kristjanson, and A. Morgan. 2000. "Palliative Care Nursing in Rural Western Australia." *International Journal of Palliative Nursing* 6, 2: 80-90.

McKee, M., M.L. Kelley, and M. Guirguis-Younger. 2007. "So No One Dies Alone: A Study of Hospice Volunteering with Rural Seniors." *Journal of Palliative Care* 23, 3: 163-72.

Ministerial Advisory Council on Rural Health. 2002. *Rural Health in Rural Hands: Strategic Directions for Rural, Remote, Northern, and Aboriginal Communities.* Ottawa: Office of Rural Health Canada.

Minkler, M., V. Breckwich, T. Mansoureh, and D. Peterson. 2008. "Promoting Environmental Justice through Community-Based Participatory Research: The Role of Community and Partnership Capacity." *Health Education and Behaviour* 35, 1: 119-37.

Minkler, M., and N. Wallerstein. 2002. "Improving Health through Community Organization and Community Building." In *Health Behaviour and Health Education: Third Edition,* edited by M. Minkler, B.K. Rimer, and F.M. Lewis, 279-311. San Francisco: Jossey-Bass.

Molinari, D.L., and M.A. Monserud. 2008. "Rural Nurse Job Satisfaction." *Rural and Remote Health* 8: 1055, http://www.rrh.org.au/.

Morgan, P. 1998. *Capacity and Capacity Development: Some Strategies.* Hull, QC: Policy Branch, CIDA.

Murtagh, F.E., M. Preston, and I. Higginson. 2004. "Patterns of Dying: Palliative Care for Non-Malignant Disease." *Clinical Medicine* 4, 1: 39-44.

North West Local Health Integration Network (NWLHIN). 2005. *North West Local Health Integration Network: Opportunities for Health System Integration.* Thunder Bay: NWLHIN, http://www.northwestlhin.on.ca/.

Northwestern Health Unit. 2007. *Northwestern Health Unit: Uniquely Situated and Distinctly Different.* Kenora, ON: Northwestern Health Unit, http:/www.nwhu.on.ca/.

Northwestern Ontario Municipal Association (NOMA). 2007. *Enhancing the Economy of Northwestern Ontario.* Thunder Bay: NOMA, http://www.noma.on.ca/.

Norton, B.L., K.R. McLeroy, J.N. Burdine, M.R.J. Felix, and A.M. Dorsey. 2002. "Community Capacity: Concept, Theory, and Methods." In *Emerging Theories in Health Promotion Practice and Research,* edited by R.D. Clementi, R. Crosby, and M. Kegler, 194-227. San Francisco: Jossey-Bass.

O'Toole, K., A. Schoo, K. Stagnitti, and K. Cuss. 2008. "Rethinking Policies for the Retention of Allied Health Professionals in Rural Areas: A Social Relations Approach." *Health Policy* 87, 3: 326-32.

Pong, R. 2008. "Strategies to Overcome Physician Shortages in Northern Ontario: A Study of Policy Implementation over 35 Years." *Human Resources for Health* 6, 24: 9 pp. + appendix, http://www.human-resources-health.com/.

Raeburn, J., M. Akerman, K. Chuengsatiansup, F. Mejia, and O. Oladepo. 2006. "Community Capacity Building and Health Promotion in a Globalized World." *Health Promotion International* 21, S1: 84-90.

Ramsden, V.R. 2003. "Learning with the Community: Evolution to Transformative Action Research." *Canadian Family Physician* 49: 195-97.

Ramsden, V.R., and A.J. Cave. 2002. "Participatory Methods to Facilitate Research." *Canadian Family Physician* 48: 548-49.

Robinson, C., B. Pesut, J. Bottorff, A. Mawry, S. Broughton, and G. Fyles. 2009. "Rural Palliative Care: A Comprehensive Review." *Journal of Palliative Medicine* 12, 3: 253-58.

Romanow, R.J. 2002. *Building on Values: The Future of Health Care in Canada*. Saskatoon: Commission on the Future of Health Care in Canada.

Sach, J. 1997. "Issues for Palliative Care in Rural Australia." *Collegian* 4, 3: 22-27.

Seamark, D.A., and D.J. Seamark. 2004. "Palliative Care in Rural Areas." *Family Practice* 12, 1: 114.

Sedgwick, M.G., and O. Yonge. 2008. "'We're It,' 'We're a Team,' 'We're a Family' Means a Sense of Belonging." *Rural and Remote Health* 8: 1021, http://www.rrh.org.au/.

Senate Committee on Social Affairs, Science and Technology. 2000. *Quality End-of-Life Care: The Right of Every Canadian*. Ottawa: Government of Canada.

Seow, H., S. King, and V. Vaitonis. 2008. "The Impact of Ontario's End of Life Care Strategy on End of Life Care in the Community." *Healthcare Quarterly* 11, 1: 56-62.

Skilbeck, J., and S. Payne. 2005. "End of Life Care: A Discursive Analysis of Specialist Palliative Care Nursing." *Journal of Advanced Nursing* 51, 4: 325-34.

Statistics Canada. 2008. *2006 Community Profiles*. Ottawa: Statistics Canada, http://www12.statcan.ca/.

Strasser, R.P. 1999. "Teams in Rural Health." *Health Care and Informatics Review Online* 4, 1, http://www.hinz.org.nz/.

–. 2003. "Rural Health around the World: Challenges and Solutions." *Family Practice* 20, 4: 457-63.

Wilson, D.M., C. Justice, S. Sheps, R. Thomas, P. Reid, and K. Leibovici. 2006. "Planning and Providing End-of-Life Care in Rural Areas." *Journal of Rural Health* 22, 2: 174-81.

Chapter 13   **Rural Mental Health Services in Canada: A Model for Research and Practice**

C. Brannen, K. Dyck, C. Hardy,
and C. Mushquash

Key Points

- Overall, rural Canadians are less likely than urban Canadians to experience mental illness and more likely to experience social support, belonging in community, and low stress. However, young rural Canadians, especially males, are at greater risk of completed suicide, and there is considerable variability across rural communities.
- Personal barriers, such as concerns about stigma and low mental health literacy, and public barriers, such as insufficient professional resources, prevent rural residents from accessing mental health services.
- Mental health programming and services for rural communities must include health promotion, illness prevention, early intervention, and treatment, with the type of intervention suited to the person's level of distress or functional impairment.
- Technological (e.g., telepsychiatry) and community-based (e.g., networks for information sharing and support) solutions can overcome barriers to accessing mental health services in rural communities.
- Rural communities are diverse, and people living in rural communities must be consulted regarding the design and delivery of mental health services in order to develop services that are meaningful and useful to rural residents.

Mental health services in Canada are sorely lacking in general and more so in rural communities (Kirby and Keon 2006). Mental health intervention research with rural Canadians also lags far behind general population research and that with other identifiable groups, such as women and visible minorities. In this chapter, we review evidence from research in which authors identified their subject matter as relevant to mental health in rural and remote communities. Most of the research was conducted in communities that fit the "Rural and Small Town" definition outlined in Chapter 1 of this volume.

Summary of Mental Health Research in Rural Canada

Overall, rural Canadians are less likely than urban Canadians to have any mental disorder and are more likely to experience the protective benefits of social support, feelings of belonging in their community, and low stress (Canadian Institute for Health Information [CIHI] 2006). However, young rural Canadians, especially young men, are at greater risk of completed suicide compared with urban age mates. These and other findings from the 2002 Canadian Community Health Survey (CCHS), a nationally representative survey conducted by Statistics Canada, are discussed in detail in Chapters 3 and 8 of this volume. Furthermore, studies of particular subgroups of rural Canadians reveal a high degree of variability in mental health disorders and risk factors across rural communities. For example, Leipert (2002) states that despair, depression, and psychological distress are becoming increasingly common for women in rural Canada. Family violence is another significant issue impacting the well-being of rural residents (Thurston, Patten, and Lagendyk 2006). Masley and colleagues (2000) reported a greater frequency of depression and insomnia among rural women, whereas men were more likely to report being highly stressed.

Rural mental health problems can arise from a complex interplay of stressors unique to particular communities, including unpredictable employment, out-migration, loss of social capital (e.g., closure of hospitals, schools, banks), and weakening social support networks. Chapters 11 and 25 in this volume detail the unique stressors facing people living in northern resource towns and prairie towns, respectively. A recent survey commissioned by the Canadian Agricultural Safety Association (2005) indicated that almost two-thirds of Canadian farmers are feeling stressed. One in five farmers self-described as being "very stressed."

The farmers surveyed attributed very high levels of stress to poor harvests or poor production, government policies, and farm finances and attributed high stress levels to weather, the bovine spongiform encephalitis (BSE) crisis, and the pressure to maintain the family farm. The above findings highlight the considerable need for timely and appropriate mental health services in rural Canada despite lower overall rates of mental illness in rural Canada compared with urban Canada.

Overview of Mental Health Service Provision

Mental health service provision in rural Canada exists within the framework of lower service utilization rates and significant mental health problems. This chapter focuses on programs rather than individual practices given the diversity of the latter. The topics reviewed in Chapter 5 of this volume are equally applicable to the realities of rural mental health service providers. Psychiatrists, psychologists, social workers, and other mental health service providers are scarce in rural areas. Those practising in rural Canada often have large caseloads and, by necessity, have to provide a vast array of treatments to diverse patients. In addition, many rural mental health service provider positions remain unfilled due to inadequate compensation. For those who do choose to practise in rural areas, there are challenges, including a sense of isolation from their colleagues, burnout from overwork, and lack of resources (Fennell and Hovestadt 2004; Rohland 2000).

Utilization of Mental Health Services

Data from the Canadian National Population Health Survey indicate that rural participants with at least one major depressive episode are less likely than urban participants to contact health professionals for their mental health difficulties (Wang 2004). Studies in Ontario (Parikh et al. 1996) and Manitoba (Manitoba Centre for Health Policy 2004) report lower rates of mental health-related physician and psychiatrist visits among rural clients compared with urban clients. As shown in Chapter 8 in this volume, data from the CCHS suggest that the relationship between location of residence and service utilization might not be straightforward. Additional factors such as level of income, age, marital status, gender, and co-morbidity might also be related to low rates of service utilization and can interact with location of residence to predict service utilization. In these surveys, and as noted in Chapter 8, service utilization rates measured in the CCHS confound availability of particular types of professional services with personal preferences for type of service accessed. Individual characteristics endorsed and valued by rural dwellers might act as roadblocks to their access to mental health services, as might features of the service delivery system itself.

Barriers to Rural Mental Health Services

As outlined in Chapter 9 of this volume, the concept of access to health services is a multidimensional concept reflecting the fit between clients' characteristics and needs and the characteristics of the health-care delivery system. Barriers are factors that interfere with delivery of care to those who need it. In the following sections, we review two categories of barriers that reduce access to mental health services in rural communities: personal (e.g., low mental health literacy) and public (e.g., lack of training programs). A model summarizing the different barriers is presented in Figure 13.1.

Personal Barriers to Mental Health Services
Personal barriers are factors that interfere with an individual's ability to seek help for a mental health problem. These barriers can include knowledge of mental illness, economic resources (e.g., working seasonally might reduce the economic resources needed to seek help), lack of supports (e.g., child care), and individual characteristics. Prior research based on survey and focus group data obtained from mental health providers, consumers, and families suggests that stigma, lack of anonymity, lack of information, and travel costs are commonly identified personal barriers to accessing mental health services in rural and remote communities (Boydell et al. 2006; Ryan-Nicholls and Haggarty 2007; Ryan-Nicholls, Racher, and Robinson 2003; see also Chapter 9, this volume). As discussed in Chapter 16 in relation to HIV/AIDS, the stigma associated with some illnesses can lead to misinformation, lack of openness with family and friends, and reluctance to use local services. Based on her qualitative research, Leipert (2002) contends that norms and values associated with hardiness and self-reliance can perpetuate the stigma associated with mental illness and prevent rural women from seeking help. Similarly, pride and independence were found to be the most important reasons that Canadian farmers gave for not seeking more help

Figure 13.1   Barriers to mental health services faced by rural Canadians

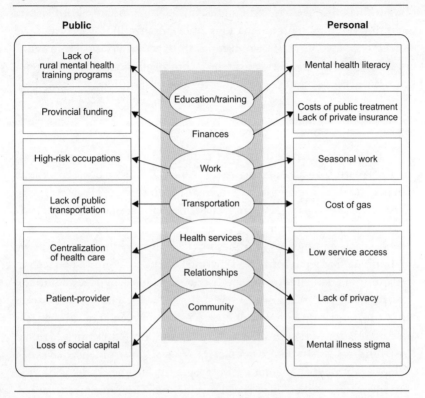

in dealing with stress and mental health concerns (Canadian Agricultural Safety Association 2005).

Public Barriers to Mental Health Services
Barriers are "public" when they relate to the provision of services rather than the individual's personal ability to obtain services. Providers and consumers of mental health care residing in rural and isolated areas of Canada have identified the following public barriers: insufficient resources, staff shortages, ineffective communication between service providers and consumers/families, insufficient mental health consumer involvement, interagency communication/referral issues, challenges related to discharge from in-patient facilities (e.g., premature discharge, housing issues), legal issues (e.g., confusion regarding various health information acts), and lack of clarity regarding program mandates (Boydell

et al. 2006; McGee et al. 2004; Ryan-Nicholls and Haggarty 2007; Ryan-Nicholls, Racher, and Robinson 2003). As discussed in Chapter 9 of this volume, small populations and centralization of services have forced residents of small communities to travel to services or go without care, while steady turnover in health professionals leads to poor continuity of care and poor client-provider relationships.

Cultural Considerations

The limited research with specific ethnic and cultural groups in rural and northern Canada suggests the presence of similar but also unique barriers to accessing appropriate mental health services. Research with First Nations peoples and Asian Canadians residing in northern Canada suggests similar barriers related to limited resources, disconnected systems of care, staffing deficits (e.g., shortages, turnover, inadequate preparation), ineffective information sharing, stigma, and limited education regarding mental illness; unique barriers include language, culturally determined interpretation of mental illness, and racial discrimination (Li and Browne 2000; Schmidt 2000). Access to mental health services in First Nations communities is further complicated by jurisdictional and funding issues. For example, provincial governments have developed community mental health programs, but the residents of First Nations communities must travel outside their communities to access these services (Schmidt 2000). Alternatively, they can access short-term crisis intervention mental health counselling services through the First Nations and Inuit Health Branch of the federal government. These services might or might not be available in the community in which they reside.

Adequate and Appropriate Services

Adequate service provision includes specialized care for mental health disorders that is reflective of the needs of the community and delivered in a timely fashion. Appropriate services include treatment options that are affordable for patients and families and that do not require the patient to leave his or her support network (Romanow 2002). Having to access expensive treatment in an unknown environment is an extremely stressful situation that can worsen mental health problems. The barriers that we have discussed can be even greater for vulnerable populations such as the elderly, the poor, the disabled, young children, and pregnant women. The challenge is this: how can the health-care system over-come these barriers and provide adequate and appropriate services for rural Canadians?

Methods to Overcome Barriers

In the remainder of this chapter, we discuss a model for conceptualiz-ing delivery of rural mental health services. The model highlights strat-egies for overcoming barriers and is grounded in the reality that rural communities are limited in their capacity to offer specialized health services, as highlighted in Chapters 9 and 25 of this volume. The model is devised from the review of rural mental health services that we con-ducted in developing this chapter but could apply to urban-based servi-ces as well. We present various examples from the review throughout the chapter. Our argument is that, by providing cost-effective and ap-propriate mental health services, especially with interventions that offer support before individuals are in crisis, there can be a redistribution of services that would allow specialists to care for those suffering the most. Health promotion, illness prevention, and early intervention are inte-gral to our approach. The model consists of a series of indicators relat-ing to services required to address mental health needs. These indicators are individual distress or functional impairment (low to high), level of intervention (population to individual), provider training (paraprofes-sional to specialized professional), delivery method (self-care at home to specialized care at clinic), and intervention timing (prevention to treat-ment). Each indicator is conceptualized as falling on a continuum, with positions on the continuum reflecting implications for the most appro-priate use of resources. For example, low distress might be best man-aged through population-based self-care with paraprofessional providers as a means of preventing the person's distress from increasing. A lack of intervention at the low distress level can lead to higher distress, re-sulting in increased likelihood that the person will require specialized care in a clinical setting. We propose that specialized care is most ap-propriate for those experiencing high levels of distress, whereas those with mild to moderate symptoms might be better served by self-directed programs or paraprofessional support. In addition, we posit that community-based approaches are the best model for overall care, with decision making for type of treatment made by collaborative teams. We offer that population-level approaches designed to educate the public about mental illness and provide skills training, such as stress management techniques, must also occur in order to prevent significant mental health problems and increase mental health literacy. Although we believe that this model is also applicable to urban-based services, contextual differences between urban and rural communities (e.g., availability of specialists, access to the Internet, access to transportation, concerns about anonymity, norms and values, culture) would impact aspects of service provision in unique ways. For example, the heightened concern that rural Canadians have reported regarding anonymity, and the rural values of hardiness, self-reliance (for rural women), and pride and independence (for Canadian farmers), suggest that rural Canadians might be most receptive to self-directed treatments and mental health services housed in a facility where the purpose of their visit is not apparent to others. The ability of rural Canadians to access transportation as well as Internet services would further influence the development of rural mental health services in ways that would be unique and specific to each community's context.

Using Technology to Provide Services

Telehealth as described in Chapter 10 of this volume refers to healthcare services provided to patients from a distance. Mental health services delivered over the Internet and/or telephone provide promise for rural residents. These interventions fall into two broad categories: specialized individual care and self-directed programs. Such programs overcome many of the barriers to traditional service provision, such as travelling, arranging child care, and receiving treatment based on the schedule of the service provider. Self-directed programs such as those offered by Here to Help in British Columbia (http://www.heretohelp. bc.ca) offer empowerment to individual clients and participants because they provide them with a sense of accomplishment as they work through the modules at their own pace while learning the skills to manage their particular mental health problem. Self-directed treatment programs have been effective in addressing a number of mental health conditions, including depression and anxiety (for a review, see Vincent, Walker, and Katz 2007). However, such programs are not without disadvantages. In particular, Internet use is much lower in rural areas (McKeown, Noce, and Czerny 2007) compared with urban areas; this might be due to a combination of limited availability of Internet access in many rural and remote areas in Canada and the lower socio-economic status of rural residents. Additionally, strong health literacy skills (discussed in

Chapter 14 of this book) are required to partake successfully in self-directed interventions.

Telepsychiatry for Specialized Care

"The use of interactive videoconferencing to provide psychiatric services to geographically remote regions" (O'Reilly et al. 2007, 836), or telepsychiatry, has been identified as one potential means of addressing the geographical and economic barriers to accessing mental health services in rural and northern communities. Health-care providers and consumers have reported being satisfied with many aspects of telepsychiatry when it is used in conjunction with adequate community-based mental health services (Greenberg, Boydell, and Volpe 2006; Jong 2004; Simpson et al. 2001a, 2001b). Based on feedback from caregivers and mental health service providers working with pediatric patients, Greenberg, Boydell, and Volpe (2006) concluded that availability of telepsychiatry and increased efforts toward building community-based expertise in rural areas need to coexist. Although this lofty goal is the ideal, it might be difficult to attain. Within this framework, we propose that individualized telepsychiatry is best suited to individuals experiencing higher levels of distress.

Self-Directed Skills-Building Programs

Educational and support programs, including parent training and stress management, are proposed to be best used for health promotion at the population level and for prevention of worsening distress in individuals and families experiencing mild to moderate mental health problems. Psycho-educational programs for population-level health promotion or for those with mild to moderate mental health problems have not been widely adapted in Canada. However, Australia has developed a comprehensive system of programs that address population health promotion (for an overview of services, see http://www.ausienet.com) and provides programs for individuals suffering from mild to moderate mental health problems (http://www.beyondblue.org.au). In Canada, the Manitoba Farm and Rural Stress Line offers counselling and support for farmers (http://www.ruralstress.ca). An evaluation of this service conducted in 2005 indicated that it is well utilized (1,857 phone calls in 2005) and that clients report a high level of satisfaction with the services provided (Manitoba Farm and Rural Stress Line 2005). This service is valuable for farmers and provides an example of the type of rural telephone support programs that should be available nation-wide. The next section describes a randomized controlled trial supporting the use of a telephone-based, self-directed treatment for rural women suffering from postpartum depression.

Distance Telephone Support for Depressed Mothers in Nova Scotia

Maternal depression is a significant population health problem. Numerous studies have reported the negative outcomes for children with depressed mothers, ranging from poorer cognitive achievement to transmission of mental health problems. However, the stigma surrounding depression, particularly depression in mothers, is a strong and persistent presence in Canada (Elgar et al. 2004). This stigma can be compounded in rural communities by factors such as the lack of anonymity when seeking treatment for mental health problems (Boydell et al. 2006) and rural women's norms and values associated with hardiness and self-reliance (Leipert 2002). These variables are barriers to treatment access in rural communities. Factors that can decrease the likelihood of a rural mom seeking treatment include stigma surrounding treatment, low population-level health literacy for depression, her personal health literacy for depression, availability of appropriate services, and costs associated with treatment. Coupled with the symptoms of depression (e.g., low energy) and the demands of looking after young children, these barriers make standard mental health treatment inaccessible to many depressed rural mothers.

The Managing Our Mood (MOM) research project consisted of a pilot study of twenty-seven participants (Brannen et al. 2006) and a randomized controlled trial, both of which were designed to provide appropriate and accessible treatment for mothers with postpartum depression (PPD). MOM consisted of a telephone-based, self-directed program with a trained coach providing support. Mothers were provided with a manual and DVDs to provide information about PPD and cognitive-behavioural techniques for managing symptoms. The program consisted of twelve sessions during which the mother worked through various cognitive-behavioural techniques alone and then reviewed her progress through each session with a trained non-professional coach. Weekly evaluations of PPD symptoms were undertaken as well as baseline, end of treatment, and twelve-month follow-up by a trained assessment assistant over the telephone. Results from the pilot study were promising: all participants reported significant improvements in their symptoms, and all but one had resolved their clinical depression. In addition, moms reported that they liked the program content and the in-home, self-directed delivery method. Although the MOM program appears to be a successful treatment for PPD, the individual, self-directed format does little to draw mothers out into their communities, where they could develop support networks vital to managing the on-going cycle of depression.

Community-Based Approaches to Improving Access to Mental Health Services

In the previous section, we argued for the appropriate use of Internet or telephone technology to help those with mild to moderate distress or functional impairment, but we also pointed out that "in-home" approaches do little to foster support networks. We view collaborative teams as the core of rural mental health treatment (Canadian Collaborative Mental Health Initiative 2006). The composition of such teams will vary depending on the size of the community and its health human resources and might consist, for example, of a general physician, a nurse, and/or a mental health or addictions counsellor. Collaborative teams provide the opportunity for individuals to connect with both community services and other individuals with similar problems. Teams also serve as supports for practitioners who might need specialized training and information resources that are lacking or hard to access in rural communities. We propose that these teams are where the decisions for level of support, whether self-directed telephone programs or individualized treatment, should be made. In this section, we profile two community-based approaches for improving access to mental health services. In keeping with our theme of a continuum of services, one case study highlights a professional training program designed to reduce barriers to accessing psychological services in rural and northern Manitoba; the other highlights a knowledge translation and resource-sharing network designed to support service providers working with children and families in northern British Columbia.

The Rural and Northern Psychology Program

The Rural and Northern Psychology Program (RandNP) of the University of Manitoba's Department of Clinical Health Psychology is a community-based training and service delivery platform developed in an effort to reduce barriers to accessing psychological services in rural and northern Manitoba. K. Dyck has been a faculty member with this program since 1997. Since the time of its initial funding from

Manitoba Health in 1996, the RandNP has grown from three community-based psychologist positions to a total of nine. There are three funded training positions (one postdoctoral and two predoctoral residency positions). Although we are focusing on the role of the staff psychologists, rather than on the training component of this program (McIlwraith et al. 2005), the training component is an integral part of the RandNP and considered key to the recruitment and retention of doctoral-level psychologists in the rural and northern areas of Manitoba. Also, though the focus here is on mental health services, staff psychologists might provide services beyond what is traditionally defined as "mental health" (e.g., chronic pain management, health behaviour change).

Psychologists in the RandNP have the same academic rank, benefits, and privileges as faculty members in Winnipeg. They work within a collaborative, community-based service delivery model including a range of professionals and paraprofessionals providing consultation, assessment, and treatment (individual, family, and group) services to a broad client base that ranges in age, ethnicity, culture, and presenting concerns. This might involve in-patient and out-patient services or out-patient services only. The psychologists are based full time in a regional community and might travel to several health offices throughout the region, thereby enabling service delivery close to the client.

Given the large geographical area and population base inherent in these positions, staff members are also involved in activities aimed at supporting regional health-care providers and paraprofessionals and addressing mental health issues on a larger scale. For example, staff members have provided presentations to community, professional, and paraprofessional groups; supervised and consulted with mental health providers and health-care staff; collaborated on the development and evaluation of programs; and participated in health promotion, stigma reduction, and illness prevention programs. An effort has been made to become involved in broader population health interventions such as the Positive Parenting Program (Triple P) from Australia (Sanders 1999). This program is a multi-level, prevention-oriented parenting and family support strategy aimed at preventing severe behavioural, emotional, and developmental problems in children. Staff members also work toward identifying ways of implementing and evaluating the use of self-directed treatment programs that allow individuals to help themselves with minimal assistance from a health-care provider. Involvement in these types of activities is viewed as essential to enhancing the availability of a continuum of mental health services and reducing barriers to accessing these services.

The Northern Attachment Network

In northern British Columbia, an engaged group of health and social service providers working with young children and their families have formed the Northern Attachment Network (NAN). NAN's vision is one of healthy family development that values infant and child mental health. Its mission is to promote awareness of parent–child (caregiver–child) attachment with families and professionals in northern British Columbia and to build capacity for community organizations and service providers to provide education and interventions for families in which parent–child relationships are in need of support. NAN intends to enact its vision by influencing policy and funding decisions, by developing collaborative relationships that support partner agencies in meeting the needs of the families whom they serve, by promoting and providing education, and by connecting with practitioners, communities, and families.

NAN's work is founded on the premise that positive attachment experiences in the first years of life lay the foundation for life-long mental health and resilience in the face of stress (Svanberg 1998) and, conversely, that adverse early attachment experiences lay the foundation for psychological difficulties such as depression, anxiety, and problematic interpersonal relationships (Carlson 1998; van Ijzendoorn, Schuengel, and Bakermans-Kranenburg 1999). Over the past decade, various interventions focused on supporting and/or modifying parent–child attachment relationships have been developed and shown to be effective (Cohen et al. 1999; Hoffman et al. 2006; Madigan et al. 2006). These interventions have been developed and disseminated widely by practitioners based in urban settings, for example by Infant Mental Health Promotion (IMP) at the Hospital for Sick Children in Toronto. NAN formed because its members were interested in adopting and adapting these interventions in their work with families living in northern and rural communities of British Columbia. Attachment-focused interventions range from primary to tertiary in focus, and we have found it important, for reasons of child and parent well-being, to match the type of intervention to the type of work (e.g., psychotherapy versus parent education) typically done by practitioners.

Since its formation in 2005, NAN has sponsored a number of skills development workshops for professionals and paraprofessionals, and a small group of practitioners received case supervision in attachment-focused interventions using telephone and videotape to communicate with their clinical supervisor, located in an urban centre. NAN members have offered workshops on basic information about parent-child attachment to a variety of agencies in northern British Columbia, and practitioners in some northern communities have come together over lunch at "attachment cafés" to discuss attachment-focused work and provide each other with peer support. To increase awareness of the importance of positive parent-child attachment relationships, NAN has produced two brochures, one for parents and one for professionals. These brochures have been distributed widely throughout northern British Columbia. Approximately seventy-five members currently belong to NAN's electronic mailing list, used to share information about workshops and training opportunities and to circulate relevant resources. Brief literature reviews about attachment-relevant topics are an example of the resources sent out via the list. These reviews are prepared by C. Hardy and senior psychology students at the University of Northern BC and are written on topics suggested by NAN members based on their needs for information. NAN is an example of a community-based initiative intended to promote and enable individual and family mental health and resilience through peer support of service providers working with children and families. It is, by necessity, interagency and interdisciplinary, and it is responsive to the rural and northern context from which it comes.

Appropriate Assessment for Rural Residents

A final issue for mental health service delivery and intervention research is the use of appropriate mental health assessments that might be unavailable or inaccessible to rural residents due to wait times. The availability of telephone assessment alleviates the shortage of assessment specialists. In Ontario and parts of Nova Scotia, pediatric mental health assessment is conducted over the telephone using a tool specifically designed for this format. The Brief Child and Family Phone Interview (BCFPI; Cunningham, Pettingill, and Boyle 2005) provides a comprehensive evaluation of the child's problems and family's functioning and has proven to be very appropriate and cost effective. Beyond the availability of appropriate assessment, there is also the problem of the appropriateness of measures developed for urban populations for use with rural residents (Brannen, Johnson-Emberly, and McGrath 2009). Most assessment and intervention approaches are applied in a non-context-specific manner. That is, the same approaches are used without considering the differences that might exist between the population used during the design of these assessment and intervention approaches and the population to which they are applied. Little attention is paid to tailoring assessment and intervention approaches to create meaningful content that speaks to the specific situations and contexts in which rural and remote residents live.

One way to approach the tailoring of assessment and intervention approaches is through active community partnership. By identifying and engaging in consultation with key people in the communities from various perspectives (professional, paraprofessional, and consumer), various issues and potential barriers to appropriate services can be identified. As well, community-specific content can be inserted into assessment and intervention approaches, thereby allowing the community to have access to services designed to meet its specific needs. Once adaptations have been made based on the recommendations of key community members, the resultant assessment and intervention approaches must be presented to ensure that the needs identified during the consultation process were met. Through open dialogue, respect is fostered, and working relationships can be built. When a new mental health service approach is being developed for delivery in a rural or remote community, this approach will help to make it as meaningful as possible, and the likelihood of the approaches being successful is increased.

An important note with regard to assessing the mental health needs of a community comes directly from the community-based approach outlined above. Community members know themselves better than service providers do, and though specific major issues can be identified by non-community members the nuances of these issues cannot be understood. The importance of community context cannot be understated. Although blanket approaches have not been successful in meeting the needs of rural and remote communities, this is not to say that service providers must invent entirely new approaches when working with rural populations; in fact, evidence-based approaches can and should be used in rural communities with particular attention paid to the adaptation for meaningfulness in the rural context.

Discussion

In this chapter, we have outlined an argument that mental health services need to be both appropriate for rural residents and realistic. The traditional model of individual, face-to-face mental health service provision by a psychologist or psychiatrist in person is not realistic for many rural Canadians. This approach is not cost effective for either the system or the client. We have argued for a continuum of services matched to the level of distress or functional impairment of the person or family that includes prevention as well as treatment and uses individual- as well as population-based interventions. Adherence to this model would free limited specialist care for those most in need while providing general practitioners with resources for their patients via collaborative teams. We acknowledge that there are considerable challenges for the implementation of our model. Notably, health-care service delivery is managed at the level of regional health regulatory authorities in most provinces. Implementation of services is often decided at the level of these authorities, making population health initiatives difficult to organize and fund. In addition, our health system is designed to treat the sick, not protect health or support those at risk for significant distress or functional impairment. Finally, mental health services are viewed as the "poor cousin" of the health-care system in Canada (Kirby and Keon 2006). We hope that the recently established Mental Health Commission will raise the profile of mental health services across the country and include rural needs.

Although technological solutions such as telepsychiatry can increase access to mental health services in rural and northern Canada, such services should be viewed as supplements to rather than replacements for high-quality, community-based mental health services. The recruitment and retention of mental health professionals in rural and northern communities will undoubtedly require a broad, multi-level approach involving educational and training strategies designed to stimulate students' interest in rural and northern mental health and raise the profile and highlight the many positive aspects of this particular career path. Developing training programs that prepare students for the uniqueness of rural and northern practice and offer appropriate support and incentives (e.g., collegial support, access to supervision and consultation, library services, continuing educational opportunities, financial incentives) will also be important steps in recruiting and retaining well-qualified service providers in rural and northern communities.

We present this chapter as both a review and a call to action for those involved in service provision and/or research. Rural and northern Canadians are not a homogeneous group but consist of diverse groups of people with a variety of mental health needs and service requirements. The model proposed in this chapter offers a potential means of addressing these needs, though additional research is necessary to guide us. We need to know more about the complex interplay between residence in rural places and issues related to mental health, such as prevalence of mental illness, presence and role of protective factors, and access to services. We need to know more about rural communities' successful strategies for organizing mental health care and overcoming barriers to using mental health services. Due to the diversity of rural communities in Canada, both large-scale national surveys and smaller-scale community studies are needed.

It is imperative that rural mental health researchers and service providers (professionals and paraprofessionals) work with each other and with the residents of rural and northern communities to ensure that research projects and services are appropriate, effective, and meaningful to the community. Within this context, researchers and service providers are in an excellent position to identify and address community concerns and to document and build on community strengths in a manner that promotes capacity building. Collaborative efforts to address the recruitment and retention of professionals in rural and northern Canadian communities are equally important to the successful implementation of the model proposed in this chapter.

Acknowledgments

C. Brannen and K. Dyck contributed equally to this chapter. They wish to thank Laura Hambleton for her assistance with revisions to the chapter.

References

Boydell, K.M., R. Pong, T. Volpe, K. Tilleczek, E. Wilson, and S. Lemieux. 2006. "Family Perspectives on Pathways to Mental Health Care for Children and Youth in Rural Communities." *Journal of Rural Health* 22, 2: 182-88.

Brannen, C., D. Johnson-Emberly, and P.J. McGrath. 2009. "Stress in Rural Canada: A Structured Review of Context, Stress Levels, and Sources of Stress." *Health and Place* 15, 1: 219-27.

Brannen, C., P.J. McGrath, C. Johnston, D. Dozois, F. Elgar, and M. Whitehead. 2006. "Managing Our Mood (MOM): Distance Treatment for Post-Partum Depression in Rural Nova Scotia." Paper presented at the annual conference of the Canadian Rural Health Research Society, Prince George, BC.

Canadian Agricultural Safety Association. 2005. *National Stress and Mental Survey of Canadian Farmers: Report to the Canadian Agricultural Safety Association.* Winnipeg: Canadian Agricultural Safety Association, http://www.ruralsupport.ca/.

Canadian Collaborative Mental Health Initiative. 2006. *Establishing Collaborative Initiatives between Mental Health and Primary Care Services for Rural and Isolated Populations: A Companion to the CCMHI Planning and Implementation Toolkit for Health Care Providers and Planners.* Mississauga: Canadian Collaborative Mental Health Initiative, http://www.ccmhi.ca/.

Canadian Institute for Health Information (CIHI). 2006. *How Healthy Are Rural Canadians? An Assessment of Their Health Status and Health Determinants.* Ottawa: CIHI, http://secure.cihi.ca/.

Carlson, E.A. 1998. "A Prospective Longitudinal Study of Attachment Disorganization/ Disorientation." *Child Development* 69, 4: 1107-28.

Cohen, N.J., E. Muir, M. Lojkasek, R. Muir, C.J. Parker, M. Barwick, and M. Brown. 1999. "Watch, Wait, and Wonder: Testing the Effectiveness of a New Approach to Mother-Infant Psychotherapy." *Infant Mental Health Journal* 20, 4: 429-51.

Cunningham, C.E., P. Pettingill, and M. Boyle. 2005. *The Brief Child and Family Phone Interview (BCFPI-3): A Computerized Intake and Outcome Assessment Tool.* Nanaimo, BC: BCFPI, http://www.bcfpi.com/.

Elgar, F.J., P.J. McGrath, D.A. Waschbusch, S.H. Stewart, and L.J. Curtis. 2004. "Mutual Influences on Maternal Depression and Child Adjustment Problems." *Clinical Psychology Review* 24, 4: 441-59.

Fennell, D.L., and A.J. Hovestadt. 2004. "Rural Mental Health Services." In *Handbook of Mental Health Services for Children, Adolescents, and Families (Issues in Clinical Child Psychology)*, edited by R.G. Steele and M.C. Roberts, 245-58. New York: Plenum.

Greenberg, N., K.M. Boydell, and T. Volpe. 2006. "Pediatric Telepsychiatry in Ontario: Caregiver and Service Provider Perspectives." *Journal of Behavioral Health Sciences and Research* 33, 1: 105-11.

Hoffman, K.T., R.S. Marvin, G. Cooper, and B. Powell. 2006. "Changing Toddlers' and Preschoolers' Attachment Classifications: The Circle of Security Intervention." *Journal of Consulting and Clinical Psychology* 74, 6: 1017-26.

Jong, M. 2004. "Managing Suicides via Videoconferencing in a Remote Northern Community in Canada." *International Journal of Circumpolar Health* 63, 4: 422-28.

Kirby, M.J.L., and W.J. Keon. 2006. *Out of the Shadows at Last: Transforming Mental Health, Mental Illness, and Addiction Services in Canada.* Ottawa: Standing Senate Committee on Social Affairs, Science and Technology.

Leipert, B. 2002. "Developing Resilience: How Women Maintain Their Health in Northern Geographically Isolated Settings." PhD diss., University of Alberta.

Li, H.Z., and A.J. Browne. 2000. "Defining Mental Illness and Accessing Mental Health Services: Perspectives of Asian Canadians." *Canadian Journal of Community Mental Health* 19, 1: 143-59.

Madigan, S., E. Hawkins, S. Goldberg, and D. Benoit. 2006. "Reduction of Disrupted Caregiver Behavior Using Modified Interaction Guidance." *Infant Mental Health Journal* 27, 5: 509-27.

Manitoba Centre for Health Policy. 2004. *Patterns of Regional Mental Illness Disorder Diagnosis and Service Use in Manitoba: A Population-Based Study.* Winnipeg: Manitoba Centre for Health Policy.

Manitoba Farm and Rural Stress Line. 2005. *2005 Annual Report.* Brandon: Manitoba Farm and Rural Stress Line.

Masley, M.L., K.M. Semchuk, A. Senthilselvan, H.H. McDuffie, P. Hanke, J.A. Dosman, et al. 2000. "Health and Environment of Rural Families: Results of a

Community Canvass Survey in the Prairie Ecosystem Study (PECOS)." *Journal of Agricultural Safety and Health* 6, 2: 103-15.

McGee, P., H. Tuokko, P. Maccourt, and M. Donnelly. 2004. "Factors Affecting the Mental Health of Older Adults in Rural and Urban Communities: An Exploration." *Canadian Journal of Community Mental Health* 23, 2: 117-26.

McIlwraith, R.D., K.G. Dyck, V.L. Holms, T.E. Carlson, and N.G. Prober. 2005. "Manitoba's Rural and Northern Community-Based Training Program for Psychology Pre-Doctoral Residents and Residents." *Professional Psychology: Research and Practice* 36, 2: 164-72.

McKeown, L., A. Noce, and P. Czerny. 2007. "Factors Associated with Internet Use: Does Rurality Matter?" *Rural and Small Town Canada Analysis Bulletin* 7, 3: 1-15. Catalogue No. 21-006-XIE.

O'Reilly, R., J. Bishop, K. Maddox, L. Hutchinson, M. Fisman, and J. Takhar. 2007. "Is Telepsychiatry Equivalent to Face-to-Face Psychiatry? Results from a Randomized Controlled Equivalence Trial." *Psychiatric Services* 58, 6: 836-43.

Parikh, S.V., D. Wasylenki, P. Goering, and J. Wong. 1996. "Mood Disorders: Rural/Urban Differences in Prevalence, Health Care Utilization, and Disability in Ontario." *Journal of Affective Disorders* 38, 1: 57-65.

Rohland, B.M. 2000. "A Survey of Burnout among Mental Health Center Directors in a Rural State." *Administration and Policy in Mental Health* 27: 221-37.

Romanow, R.J. 2002. *Building on Values: The Future of Health Care in Canada.* Saskatoon: Commission on the Future of Health Care in Canada.

Ryan-Nicholls, K.D., and J.M. Haggarty. 2007. "Collaborative Mental Health Care in Rural and Isolated Canada: Stakeholder Feedback." *Journal of Psychosocial Nursing* 45, 12: 37-45.

Ryan-Nicholls, K.D., F.E. Racher, and J.R. Robinson. 2003. "Providers' Perception of How Rural Consumers Access and Use Mental Health Services." *Journal of Psychosocial Nursing* 41, 6: 34-43.

Sanders, M.R. 1999. "The Triple P – Positive Parenting Program: Towards an Empirically Validated Multilevel Parenting and Family Support Strategy for the Prevention of Behavioral and Emotional Problems in Children." *Clinical Child and Family Psychology Review* 2, 2: 71-90.

Schmidt, G. 2000. "Barriers to Recovery in a First Nations Community." *Canadian Journal of Community Mental Health* 19, 2: 75-87.

Simpson, J., S. Doze, D. Urness, D. Hailey, and P. Jacobs. 2001a. "Evaluation of a Routine Telepsychiatry Service." *Journal of Telemedicine and Telecare* 7, 2: 90-98.

–. 2001b. "Telepsychiatry as a Routine Service: The Perspective of the Patient." *Journal of Telemedicine and Telecare* 7, 3: 155-60.

Svanberg, P.O.G. 1998. "Attachment, Resilience, and Prevention." *Journal of Mental Health* 7, 6: 543-78.

Thurston, W.E., S. Patten, and L. Lagendyk. 2006. "Prevalence of Violence against Women Reported in a Rural Health Region." *Canadian Journal of Rural Medicine* 11, 4: 259-67.

van Ijzendoorn, M.H., C. Schuengel, and M.J. Bakermans-Kranenburg. 1999. "Disorganized Attachment in Early Childhood: Meta-Analysis of Precursors, Concomitants, and Sequelae." *Development and Psychopathology* 11, 2: 225-49.

Vincent, N., J. Walker, and A. Katz. 2007. "Self-Administered Therapies in Primary Care." In *Handbook of Self-Help Therapies,* edited by P.L. Watkins and G. Clum, 387-417. New York: Routledge.

Wang, J.L. 2004. "Rural-Urban Differences in the Prevalence of Major Depression and Associated Impairment." *Social Psychiatry and Psychiatric Epidemiology* 39, 1: 19-25.

Chapter 14   **Health Literacy in Rural Communities: Challenges and Champions**

D. Gillis and S. Sears

Key Points

- Health literacy is a pressing population health concern with relevance to those living in rural Canada.
- A participatory research process exploring the links between literacy and health through the lived experiences of people with low literacy helped to build capacity for meaningful change in practices and policies in one rural health district in Nova Scotia.
- By sharing their knowledge and perspectives, community members, practitioners, managers, and policy makers from the fields of health and literacy developed a shared understanding of the emerging concept of health literacy, identified priorities for action to reduce the impact of low literacy on health, and championed system-wide change to improve health literacy.

Literacy has long been considered a necessary resource for everyday living and for achieving one's aspirations in life. In addressing the daunting challenges facing rural Atlantic Canadians in the 1930s and 1940s, social justice champion Dr. Moses Coady considered literacy fundamental to "a full and abundant life for everyone in the community." Despite this fundamental premise, literacy is not at the forefront of Canadian public policy. Indeed, policy analyst Judith Maxwell has referred to low literacy as Canada's "hidden deficit" (Maxwell and Teplova 2005).

Although low literacy is often pointed to as one of many barriers faced by people living in rural communities, little attention has been directed to the impact of literacy on health. Over the past two decades, growing evidence of direct and indirect effects of literacy on health has positioned literacy as an important determinant of health in Canada (Ronson and Rootman 2008). Recently, the concept of health literacy has captured the attention of researchers, policy makers, and practitioners. Drawing from our experience in addressing the links between literacy and health in rural Nova Scotia, we focus on the implications for health literacy policy and practice in a rural Canadian context. In this chapter, we describe a community-university participatory research project, key findings from this collaborative research, and the system-wide response to a call for action. We begin by examining health literacy – an evolving concept of increasing policy and practice relevance in Canada.

Understandings of Education, Literacy, and Health Literacy

Levels of education are consistently reported to be lower among rural residents than among non-rural dwellers (Canadian Institute for Health Information [CIHI] 2006). Although the two are closely connected, the level of literacy is not the same as the level of educational attainment. Estimating literacy by years of schooling does not reflect quality of schooling, jurisdictional variations in schooling standards across Canadian provinces and territories, or the influence of broader socio-demographic factors. In particular, the degree of rurality affects one's access to schooling and opportunities for informal learning. Although some individuals might not attain high levels of education, as measured by credentials, they might have adequate skills to meet the literacy demands of workplace and community. Others might progress through school yet not acquire the literacy skills needed to function fully in their community and society. Moreover, the demand for both level and type of literacy changes over time. This is the case in rural communities transitioning from resource-based occupations such as forestry, fishing, mining, and farming to more information- and technology-dependent occupations. More sophisticated literacy skills are increasingly needed to operate in all areas of society, from managing one's finances, to making food choices in the marketplace, to navigating complex health-care systems.

In recent years, descriptions of literacy have been expanding from a traditional focus on reading and writing skills to include a wider range of abilities needed for life in an increasingly complex information-based society. Most definitions began with the fundamental require-ment for a command of the written word and emphasized the instrumental, or *functional,* value of literacy. According to Quigley et al. (2006, 12), the definition commonly accepted by provincial literacy coalitions across Canada is that used by Statistics Canada and Human Resources and Skills Development Canada. Literacy is described as "the ability to understand and employ printed information in daily ac-tivities at home, at work and in the community – to achieve one's goals, and to develop one's knowledge and potential."

A current and more culturally responsive view of literacy suggests that literacy practices vary from one context to another and that to be literate requires one to apply not one but multiple literacies. Instead of speaking of literacy as a commodity and discrete ability that one has or does not have, one frequently hears reference to various literacies, such as computer literacy, financial literacy, media literacy – and health lit-eracy. The idea of the plurality of literacy reflects its dynamic nature "based on manifold communicative and social practices" (UNESCO 2004, 29). This more complex notion of literacy represents a shift in thinking away from what literacy *does to* people toward what people *can do with* literacy. From a practice perspective, this approach refocuses the target of interventions to advance literacy from changing individ-uals to creating supportive literacy environments. For example, the extent to which varied settings support individuals in accessing, under-standing, and using information for their health frames health literacy from a social-cultural perspective and not solely as a distinct set of cog-nitive skills that one might or might not have.

Given the ambiguous nature of the concept of literacy, it is not sur-prising that many definitions of health literacy appear in the current literature and that no universal definition is shared among health prac-titioners and policy makers. Although some view health literacy as a domain of literacy, others see it as a separate concept (Rootman 2004). Diverse understandings of health literacy reflect not only pedagogical debates within the field of literacy but also the tensions between indi-vidual and population approaches within the health field. Definitions of health literacy in the literature span the spectrum from a focus on health literacy as the ability of individuals to access, understand, and use information within health-care settings to broader notions reflect-ing the interactions of individuals with systems.

A narrower view is reflected in the American Medical Association (AMA) reference to health literacy as "a constellation of skills including the ability to perform basic reading and numerical tasks required to function in the health care environment" (Ad Hoc Committee on Health Literacy 1999, 533). Ratzan and Parker (2000, 3) extended the application beyond health care by describing health literacy as "the degree to which individuals have the capacity to obtain, process, and understand basic health information and services needed to make appropriate health decisions." This definition was later adopted in 2004 by the Institute of Medicine (IOM) in *Health Literacy: A Prescription to End Confusion*. This landmark report emphasized that individuals obtain information from many sources and make health-relevant decisions in a wide range of contexts. Health literacy was therefore framed as a "mediator between individuals and the health context" (IOM 2004, 32).

In keeping with the ideals of capacity building and empowerment, the World Health Organization (WHO) depicted health literacy as more than one's ability to read a medicine bottle or a consent form. The WHO definition considered health literacy as "the cognitive and social skills which determine the motivation and ability of individuals to gain access to, understand and use information in ways which promote and maintain good health." Accordingly, "by improving people's access to health information and their capacity to use it effectively, health literacy is seen as critical to personal empowerment" (1998, 10). In arguing for a capacity-building and empowerment approach consistent with the WHO definition of health literacy, Nutbeam (2000, 382) introduced the idea of three levels of health literacy – functional, interactive, and critical – which he said "progressively allow for greater autonomy in decision-making and personal empowerment, demonstrated through the actions of individuals and communities." Nutbeam challenged practitioners to refocus their efforts from primarily transmitting information to people toward applying ways of practice that strengthen people's capacity to use the information provided to enhance their health. The notion of empowerment is particularly evident in Nutbeam's concept of critical health literacy, which reflects an emancipatory approach to change in calling for action to address the socioenvironmental conditions determining one's capacity for health. Although the lively international debate in the literature about the nature of health literacy might frustrate practitioners and policy makers seeking one universal definition, it speaks to the inherent tensions in framing complex health issues today (Nutbeam 2008).

The concept of health literacy appeared relatively recently in Canada, where it has tended to be situated within the context of health promotion and population health. This broader approach is reflected in a recent report by the Expert Panel on Health Literacy, convened by the Canadian Public Health Association (CPHA) and funded by the Canadian Council on Learning (CCL) through its Health and Learning Knowledge Centre at the University of Victoria. The panel defined health literacy as the "ability to access, understand, evaluate and communicate information as a way to promote, maintain and improve health in a variety of settings across the life-course" (Rootman and Gordon-El-Bihbety 2008, 11). In this instance, health literacy is recognized as ability needed over the life course, not just in dealing with episodic health concerns and medical encounters. Moreover, this definition implies that health literacy is mediated by "education, culture and language, by the communication skills of professionals, by the nature of materials and messages, and by the settings in which health-related support are provided" (Rootman and Gordon-El-Bihbety 2008, 11). The wider lens considers health literacy pertaining not just to the abilities of individuals but also to the interactions of individuals and the systems through which they access information. In its report, Canada's Expert Panel on Health Literacy addressed individual and systemic barriers to health literacy, recommended the development of a pan-Canadian strategy for health literacy, and proposed the following vision for a health-literate Canada: "All people will have the capacity, opportunities and support they need to obtain and use health information effectively, to act as informed partners in caring for themselves, their families and communities, and to manage interactions in a variety of settings that affect health and well-being" (Rootman and Gordon-El-Bihbety 2008, 23). This vision is clearly grounded in a capacity-building, as opposed to a deficit, approach to addressing health literacy.

The variety of contexts in which people access and use health information underscores the importance of examining issues of place as people interact with health-relevant services. In this chapter, we suggest that the conditions and life realities of rural Canadians illustrate the importance of context in addressing health literacy. Issues of access to health information and services in rural communities and their special health risks require prevention and promotion interventions specific to these concerns (CIHI 2006).

Health Literacy in Practice

Evaluation reports about the effectiveness of health literacy interventions are limited (Berkman et al. 2004). In a Canadian review of interventions to improve health literacy, King (2007) reported little evidence of evaluation. From her interviews with key informants involved in health literacy research and evaluation in Canada and abroad, King found widely differing views on the meaning of health literacy. In addition, many informants contended that health practitioners needed to become more aware of health literacy. Despite the growing concern about health literacy as a population health issue, Canadian health practitioners are reported to lack awareness of health literacy (Rootman and Gordon-El-Bihbety 2008). Results from a survey of some 700 professionals and policy makers undertaken for the Expert Panel on Health Literacy (CPHA 2007) found that almost 30 percent were unaware of health literacy, and only 34 percent said that the term was used in their organizations. Although 68 percent reported that their organizations provided direct services, more than 30 percent were unsure of their clients' levels of literacy. Only 7 percent of respondents reported that their organizations had policies on health literacy.

Health Literacy as a Population Health Problem in Canada

Recent evidence from the 2003 International Adult Literacy and Skills Survey (IALSS)[1] has suggested that low health literacy is a serious population health concern in Canada (CCL 2007). In its February 2008 report, *Health Literacy in Canada: A Healthy Understanding,* the CCL drew the following conclusion about the health literacy status of Canadians: "If it is assumed that, as in prose literacy, Level 3 (276-325) on the health-literacy scale is the minimum required in order to participate fairly and fully in society, Canada has a significant percentage of adults (60 percent) who lack the skills to manage their health-literacy needs" (20). Compared with those at Level 4 and Level 5, Canadian adults with the lowest health literacy skills were 2.5 times as likely to report being in fair to poor health, less likely to participate in a community group, and more than 2.5 times as likely to be receiving income assistance.[2]

These findings held when the impacts of age, gender, education, first language, immigrant status, and Aboriginal status were controlled. Seniors, immigrants, and the unemployed were considered the most vulnerable. The report concluded that mastering health literacy tasks appears even more demanding than mastering general literacy. Requirements for health literacy often entail the simultaneous use of prose, document, and numeracy skills. Not surprisingly, health literacy scores increased with the level of formal education attained (CCL 2007). Notably, the strongest factor predicting higher levels of health literacy was daily reading.

Although health literacy scores vary considerably across Canadian provinces and territories, there is "a large proportion of adults in every jurisdiction with literacy skill levels that put them at risk of poor health" (CCL 2008, 20). Informed by these findings, the Expert Panel on Health Literacy concluded that "low health literacy is a serious and costly problem that will likely grow as the population ages and the incidence of chronic disease increases" (Rootman and Gordon-El-Bihbety 2008, 41). Although no significant difference in health literacy scores between urban and rural areas at the national level was reported by the CCL, there is evidence of health literacy differences within several provinces that have implications for rural health practice. Health literacy is a health disparities issue demanding the attention of practitioners and policy makers, as described in the following case study set in rural Nova Scotia.

Health Literacy as a Rural Health Disparity

The Guysborough Antigonish Strait Health Authority (GASHA) covers the northeastern part of mainland Nova Scotia and the neighbouring part of Cape Breton Island, as shown in the map of Nova Scotia in Figure 14.1. GASHA is one of nine District Health Authorities (DHAs) created in 2000 as part of the restructuring of the provincial health system. Its population, according to the latest available census data (2006),[3] is 44,815, which represents almost 5 percent of Nova Scotia's total population of 913,462. GASHA includes the counties of Antigonish and Guysborough on the mainland as well as Richmond and a small part of Inverness on Cape Breton Island. Most people here are Canadian born, with the predominant heritage being Scottish and Irish. Communities of Acadian, Mi'kmaq, and black African Nova Scotians are scattered throughout the region.

Figure 14.1   Map of Nova Scotia with District Health Authorities (DHAs)

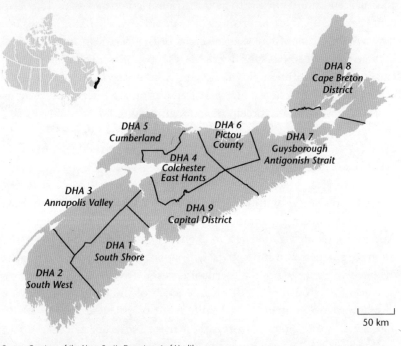

Source: Courtesy of the Nova Scotia Department of Health.

The livelihood of people in northeastern Nova Scotia, as in many parts of Atlantic Canada, until recently has depended heavily on resource-based industries such as fishing, forestry, and mining. Over the past few decades, communities have faced dramatic changes. Most striking are shifts in population demographics, with out-migration of working-aged people to Halifax and other parts of Canada where employment opportunities are more plentiful. Coastal communities have been particularly vulnerable to poor economic and social conditions due to a decline in off-shore fishing and processing.

Evidence of health disparities is striking when GASHA is compared with the province. Mortality and morbidity rates are higher in GASHA than in Nova Scotia and Canada.[4] Total age-standardized mortality data reveal a rate of 938.7 per 100,000 in GASHA compared with a provincial rate of 895.2 per 100,000. Residents of GASHA have the second highest diabetes rates in Nova Scotia. According to self-reported health data, only 16.3 percent of GASHA residents rate their health as excellent compared with 18.4 percent in the province. Moreover, 15.6 percent rate their health as fair to poor compared with 13.8 percent provincially. Not surprisingly, the population of GASHA does not fare well in terms of key determinants of health. Mean total personal income from all sources for district residents is lower than the provincial average. The unemployment rate is consistently higher than for other parts of Nova Scotia. Levels of education are lower than provincial averages, with 44 percent of residents between 45 and 64 years of age having less than a high school diploma compared with 33.7 percent of all Nova Scotians. On a positive note, self-perceived levels of social support are higher among GASHA residents at 88.4 percent compared with 85.1 percent of Nova Scotians. There are also notable socioeconomic disparities within the health district.[5] For example, household income and levels of education within GASHA tend to be highest in Antigonish County and lowest in Guysborough County. The latter, the province's largest and most sparsely populated county, has the highest mean age, largely attributed to out-migration of working-age adults.

Recent data on the health literacy levels of the population provide insight into health literacy as a health disparity issue (CCL 2007, 2008). The mean health literacy score is higher for Nova Scotia (258.7) than for Canada (255.7). Such is not the case in the other Atlantic provinces. However, this finding does not reveal the full picture with regard to health literacy levels in rural Nova Scotia. The mean health literacy score is lower in rural Nova Scotia (254.7) than in urban areas (261.8).[6] The proportion of adults performing at Level 2 or below who live in urban areas is 55 percent[7] compared with 60 percent of those living in rural areas. Moreover, low health literacy scores are more prevalent within GASHA compared with the province and Canada, as shown in Table 14.1. Health literacy disparity is striking when one looks at the CCL (2007) map of Canada's health literacy.[8] Using geographical information systems (GIS), interactive health literacy maps depict health literacy performance in District Health Authorities across Canada. Within GASHA, there is a pronounced increase in the distribution of low health literacy in communities outside Antigonish – the district's centre for medical, educational, and professional services.

The Health Literacy in Rural Nova Scotia Research Project

The Health Literacy in Rural Nova Scotia Research Project (HLRNSRP), a participatory action research (PAR) project funded in 2001 by the

Table 14.1   Distribution of low health literacy: GASHA compared with
Nova Scotia and Canada

Distribution of low health literacy	GASHA	Nova Scotia	Canada
Proportion at level 2 and below	68%	57%	59.5%
Proportion at level 1 and below	38%	25.3%	25.9%
Number at level 2 and below	26,500	426,003	14,814,623
Number at level 1 and below	12,500	188,998	6,450,844
Mean health literacy score	240	258.7	255.7

Source: Data from the 2003 IALLS survey and the 2001 Canadian Census.

Social Sciences and Humanities Research Council of Canada (SSHRCC), explored links between literacy and health through the experience of people in rural northeastern Nova Scotia. The study was conducted by a multidisciplinary research team from St. Francis Xavier University partnering with five community-based literacy and health organizations within GASHA.

Although the current evidence is compelling that health literacy is of high relevance to rural health, no such data were available in 2001 when a citizen-led health-planning organization in northeastern Nova Scotia identified the literacy level of residents as a population health concern. The Antigonish Town and County Community Health Board (ATCCHB), one of three Community Health Boards in GASHA, was a product of the restructuring of health services and the decentralizing of health planning in the late 1990s. From the onset, the ATCCHB took on its health-planning role with an understanding that non-medical determinants, such as income, employment, social support, education, and literacy, were fundamental to health in their communities. Early in its mandate, the ATCCHB conducted group interviews with residents to determine what they considered important determinants of their health. Findings revealed that education and literacy were considered key. The relevance of low levels of literacy among the population came to the forefront when the ATCCHB initiated an evaluation of a health services directory that had been distributed to every household in the county. It became apparent that low literacy levels could limit not only residents' ability to respond to an evaluation questionnaire but also their access to and use of health information and services. Members of the Community Health Board brought their concerns to researchers from the Faculties of Human Nutrition, Adult Education, and Nursing at St. Francis Xavier. Workshops were held in the district to explore the need for, and interest in, exploring the links between literacy and health. A research proposal was developed and funding secured. A community-university partnership of adult learning and health organizations from throughout the health district were involved in the research from development of the proposal to dissemination of the findings.

The central aim of the participatory research project was to learn more about the experiences of people in this rural area who had literacy difficulties and the challenges faced by practitioners while working with them to address their health issues. The research asked which factors influence how less literate adults living in northeastern Nova Scotia access and act on health information and services and which strategies for change will build upon existing capacities for achieving health. Community partners were adamant that findings be directed at effecting change in policies and practices in order to build capacity for health among residents in their communities (Gillis 2007).

Although the researchers were familiar with definitions of health literacy in the literature, they did not adopt one. Rather, by drawing on the knowledge of the community partners, together they developed a shared understanding of health literacy. As described on the project website (http://www.nald.ca/healthliteracystfx), health literacy means "working together to enable all people to find, understand, and use the information they need to stay healthy; get the services and supports that they need; make choices in their own lives that help keep them healthy; speak up about their own health needs and have more control over the things that make and keep them healthy." This understanding of health literacy is in keeping with a health promotion approach and consistent with Nutbeam's (2000) broad notion of health literacy.

Using a reflective adult education process, a research assistant experienced in family literacy interviewed forty-six adults with limited literacy. This sample was purposefully selected with the assistance of practitioners in various adult-learning and health settings who had been identified by members of the community-university partnership. These practitioners selected individuals whom they knew from repeated contact had literacy difficulties. They told them about the research project and asked them if they were interested in participating in the study. If interested, individuals signed a consent form agreeing to be contacted by the research assistant. The assistant then contacted them and invited them to participate. Although she provided a letter of information about the study written in plain language, she orally explained its content and addressed any questions. All participants signed a written consent form prior to being interviewed.

Of the forty-six participants with limited literacy, twenty-five were enrolled in adult-learning programs, and twenty-one were recruited through the diabetes out-patient clinic and community-based agencies. The fifteen males and thirty-one females ranged in age from eighteen to over fifty-five, had from grade 1 to grade 12 education, and included Acadian, Mi'kmaq, and African Nova Scotians. Twenty community leaders were identified by the community partners for interviews as key informants. In addition, seven group interviews were held with sixty-four health and literacy practitioners. All interviews were audiotaped and transcribed. Thematic analysis was conducted by the research team, and emerging themes were presented to members of the community-university partnership for feedback.

Participants gave poignant accounts reflecting how closely literacy interconnects with other determinants of rural health (Gillis, MacIsaac, and Quigley 2005). Difficulty in accessing appropriate and timely services to meet their health-care needs was a common theme. Although travel distances to service providers are not as great as in the northern communities described in Chapter 9 of this volume, people living in rural northeastern Nova Scotia lack public transportation, face treacherous winter driving conditions, and have few outreach services. Their stories emphasized the challenges of rural life, including lack of employment opportunities, accessible and affordable health-care resources, social supports, and transportation. The profound influence that the social stigma associated with low literacy has on people's lives spoke to how deeply embedded within the socio-economic conditions of everyday living are challenges related to health literacy. The story of Gerald (see Box 14.1) provides a glimpse into the difficulties of one man as he attempts to access, understand, and use information needed to manage diabetes within the context of limited literacy and many interrelated socio-economic determinants of health.

Health providers talked about the dilemmas they faced when working with people with limited command of the written word. Their identification of the difficulties in talking about and addressing low literacy in their practice was particularly striking. As noted by one health practitioner, "the words can only take you so far. It is the experience of being in health care and coming up against that literacy issue

BOX 14.1   Gerald's Story

Gerald, in his mid-sixties, lives in an old, drafty trailer with his wife and their sixteen-year-old granddaughter. He is diabetic and has high blood pressure. He began working in the woods at age sixteen. After years of work-related injuries to his hands, he couldn't use a power saw at all. Working in the woods was his only source of income, and, because he was not educated enough to get any other form of employment, he ended up on a disability pension at an early age. Gerald sums up his current literacy level by saying, "well, I can't read, and I can't write. I can just sign my own name ... That is about it." As a child, his school attendance was sporadic, and he finally quit altogether in grade 4. To quote him,

> Back then, that was in the '30s and '40s, and there wasn't too much money coming in. I lived on a farm, and I had twelve kids in the family, so you only go to school once or twice a week ... if you went then ... See, I was the oldest in the family, and the rest of them were younger than I was.

Gerald admits that he has not disclosed his literacy difficulties: "Even your own people don't know you can't read, ... and you don't even tell your own ... If you asked one of my brothers and sisters if I could read, they would probably say, 'oh, yeah, he can read.'"

About twenty-five years ago, Gerald discovered that he had diabetes when, as he says, he "started passing out and having blackouts." He still feels quite tired and rundown. When asked how he manages his diabetes, he says,

> I should be on the needles by rights. I don't figure I could be able to afford it ... To be on medicine like that and stuff, you stay on until you can't get the money to buy it ... I can't get enough to get the food I am supposed to get. You need a lot of certain stuff ... I get the cheap stuff ... and whatever is the cheapest. I don't get no quality stuff. Certain things I have to eat ... like low fat and not too much sugar and stuff like that ... Like after a while you just forget about your diet, and you eat a little more of this and a little more of that.

Gerald goes on to say that the people at the diabetes clinic try to help him as much as they can; however, "by the time you get out of the hospital [clinic], you forget it ... I don't imagine there is too much they could do ... if you can't read." Although he has never told them at the clinic that he doesn't know how to read, he suspects that they have figured it out.

When asked how his situation would change if he knew how to read, Gerald replies, "well, first getting the trailer fixed and going to the [tenancy] board and all that ... and knowing what you are doing ... I would be looking up a lot of things – diabetic stuff." He admits that he wishes someone would "help me a little bit." He also comments, however, "you don't know what you want, ... so how are they going to help you? ... You feel uncomfortable, and you don't know what to ask for ... See, we are kind of like blindfolded, ... just like you are in the dark ... A lot of people, you know, can't read." His advice to others is "go to school and get your reading so you can help yourself ... You ought to be able to learn how to read and write in this world, or you are done for." When asked if he is interested in a program that will help him learn to read and write, Gerald replies, "if you can't read and write, how can you get in touch with them? They tell you to come to a certain office in a certain place ... You wouldn't know how to get there."

---

that makes you experience and understand it ... but I could never put it into words." For many health practitioners, the stigma of low literacy was a barrier to addressing health literacy concerns in their practice – a point well supported in the literature (Parikh et al. 1996; Wolf et al. 2007). In discussing the information needs of people living with HIV/ AIDS in Chapter 16, Harris describes the effects of social isolation and stigma in rural settings in other regions of Canada. Not surprisingly, the stigma associated with low literacy combined with hesitancy to discuss sensitive issues was considered particularly challenging by these Nova Scotia practitioners.

Determining Priorities for Action from the Findings

In the fall of 2003, key research findings and a call for action stemming from the findings were presented in a clear-language discussion paper entitled "Taking Off the Blindfold: Seeing How Literacy Affects Health in Rural Nova Scotia." This document served as the focal point for developing priorities for action at roundtable consultations held with a wide array of research participants and other stakeholders, including district- and province-level program and policy managers. Priorities, summarized in Box 14.2, were incorporated into an updated report in

BOX 14.2   Priorities for Action Determined by Participants

- Increase awareness of literacy as a determinant of health and well-being.
- Increase awareness of health literacy issues among service providers.
- Find ways to reduce barriers to enrolling in and attending literacy programs.
- Increase networking among service providers to reach those who may "slip through the cracks."
- Make health information more accessible to everyone.
- Take health information and services to the people: for example, drop-in health centres and health-mobiles.
- Support the use of client advocates to help people move through the health-care system and to determine when English is not the first language.
- Support community-based organizations and services in fostering health and literacy.
- Develop health and literacy promotion strategies that address needs in rural areas, including the lack of public transportation.

June 2004 (Gillis and Quigley 2004) and served as a focus for effecting change in district-wide policies and practices.

Championing Change in Practice and Policy

In response to the call for action, GASHA initiated a project in June 2004 with support from the Primary Health Care Transition Fund. It began with an environmental scan of practices and policies conducted with health practitioners and managers throughout GASHA. Although 70 percent of the participants reported having heard of the health literacy research project, few identified policies or programs to address health literacy issues in their practice settings. They did, however, report individual practices used when working with clients limited in literacy. These practices included checking for a patient's understanding of information and using plain-language print materials.

"Health Literacy Awareness" sessions were developed by the GASHA primary health-care manager (S. Sears) and conducted throughout GASHA to address two priority actions from the HLRNSRP. They were aimed at increasing primary health-care providers' awareness of literacy as a determinant of health and well-being and their awareness of health literacy. Some 185 staff and physicians, almost one-quarter of the total GASHA workforce of 800, participated in one of the five noon-hour sessions, either in person or via telehealth in the more rural sites. The Health Literacy Awareness session was offered once a day for a week in September 2004. Each session provided background on the links between literacy and health, the concept of health literacy, findings from the HLRNSRP, the GASHA environmental scan, and a twenty-minute popular education dramatization.

The dramatization was particularly effective in capturing the attention of health practitioners. It had been successfully used during the roundtable sessions in the dissemination and discussion of findings from the HLRNSRP. The dramatization was developed by a popular theatre group working with the principal investigator (D. Gillis) and the research assistant. Using excerpts from the transcribed interviews, they developed a skit about the experiences of a single mother with an adolescent child and grandfather living in a community characteristic of many in the health district. The challenges faced by this family mirrored themes from the research related to literacy and determinants of health, in particular income, employment, rural geography, and social support. Three actors from the theatre group, the Irondale Ensemble Project (http://www.irondale.com), played the various roles without props or staging. The popular theatre approach not only highlighted the story line and underpinned themes relevant to health literacy but also made the production easily transportable and cost efficient. The logistical appropriateness of this approach was paramount given the rural health settings and distances between sites.

Freeing up staff from service, engaging a wide range of practitioners in topics directly relevant to their practice, overcoming long travel distances to training sites, and finding replacement staff are a few of the challenges in providing continuing education for rural practitioners. Presenting local research findings through the dramatization was particularly effective in engaging practitioners in reflecting on the literacy and health literacy challenges faced by people in their communities and the implications for their practice.

The awareness sessions were evaluated by interviewing practitioners and managers six months after their attendance at the sessions. A part-time health literacy coordinator conducted telephone interviews using a combination of open- and closed-ended questions. Findings were analyzed by the coordinator and the primary health-care manager (S. Sears). Nearly all (97 percent) of the fifty-eight respondents indicated that their awareness of health literacy issues had been raised. One practitioner made the following observation: "I always had a more shallow definition of health literacy that it was about reading and writing. The session helped me to have a more in-depth understanding of how people access, understand, and use the information related to health." Another practitioner reported being "more conscious of how I communicate with people and not making assumptions." Several respondents referred to their heightened awareness of the social stigma associated with low literacy and their difficulty in identifying whether individuals have literacy difficulties. For example, one practitioner reported being "more aware of the embarrassment that people may feel and how we ask about education level, but that is not indicative of literacy level. More clued in to actions they may show."

Close to 70 percent of respondents reported changing their behaviour as a result of the awareness session. Examples of reported changes in health literacy practices included improving signage to help people better navigate health facilities, assessing and improving the level of readability of print materials, changing how people are asked to complete forms, and asking patients how they prefer to receive health information. As one practitioner said, "I give verbal directions to patients, not just written. I use teach back and go over the info with them. Now I make sure I take the time to ensure clients understand, and if not I get the family involved as well." According to another practitioner, "now we don't assume that people can read, and now we offer to give assistance to all people to fill out forms."

Both practitioners and managers described a number of benefits of addressing health literacy in their practice, in particular by making their health settings more supportive for clients limited in literacy. Some suggested that there was better compliance with advice, decreased stress, and more confidence among their patients. As one practitioner said, "clients feel less intimidated. They are more likely to ask questions and have less anxiety when approaching the health-care system or worker."

Many of the suggestions for improvement were followed up by GASHA managers. Business-style cards with information about local adult learning programs were developed for practitioners to distribute, health literacy awareness was integrated into the orientation of new staff, written patient education materials were reviewed and revised, and signs and forms used in the workplace were made clearer. A plain-language specialist conducted a skill-building workshop for practitioners, and a network of literacy and health organizations and individuals was formed. Community partnerships resulted in other activities as well. For example, literacy network leaders in Richmond County engaged citizens in assisting seniors with using medications and accessing services. In partnership with the regional library, GASHA developed a health resource centre called Health Connections.

A health literacy policy was developed by GASHA and linked in 2006 to quality improvement recommendations directed to the senior leadership team. The policy called for the completion of a health literacy audit annually by staff and managers in all program areas. The audit was developed to engage staff and managers in assessing the extent to which their services and workplaces are in keeping with the policy objective to accommodate clients better at all literacy levels. The policy and audit tool were posted with other health literacy resources on the GASHA website (http://www.gasha.nshealth.ca).

In 2006, GASHA opened Health Connections, a health resource centre for community members to have better access to health information, programs, and services. In 2011, the value placed on literacy, health, and health literacy by organizations and citizens was reflected in the creation of a new gathering place called People's Place (http://www.peoplesplace.ca). People's Place houses the public library, ACALA's adult learning centre, and GASHA's Health Connections.

The interventions undertaken by GASHA created interest in taking action on improving health literacy in other district health authorities, the provincial health department, and other provinces. In 2005, the Health Literacy Awareness Initiative was created by the Nova Scotia Department of Health to facilitate awareness of health literacy among primary health-care providers across the province. The Nova Scotia Departments of Health and Education partnered with Communications Nova Scotia to create a health literacy DVD that highlights the participatory research and follow-up initiatives undertaken by GASHA.

Implications for Practice

Many lessons learned from this rural Nova Scotia experience have implications for advancing health literacy practice and policy in other rural communities. First and foremost was the importance of recognizing and respecting knowledge about the determinants of health held by community members. Although they did not have hard data on literacy and health, their intuitiveness and indigenous knowledge led members of the Community Health Board to ask critical questions that resulted in insightful and innovative ways to address what they saw as a serious problem relevant to the health of their population. Hearing the concerns of citizens and assisting them in finding answers to their questions was a responsibility accepted by the researchers who became partners in this effort. Citizens' identification of low literacy as a potential barrier to the health of the population, their desire to examine it through a participatory research process, and their focus on strengthening capacity throughout the district to advance health literacy policy and practice based on findings reflect Nutbeam's (2000) notion of critical health literacy, which is directed at improving individual and community capacity to address the social and economic determinants of health. According to Nutbeam, health literacy is not only of benefit to individuals but "also implies that the achievement of higher levels of health literacy among a greater proportion of the population will have social benefits, contributing, e.g., by enabling effective community action for health, and contributing to the development of social capital" (264).

Lessons were learned about the value of participatory research approaches and community-university collaboration and about the challenges of working across disciplines and fields of practice. Providing ways for partners to work and learn together to develop their understanding of health literacy as it related to the lives of people in this rural region was critical. A willingness to learn as the research process progressed was essential. For example, not adopting a definition of health literacy from the existing literature but engaging in a reflective learning process enabled partners to come to a shared understanding of health literacy as their research unfolded.

Although rigour in research was imperative, so was the need to be respectful of the skills, knowledge, and desire for ownership of findings of all participants. Important lessons were learned about identifying interview participants, enabling them to share their stories, capturing the richness and complexity of their insights in presenting findings, and continuing efforts to spur action based on the findings and calls for change. Both the researchers and the community partners had confidence in their findings and were committed to seeing the findings used to effect changes in practice and policy. Notably, the community partners were committed to disseminating and using the findings from their study to champion the change needed to address the health literacy concerns of their population and, especially among those residents facing barriers to health because of low literacy.

Acknowledgments

We acknowledge the commitment and collaboration of members from the following organizations: Antigonish County Adult Learning Association, Antigonish Town and County Community Health Board, Guysborough County Adult Learning Association, Guysborough Antigonish Strait Health Authority, and Richmond County Literacy Network. Special recognition is given to Evelyn Lindsey, former chair of the ATCCHB. The research was funded by the Social Sciences and Humanities Research Council of Canada.

Notes

1 The International Adult Literacy Survey (IALS) was conducted in 1994 by Statistics Canada and the Organization for Economic Cooperation and Development (OECD) to measure prose, document, and quantitative skills of Canadians aged sixteen to sixty-five. In 2003, the International Adult Literacy and Skills Survey (IALSS), also referred to as the Adult Literacy and Life Skills (ALLS) survey in Canada, was conducted with Canadians over sixteen years of age. It included a problem-solving component. Over 20,000 Canadians participated in the 2003 survey in either English or French.
2 To determine the relationship between health literacy and health, results from the IALLS were compared with responses to a self-reported quality-of-life tool (the SF-12) used by Statistics Canada.
3 Nova Scotia Department of Finance – Statistics 2006.
4 Unless otherwise noted, information profiling the population within GASHA is taken from the June 2005 Guysborough Antigonish Strait Health Authority Health Status and District Profile Update.
5 See http://www.targetnovascotia.com/.
6 IALLS 2003 survey data were accessed through personal communication by email with M. Lachance, Canadian Council on Learning, 4 July 2008.
7 Level 1 (0-225) reflects very low literacy skills; Level 2 (226-75) reflects a capacity to deal only with simple, clear material involving uncomplicated tasks; Level 3 (276-325) reflects adequate skills to cope with the demands of everyday life and work in an advanced society; and Level 4 (326-75) and Level 5 (376-500) reflect strong skills.
8 See http://www.ccl-cca.ca/. The analysis and mapping of the health literacy results were conducted by J. Douglas Willms, Canada Research Chair in Human Development at the University of New Brunswick (UNB), with the assistance of Teresa Tang, a GIS programmer at the Canadian Research Institute for Social Policy at UNB. The data for the local area maps are from the 2003 IALSS and the 2001 census.

References

Ad Hoc Committee on Health Literacy. 1999. "Health Literacy: Report of the Council on Scientific Affairs." *Journal of the American Medical Association* 281, 8: 552-57.
Berkman, N.D., D.A. DeWalt, M.P. Pignone, S.L. Sheridan, K.N. Lohr, L. Lux, et al. 2004. *Literacy and Health Outcomes Evidence Report/Technology Assessment No. 87.*

Agency for Healthcare Research and Quality (AHRQ) Publication No. 04-E007-2. Rockville, MD: AHRQ.

Canadian Council on Learning (CCL). 2007. *Health Literacy in Canada: Initial Results from the International Adult Literacy and Skills Survey.* Ottawa: CCL, http://www.ccl -cca.ca/.

– 2008. *Health Literacy in Canada: A Healthy Understanding.* Ottawa: CCL, http://www. ccl-cca.ca/.

Canadian Institute for Health Information (CIHI). 2006. *How Healthy Are Rural Canadians? An Assessment of Their Health Status and Health Determinants.* Ottawa: CIHI.

Canadian Public Health Association (CPHA). 2007. "Summary of Preliminary Findings of an Electronic Scan on Health Literacy." Unpublished report for the Expert Panel on Health Literacy. Ottawa: CPHA, http://www.cpha.ca/.

Gillis, D. 2007. "A Community-Based Approach to Health Literacy Using Participatory Research." *Adult Learning* 15, 1-2 [special issue on health literacy]: 14-17.

Gillis, D., A. MacIsaac, and B.A. Quigley. 2005. "If You Were Me, How Could You Make It Better? Responding to the Challenge of Literacy and Health." *Literacies* 5: 28-31.

Gillis, D.E., and B.A. Quigley. 2004. "Taking Off the Blindfold: Seeing How Literacy Affects Health in Rural Nova Scotia." Report of the Health Literacy in Rural Nova Scotia Research Project, http://www.nald.ca/.

Guysborough Antigonish Strait Health Authority (GASHA). 2005. Guysborough Antigonish Strait Health Authority Health Status and District Profile Update, June 2005. Antigonish, NS: GASHA.

Institute of Medicine (IOM). 2004. *Health Literacy: A Prescription to End Confusion.* Institute of Medicine (IOM) Report. Washington, DC: The National Academic Press.

King, J. 2007. *Environmental Scan of Interventions to Improve Health Literacy: Final Report.* Antigonish, NS: National Collaborating Centre for Determinants of Health, http://www.nccdh.ca/.

Maxwell, J., and T. Teplova. 2005. *Canada's Hidden Deficit: The Social Cost of Low Literacy Skills.* Canadian Language and Literacy Research Network, http://www.cllrnet. ca/.

Nutbeam, D. 2000. "Health Literacy as a Public Health Goal: A Challenge for Contemporary Health Education and Communication Strategies into the 21st Century." *Health Promotion International* 15: 359-67.

–. 2008. "The Evolving Concept of Health Literacy." *Social Science and Medicine* 67, 12: 2072-78.

Parikh, N.S., R.M. Parker, J.R. Nurss, D.W. Baker, and M.V. Williams. 1996. "Shame and Health Literacy: The Unspoken Connection." *Patient Education and Counselling* 27, 1: 33-39.

Quigley, A., S. Folinsbee, W. Kraglund-Gauthier, and L. Shohet. 2006. *The State of the Field Report: Adult Literacy.* Fredericton: University of New Brunswick National Adult Literacy Database, http://www.nald.ca/.

Ratzan, S., and R.M. Parker. 2000. "Introduction." In *National Academies of Medicine Current Bibliographies in Medicine: Health Literacy,* edited by C. Selden, M. Zorn, S.C. Ratzan, and R.M. Parker. Bethesda, MD: National Institutes of Health, US Department of Health and Human Services.

Ronson, B., and I. Rootman. 2008. "Literacy and Health Literacy: New Understandings about Their Impact on Health." In *Social Determinants of Health: Canadian Perspectives,* edited by D. Raphael, 170-85. Toronto: Canadian Scholars' Press.

Rootman, I. 2004. "Critical Issues in Literacy and Health." *Literacy across the Curriculu-media Focus* 17, 2: 8-10.

Rootman, I., and D. Gordon-El-Bihbety. 2008. *A Vision for a Health Literate Canada: Report of the Expert Panel on Health Literacy.* Ottawa: CPHA, http://www.cpha.ca/.

United Nations Educational, Scientific, and Cultural Organization (UNESCO). 2004. *The Plurality of Literacy and Its Implications for Policies and Programmes.* UNESCO Education Sector Position Paper ED-2004/WS/31. Paris: UNESCO.

Wolf, M.S., M.V. Williams, R.M. Parker, N.S. Parikh, A.W. Nowlan, and D.W. Baker. 2007. "Patients' Shame and Attitudes toward Discussing the Results of Literacy Screening." *Journal of Health Communication* 12: 721-32.

World Health Organization (WHO). 1998. *Health Promotion Glossary.* Geneva: WHO, http://www.who.int/.

Chapter 15

**Potholes along the Roads:
The Ethics of Health Research
in Rural and Remote Canada**

S. Wilson-Forsberg and J. Easley

Key Points

- People's understandings of health, illness, or ethics are naturally influenced by socio-cultural contexts. Ethics can take on different meanings in rural and remote communities, and this variance impacts the extent to which ethical dilemmas are identified and resolved by researchers.
- In rural and remote settings, disseminating research results can have major consequences for participants of the study as well as the entire community.
- To be a member of a rural community often means that close bonds exist, and there is an expectation that people involved in health research and health-care delivery engage in cultural mores and community events. It is important for the researcher to develop skills in assessing the potential harm or benefit of boundary crossings in the research and to discuss these situations with participants.
- Finley (2003) calls for research that embraces an "ethics of care." That research would deepen relationships, allow the voices of participants to be heard, and respond to culture, context, and community.

The winding roads of research are often bumpy at best. As researchers navigate their way through literature reviews, funding applications, and institutional ethics review boards, the final destination is not always close at hand or even known. Although it is only natural for a researcher to seek control and precision in analyzing and reporting phenomena, the discovery of novel or unanticipated findings makes the research journey all the more rewarding. Researchers who venture off the beaten paths and paved roads, away from urban settings, might be in for an even rougher ride. This is particularly true in the field of health research. Institutional ethics review boards are there early in the research process issuing roadmaps with travel details etched in ink. The ethics review process is clearly vital since important ethical issues need to be addressed to protect participants and carry out high-quality research; however, the urban context from which the guidelines are derived can create obstacles for rural health researchers.

Many of the ethical issues involved in rural health research are similar to those faced in an urban context, but rural and remote settings present additional challenges to researchers and require special attention. Although it is difficult to generalize about a particular culture or geographical area, a number of authors support the claim that health research in rural and remote communities presents unique ethical considerations (Cook and Hoas 2008; Fryer-Edwards 2006; Hardwig 2006; Helbok 2003; Klugman 2008; Nelson 2004; Nelson et al. 2007; Pierce and Scherra 2004; Prata Miller 2006; Simpson and Kirby 2004; Weiss Roberts, Battaglia, and Epstein 1999). Concerns such as confidentiality and anonymity pose exceptional challenges in small communities, where strangers are few and personal information seems to belong to everyone. As a result, researchers can be deterred as obstacles arise and their traditional research methods are not easily transferred to rural contexts (St. Lawrence and Ndiaye 1997). But equipped with knowledge of and respect for these qualities, they can be better prepared to avoid the "potholes" along the way and prevent making the roads worse for the people who live along them.

This chapter highlights three general areas of ethical concern when collecting health-related data in rural and remote communities and when disseminating the results of those data: (1) socio-cultural context; (2) confidentiality and anonymity; and (3) overlapping roles and relationships. The chapter is based on the published discussions and studies of researchers and practitioners in health and the social sciences supplemented by examples from my own experience as the primary author of this chapter currently in the final stages of a qualitative case study in rural New Brunswick. The case study focuses on the reception of immigrants by the residents of a small agricultural community. As immigrants arrive and integrate into the community, I document the changes that both they and the local residents undergo. Although the study is not specifically focused on health at the individual or community level, the deteriorating mental health of some of these newcomers has emerged as an important theme in the research. Although the research is uniquely Canadian, much of the literature cited is international in scope – primarily American and Australian – and, though the arguments are consistent across the literature, the chapter leaves it to readers to decide if the ethical concerns described would play out in the same way and with the same consistency in rural and remote communities throughout Canada.

As noted in Chapter 1 of this volume, "Rural and Small Town" refers to those populations living in towns and municipalities outside the commuting zones of larger urban centres in Canada. "Remote" refers to a location sufficiently far removed from the nearest community, such as a large urban centre, where out-commuting on a daily basis is impossible and where access to services, especially social and medical services, is difficult or impossible (Slack, Bourne, and Gertler 2003). Although these definitions of rural and remote are widely accepted across Canada, what they seem to be missing is a popular consciousness of "ruralness" (Halfacree 1995; Willett and Luloff 1995). Since rural communities are defined in academic literature and government reports almost strictly by comparison with non-rural communities, the socio-cultural context of what it means to be rural and remote is rarely considered. The emphasis on distinction from non-rural communities often encourages the misleading view that rural communities are homogeneous (Prata Miller 2006). Although rural and remote communities are similar in terms of low population density and distance from urban areas, they are actually very rich, diverse, and broad in culture, age, and ethnicity (Klugman 2008). The fastest-growing segments of rural communities in Canada and the United States, for example, are urbanites who choose to relocate for retirement and immigrants who follow jobs in manufacturing, forestry, and agricultural food processing. It is within this setting of rural and remote communities, with all of their richness and complexity, that researchers collect, analyze, and disseminate health-related data. And it is within this setting that the above three ethical considerations can come to light and require attention.

Rural Lives: The Socio-Cultural Context

As pointed out in Chapter 11 of this volume, shifting demographics in many rural areas have contributed to rather rapid rural changes. But despite these changes, some authors argue that people in sparsely settled and remote areas have displayed a distinctive socio-cultural pattern. Keller and Murray (1982, 8) identify three values that appear repeatedly in research on rural and remote communities: (1) an emphasis on hard work and mastery of the physical environment; (2) an emphasis on the importance of family and community ties; and (3) an orientation toward traditional moral standards and conformity to group norms.

People's understandings of health, illness, or ethics are naturally influenced by this socio-cultural context. For example, several participants in a study of the health beliefs of rural Canadians by Thomlinson and colleagues (2004, 261) equate being healthy with not having to go to physicians or hospitals. When asked about what unhealthy meant to them, many of the participants noted "not being able to do" something or "not having the strength or ability to do anything." This inability to do things is consistent with the reference in Chapter 4 of this volume to people living in rural areas defining health as the capacity to be economically productive. Likewise, Long (1993) found that rural dwellers tend to view health from a role performance perspective that meant being able to work and meet family obligations. In accordance with these findings, Klugman (2008, 57) gives the example of the farmer suffering from diabetes who does not consider himself sick because he can still get out of bed in the morning and run the farm. He is healthy as long as he can pull his weight. Rural and remote community members are also more likely to use informal supports such as family, neighbours, and the church when they are sick. "Going to the healthcare provider is considered an option of last resort," writes Klugman. "Not only does such a move have moral overtures that one lacks hardiness, but pragmatically, going to a medical practitioner often means going far from home and burdening the family" (57).

Ethics can take on different meanings in rural and remote communities as well, and this variance impacts the extent to which ethical dilemmas are identified and resolved by researchers (Cook and Hoas 2008). As Nelson and colleagues (2007, 138) point out, "ethical conflicts arise when there is insufficient recognition and respect for indigenous rural values or when the researcher overemphasizes published, traditional bioethics or personal values." In a multi-method study of what rural residents recognize as ethical dilemmas and how they resolve them, Cook and Hoas (2008) found that health researchers and health-care providers do encounter moral dilemmas but not necessarily the ones expected or described by institutional ethics review boards. Because the study participants did not refer to major bio-ethics theories, but rather to the social, political, and economic contexts in which the ethical issues unfold, the authors concluded that "discussions about moral dilemmas are not necessarily framed with the careful, formal language or methodology of ethics" (Cook and Hoas 2008, 51).

By way of illustration, Fryer-Edwards (2006) describes a radio program in rural United States called *The Hospital Report.* The announcer would mention who was in the hospital on that given day. According to Fryer-Edwards, "when they heard that Mr. Jones was in the hospital, the ranchers nearby knew to plan an extra stop at the Jones ranch to give a hand with the cattle. With many of the elderly in the community living alone, on various medications and managing chronic illnesses, they relied upon neighbours to look in on them" (55). When the program was deemed unethical and subsequently cancelled by the state government, the community protested that, on the contrary, taking the program off the air was unethical. It seems that this radio program served as a highly functional support network for this independent yet interdependent community and that cancelling it interfered with that informal support system.

Addressing health issues through informal social support networks certainly resonates with my research experience. The residents of my case community are generally very welcoming of the substantial numbers of immigrants who have recently settled there. However, they do not readily recognize or respond to the emotional and mental distress that some of these newcomers experience as they struggle to overcome their initial culture shock and attempt to integrate into the community. Like the elderly women in rural Saskatchewan and Ontario described in Chapters 22 and 26 of this volume, immigrants in rural New Brunswick experience social isolation caused by language barriers and lack of transportation. This is especially the case for women who often stay at home alone while their husbands work and children attend school. Some of these women live a lonely existence completely cut off from their new community.

According to the community residents whom I interviewed, when psychological problems such as anxiety and depression develop, individuals are expected to deal with the problems within their families or perhaps by talking with a family physician. The community residents are tightly knit and have fostered a strong support network, which the immigrants are either unaware of or unable to penetrate. Furthermore, as mentioned in Chapter 4 in this book, many health facilities and services, often taken for granted in large cities, are not available in rural communities. Because many newcomers lack the English skills and transportation necessary to access mental health services outside the community, they have nowhere to go for help. The stories that I heard from the immigrants and native-born participants in the community are consistent with the published literature, which demonstrates the difficulties of noticing and addressing the health needs of vulnerable populations in rural settings. Maddalena and Sherwin (2004), for example, demonstrate that significant and systematic health disparities exist between mainstream and vulnerable populations and that these inequities are exacerbated by the challenges associated with rural living.

Given the above situation, and others like it, Hardwig (2006, 54) suggests that researchers should view rural communities as a foreign land, to be heard and understood "without forcing it [the rural community] into our familiar language of an urban bioethics bias." Klugman (2008) recommends that as researchers we need to engage community members, asking them which health and ethical issues they perceive, how their issues are resolved, and which resources they think they need. And Lightfoot and colleagues (2008) stress that, when possible, the researcher or research team should have a regular and ongoing presence in the community during all phases of the study and include local expertise in all of its aspects.

Some authors assert that, in addition to respect, beneficence, and justice, guidelines on ethics in research involving human subjects should include *respect for community* (Levine 1991; Weijer 1999). The additional tenet implies that community concerns are distinguishable from individual ones and that communities have moral status as collectives. The authors specifically refer to Aboriginal people in Canada, who commonly see a lack of collaboration and community focus in research as a serious ethical issue, even in research designs that have received ethics approval from institutional review boards (Lightfoot et al. 2008, 163). Although the addition of a formal, community-level guideline is debatable (see Juengst 1998), the level and type of community involvement in research efforts are changing (Estroff 1999; Weijer 1999). In some cases, the role of the community has expanded to include setting the research agenda, approving the research design, monitoring implementation processes, approving publications and presentations, and requiring ownership of data and results (Kaufman and Saumya 2005).

Fishbowl Ethics: Confidentiality and Anonymity in Rural and Remote Settings

When researchers embark on a research project, it is usually with the hope of discovering new information or shedding light on a topic or population previously under-studied. To do so, the onus is on researchers to share their results with as wide an audience as possible, including the participants and their community. This is most often accomplished through academic publications, the popular press, lay research summaries, and presentations. However, in rural and remote settings, disseminating research results could have major consequences for the participants of the study as well as the entire community. It takes but a tiny stone to make big waves in a small pond. Overlapping social networks bring community members together as neighbours, sharing resources and potentially having regular contact (Nelson 2004). Along with this sharing comes the increased probability of shared information and knowledge of others. Finding the ethical balance in the context of familiarity is often difficult as respect for confidentiality and privacy becomes more complex (D'Agincourt-Canning 2004).

Researchers often protect the confidentiality of participants and their activities by making them anonymous: that is, either by not recording names and other data or by removing names and other identifying information at the earliest possible stage (Israel and Hay 2006). Although undoubtedly there are ethical justifications for making individuals anonymous in research data, the process is fraught with practical difficulties, and nowhere are these difficulties more obvious than conducting health research in a small, remote place. Life in rural and remote communities has often been compared with life inside a fishbowl, where nothing is hidden and everyone knows everything about everyone else (Weiss Roberts, Battaglia, and Epstein 1999). If confidentiality cannot be assured, then there can be serious consequences for research participants. For example, a participant can be identified as having disclosed mental health information or details about a sexually transmitted disease that might affect his or her personal and professional relationships, or a perceived lack of anonymity might bias the answers given by research participants. They might feel compelled to lie in an interview in order to protect themselves or others from potential negative outcomes of the research, which could be anything from the loss of day-care or health-care services to the loss of a job or friends within the community.

Researchers also often disguise the identity of the community being studied. In part, this is to protect participants further from being identified, but it also protects the locale from potentially negative reporting, which could perpetuate stigmatizing discourses about it (Clark 2006). Research projects undertaken in rural and remote communities might not be publishable if the population is identifiable, and this might deter researchers from undertaking rural research (Fraser and Alexander 2006). Yet confidentiality in a small community is a much bigger problem than simply using pseudonyms or ensuring anonymity (Evans 2004). A community's identity is likely to be purposefully or accidentally discovered regardless, especially if community members, government officials, and the university are aware of the research. Moreover, even if location identifiers are removed from the data, places remain identifiable because they are constructed through stories and myths, gossip, and historical events (Clark 2006).

De-identified case studies have been suggested as a way to deal with this issue; however, to take out the contextual description of an interview or observation risks losing the rich details that make the setting unique. For example, in New Brunswick, rural economies are industry driven. These industries are very much an identifying factor in the overall community and individual experiences in that community. To take away contextual details, such as the effects of mill closures or other distinctive details about the community at large, diminishes the significance of the current experiences. According to Lutz (1995, 253), de-identification "takes the focus off the community, separates stories from their origin and strips the experiences of research participants of their reference to a concrete phenomenal world of specific contexts and history." Other practical considerations here include the verification of data and potential policy implications. Among other things, triangulation of data necessitates going back to the interviewees and research setting to verify facts. It would be challenging to do so if the names of people and places were removed in the early stages of data collection. The data might also have an applied dimension, and it is very difficult to contribute to policy discourse when the name of the case study has been changed. Even if the interested parties can see through the pseudonym, they might be less likely to take the research seriously and engage with its real-life implications.

As I discovered in my research, not all individuals desire anonymity. With the authorization of the institutional ethics review board at the University of New Brunswick, many of my research participants over the age of eighteen have waived anonymity. Although the potential for doing harm to research participants in my case study is very low, I am still interested in their personal views and circumstances. The participants, however, want their stories to be read and their community to be recognized. They have explicitly requested on the individual voluntary consent forms that their real names and places of origin be used, so I have been giving them a copy of the analyzed data to ensure accuracy. At that time, I ask again if they would like to be identified and formalize their consent or refusal in writing. If I cannot meet with individuals in person before and after they read the report due to the distance of the case study community from my locale, I send it as an email attachment or through priority mail and correspond with them in the same manner.

With regard to revealing the identity of the case study community, I requested permission from all research participants and gatekeepers involved in the study to refer to the community by its actual name, and they unanimously agreed that the community should be identified. This does not constitute "community consent," but the sample does involve a substantial number of people. Place of origin is another potential identifier in my research that most participants have given me permission to use. I believe that place of origin, along with immigration and settlement history, clearly provides context for a deeper understanding of these people's stories and should not be anonymous. In an effort to conceal place of origin, researchers frequently apply broad, pan-ethnic labels, such as black, Hispanic, or Asian. Trimble (1990) refers to this attempt at anonymity as "ethnic gloss." It produces overgeneralizations about the experiences of ethnic minorities and neglects the unique differences among individuals within various racial and ethnic groups.

The Ethics of Familiarity: Overlapping Roles and Relationships

Various authors have noted that people in rural and remote communities know one another, depend on one another, and share many common relationships (see Healy 2003; Helbok 2003; Simpson and Kirby

2004; Smith and Fitzpatrick 1995; St. Germaine 1993; and Stockman 1990). To be a member of a rural community often means that close bonds exist, and there is an expectation that people involved in health research and health-care delivery engage in cultural mores and community events (Galambos et al. 2006). Again, in this situation, prevailing standards and codes of ethics cannot be applied in automatic ways.

The bulk of the literature on overlapping roles and relationships in rural and remote communities focuses on boundary crossing between mental health practitioners and their clients (see Campbell and Gordon 2003; Faulkner and Faulkner 1997; and Horst 1989). In a study of college therapists in rural communities, Sharkin and Birky (1992) found that 95 percent of therapists in their sample had accidental meetings with clients. Non-professional interactions in rural settings ran the gamut from minor accidental meetings to substantial overlapping relationships. Schank and Skovholt (1997) surveyed members of the Minnesota Psychological Association practising in rural areas and found that all respondents reported overlapping relationships. Health researchers in rural communities are not often practitioners, but many of us do have face-to-face contact with research participants through often lengthy interviews, and we possess very personal information. In these regards, the mental health literature is consistent with our reality.

Like health practitioners, researchers who are immersed in a rural and remote community while collecting qualitative or quantitative data might also experience difficulties in maintaining their own privacy when encountering research participants outside the interview setting. Even if the researcher is an outsider residing in that community temporarily to carry out research, it is important to be seen in the community and to be involved in activities that build trust and acceptance for the professional role (Horst 1989; Schank and Skovholt 1997). This "ethics of familiarity" (as referred to by Simpson and Kirby 2004) can affect the ability of the researcher to create an optimal, safe place for people to discuss the details of their life experiences. It also affects whom to approach as the gatekeeper, the person who gives consent to conduct research in a community, and whom to interview. Creating alliances exclusively with one group or upsetting the local balance by overlooking rivalries can have serious effects on the study outcomes and the study population itself. Researchers in rural settings must quickly become aware of the unspoken community rules and local hot topics, or they risk being considered untrustworthy (Glover 2001).

In my case community, the boundary lines are very blurred as multiple levels of interactions take place on a daily basis. The food-processing plant that employs most of the immigrant participants also provides them with basic settlement services and language training; it contributes funding to and oversees the local multicultural association, and it organizes many other community initiatives. The immigrant participants are clearly hesitant to relay negative stories about the community, perhaps not wanting what could be construed as complaints to be heard by their employer and caretaker, the food-processing company. As a result, they almost overwhelmingly speak of the community in positive terms. This brings to mind my exposure to multiple versions of the same story (yet another aspect of overlapping roles and relationships featured in the available literature; see, e.g., Endacott et al. 2006).

The immigrants participating in my case study claim to feel very welcome, and they refer to the community as very friendly and accommodating. Nevertheless, these positive stories are more often than not accompanied by references to culture shock, isolation, loneliness, and even depression. These stories have led me to cross boundaries on a number of occasions by playing matchmaker – finding less than subtle ways to introduce immigrant participants from the same cultural background, or to mix local residents and immigrants in one room, while at the same time seeking to remain "empathetically neutral" and attempting to "not disturb the natural surroundings of the research site" (Patton 2001, 49; Madison 2005, 121).

In short, researchers working in small, isolated rural communities usually do not have a choice about entering a dual relationship. Thus, the focus needs to be on managing the dual relationships (Endacott et al. 2006). Reamer (2003) contends that boundary crossings in such a natural setting are not always harmful; however, it is important for the researcher to develop skills in assessing the potential harms or benefits of boundary crossings that might present themselves in the research and to discuss these situations with the participants. Galambos and colleagues (2006) urge researchers to obtain informed consent, protect confidentiality, and explain the limits of confidentiality by discussing any overlapping relationships. St. Germaine (1993) suggests that these situations can even become opportunities to see participants function in the social setting. Information received in informal settings or outside the realm of the research relationship presents challenges to the researcher, but at the same time this information is a very important part of the research. Although this is true of quantitative research, qualitative inquiry is especially influenced by Lincoln and Guba's (1985) "naturalistic inquiry," which emphasizes "a commitment to studying human action in some setting that is not contrived, manipulated, or artificially fashioned by the inquirer" (Schwandt 1997, 174).

Conclusion: Research Ethics in Rural and Remote Communities

In sum, as researchers make their way along the roads of rural and remote health research in Canada, they should proceed with caution. It is important to approach these communities with knowledge of, and sensitivity to, the values that might be in place and the awkward situations that can arise. These ethical potholes might be unavoidable, but the risk of damage is lowered with due caution and awareness of the issues.

In the long term, we suggest that serious thought should be given to including a section within the *Tri-Council Policy Statement for Ethical Conduct for Research Involving Humans (TCPS)* outlining a few key points for "good ethical practices" in rural and remote communities (Canada 1998). A similar list is already in the *TCPS* (section 6B) in regard to research involving Aboriginal peoples. The list could be comprised of a number of common, reoccurring ethical considerations in relation to this special population, including the three topics addressed in this chapter. Accompanying these guidelines should be the development and implementation of ethics-training curricula and other educational resources for researchers embarking on projects in rural and remote Canada. Research ethics training is not a mandatory course for doctoral students at most universities in Canada. Those research ethics courses that have been designed for graduate students do not have a specific rural and remote community component, which is unfortunate given the large and underresearched rural and remote areas in Canada. As noted in this chapter, a research ethics agenda in the health field should include increased awareness and understanding of ethical issues as perceived by rural residents, including the contextual influences on ethical issues and how the issues are different from those in non-rural settings. It should also include increased dialogue with the general health-care ethics community regarding the unique nature of rural ethical issues and greater collaboration between rural health researchers and rural health-care professionals (Nelson et al. 2007).

In the short term, however, we realize that it is rarely possible to make all of the ethical decisions relating to the research before it begins.

As Cloke and colleagues (2000, 136) point out, "ethical issues arise or are shaped contextually, and therefore need to be addressed by researchers in a situated manner." Researchers should therefore approach these ethical concerns with flexibility. Villa-Vicencio (1994, 75) writes that "the experience of most researchers in attempting to employ ethical practices is that the demands of the actual situation or context are as important as the ethical norms on which one draws in deciding on what is morally right." Fryer-Edwards (2006) emphasizes that as rural researchers we should focus less on the rule or standard and get back to the ethical motivation for that rule or standard.

The practice of ethics, then, has to be flexible; however, for that flexibility not to be reduced to mere relativism, it becomes necessary to instill in researchers what Johnson (1993, 202) refers to as the "moral imagination": that is, "the ability to imaginatively discern various possibilities for acting in a given situation and to envision the potential help and harm that are likely to result from a given action" (see also Hay 1998; and Werhane 1999). Here "the standard ethical prompts for research have to be set against the complexities arising from the shifting multiple identities of the researchers, the multi-functional roles and positions we find ourselves in and the varying circumstances in which 'we' relate to 'them' and vice versa," write Cloke and colleagues (2000, 142). On a similar and appropriate concluding note, Finley (2003) calls for research that embraces an "ethics of care." That research would deepen relationships, allow the voices of participants to be heard, and respond to culture, context, and community. It would seek not to hide but to display the positionality of the researcher, it would allow for the blurring of roles in the research setting, and it would encourage reciprocity between researcher and participants.

References

Campbell, C.D., and M.C. Gordon. 2003. "Acknowledging the Inevitable: Understanding Multiple Relationships in Rural Practice." *Professional Psychology Research and Practice* 34, 4: 430-34.

Canada. Panel on Research Ethics. 1998. *Tri-Council Policy Statement: Ethical Conduct for Research Involving Humans 1998 (with 2000, 2002, 2005 Amendments).* Ottawa, http://www.pre.ethics.gc.ca/.

Clark, A. 2006. "Anonymizing Research Data." Real Life Methods Working Paper, University of Manchester, http://www.reallifemethods.ac.uk/.

Cloke, P., P. Cooke, J. Cursons, P. Milbourne, and R. Widdowfield. 2000. "Ethics, Reflexivity, and Research: Encounters with Homeless People." *Ethics, Place, and Environment* 3, 2: 133-54.

Cook, A.F., and H. Hoas. 2008. "Revisiting Ethics and Rural Healthcare: What Really Happens? What Might Help?" *American Journal of Bioethics* 8, 4: W3-W4.

D'Agincourt-Canning, L. 2004. "Genetic Testing for Hereditary Cancer: Challenges to Ethical Care in Rural and Remote Communities." *HEC Forum* 16, 4: 222-33.

Endacott, R., S. Kidd, M. Deacon-Crouch, F. Judd, M. Menzel, and M. Cornett. 2006. "Developing New Services for Eating Disorders: An Evaluation Study." *Australasian Psychiatry* 14: 57-62.

Estroff, S.E. 1999. "The Gaze of Scholars and Subjects: Rights, Roles, and Obligations in Ethnographic Research." In *Beyond Regulations: Ethics in Human Subjects Research,* edited by N.M.P. King et al., 72-80. Chapel Hill: University of North Carolina Press.

Evans, M. 2004. "Ethics, Anonymity, and Authorship in Community Centred Research or Anonymity and the Island Cache." *Pimatisiwin: A Journal of Aboriginal and Indigenous Community Health* 2, 1: 59-75.

Faulkner, K.K., and T.A. Faulkner. 1997. "Managing Multiple Relationships in Rural Communities: Neutrality and Boundary Violations." *Clinical Psychology: Science and Practice* 3: 225-34.

Finley, S. 2003. "Arts-Based Inquiry in QI: Seven Years from Crisis to Guerrilla Warfare." *Qualitative Inquiry* 9, 2: 281-96.

Fraser, J., and C. Alexander. 2006. "Publish and Perish: A Case Study of Publication Ethics in a Rural Community." *Journal of Medical Ethics* 32: 526-29.

Fryer-Edwards, K. 2006. "On Cattle and Casseroles." *Rural Healthcare Ethics* 6, 2: 55-56.

Galambos, C., J. Wilson-Watt, K. Anderson, and F. Danis. 2005. "Ethics Forum Rural Social Work Practice: Maintaining Confidentiality in the Face of Dual Relationships." *Journal of Social Work, Values, and Ethics* 2, 2, http://www.socialworker.com/.

Glover, J.J. 2001. "Rural Bioethical Issues of the Elderly: How Do They Differ from Urban Ones?" *Journal of Rural Health* 17, 4: 332-35.

Halfacree, K.H. 1995. "Household Migration and the Structuration of Patriarchy: Evidence from the USA." *Progress in Human Geography* 19, 2: 159-82.

Hardwig, J. 2006. "Rural Health Care Ethics: What Assumptions and Attitudes Should Drive the Research?" *American Journal of Bioethics* 6, 2: 53-54.

Hay, I. 1998. "Making Moral Imaginations: Research Ethics, Pedagogy, and Professional Human Geography." *Ethics, Place, and Environment* 1, 1: 55-76.

Healy, T.C. 2003. "Ethical Practice Issues in Rural Perspective." *Journal of Gerontological Social Work* 41, 4: 265-85.

Helbok, C.M. 2003. "The Practice of Psychology in Rural Communities: Potential Ethical Dilemmas." *Ethics and Behaviour* 13, 4: 367-84.

Horst, E.A. 1989. "Dual Relationships between Psychologists and Clients in Rural and Urban Areas." *Journal of Rural Community Psychology* 10, 2: 15-24.

Israel, M., and I. Hay. 2006. *Research Ethics for Social Scientists.* London: Sage.

Johnson, M. 1993. *Moral Imagination: Implications of Cognitive Science for Ethics.* Chicago: University of Chicago Press.

Juengst, E.T. 1998. "Groups as Gatekeepers to Genomic Research: Conceptually Confusing, Morally Hazardous, and Practically Useless." *Kennedy Institute of Ethics Journal* 8, 2: 183-200.

Kaufman, C., and R. Saumya. 2005. "Community Confidentiality, Consent, and the Individual Research Process: Implications for Demographic Research." *Population Research and Policy Review* 24, 2: 149-73.

Keller, P.A., and J.D. Murray. 1982. *Handbook of Rural Community Mental Health.* New York: Human Sciences Press.

Klugman, C.M. 2008. "Vast Tracts of Land: Rural Healthcare Culture." *American Journal of Bioethics* 8, 4: 57-58.

Levine, R.J. 1991. "Informed Consent: Some Challenges to the Universal Validity of the Western Mode." *Law, Medicine, and Health Care* 19, 3-4: 207-13.

Lightfoot, N., R. Strasser, M. Maar, and K. Jacklin. 2008. "Challenges and Rewards of Health Research in Northern, Rural, and Remote Communities." *Annals of Epidemiology* 18: 507-14.

Lincoln, Y.S., and E.G. Guba. 1985. *Naturalistic Inquiry.* Beverly Hills, CA: Sage.

Long, K.A. 1993. "The Concept of Health: Rural Perspectives." *Nursing Clinics of North America* 28: 123-30.

Lutz, C. 1995. "The Gender of Theory." In *Women Writing Culture,* edited by R. Behar and D. Gordon, 249-66. Berkeley: University of California Press.

Maddalena, V., and S. Sherwin. 2004. "Vulnerable Populations in Rural Areas: Challenges for Ethics Committees." *HEC Forum* 6, 4: 234-46.

Madison, D.S. 2005. *Critical Ethnography: Method, Ethics, and Performance.* Thousand Oaks, CA: Sage.

Nelson, W. 2004. "Addressing Rural Ethics Issues." *Healthcare Executive* 19, 4: 36-37.

Nelson, W., A. Pomerantz, K. Howard, and A. Bushy. 2007. "A Proposed Rural Healthcare Ethics Agenda." *Journal of Medical Ethics* 3, 3: 136-39.

Patton, M.Q. 2001. *Qualitative Research and Evaluation Methods.* 3rd ed. Thousand Oaks, CA: Sage.

Pierce, C., and E. Scherra. 2004. "The Challenges of Data Collection in Rural Dwelling Samples." *Online Journal of Rural Nursing and Health Care* 4, 2: 25-30, http://www.rno.org/.

Prata Miller, J. 2006. "Defining Research in Rural Healthcare Ethics." *Rural Healthcare Ethics* 6, 2: 59-61.

Reamer, F.G. 2003. "Boundary Issues in Social Work: Managing Dual Relationships." *Social Work* 48: 121-33.

Schank, J.A., and T.M. Skovholt. 1997. "Dual-Relationship Dilemmas of Rural and Small-Community Psychologists." *Professional Psychology: Research and Practice* 28, 1: 44-49.

Schwandt, T.A. 1997. *Qualitative Inquiry: A Dictionary of Terms.* Thousand Oaks, CA: Sage.

Sharkin, B.S., and I. Birky. 1992. "Incidental Encounters between Therapists and Their Clients." *Professional Psychology: Research and Practice* 23, 4: 326-28.

Simpson, C., and J. Kirby. 2004. "Organizational Ethics and Social Justice in Practice: Choices and Challenges in a Rural-Urban Health Region." *HEC Forum* 16, 4: 274-83.

Slack, E., L.S. Bourne, and M. Gertler. 2003. *Small, Rural, and Remote Communities: The Anatomy of Risk.* Panel on the Role of Government Research Report 18. Toronto: Office of the Premier.

Smith, D., and M. Fitzpatrick. 1995. "Boundary Issues in Counseling and Psychotherapy: An Integrative Review of Theory and Research. *Professional Psychology: Research and Practice* 26: 499-507.

St. Germaine, J. 1993. "Dual Relationships: What's Wrong with Them?" *American Counselor* 2, 3: 25-30.

St. Lawrence, J.S., and S.M. Ndiaye. 1997. "Prevention Research in Rural Communities: Overview and Concluding Comments." *American Journal of Community Psychology* 25, 4: 545-62.

Stockman, A.F. 1990. "Dual Relationships in Rural Mental Health Practice: An Ethical Dilemma." *Journal of Rural Community Psychology* 11: 31-45.

Thomlinson, M., K. McDonagh, K. Baird Crooks, and M. Lees. 2004. "Health Beliefs of Rural Canadians: Implications for Practice." *Australian Journal of Rural Health* 12, 6: 258-63.

Trimble, J.E. 1990. "Ethnic Specification, Validation Prospects, and Future of Drug Abuse Research." *International Journal of the Addictions* 25: 149-69.

Villa-Vicencio, C. 1994. "Ethics of Responsibility." In *Doing Ethics in Context,* edited by C. Villa-Vicencio and J. Grucy, 75-88. Maryknoll, NY: Orbis Books.

Weijer, C. 1999. "Protecting Communities in Research: Philosophical and Pragmatic Challenges." *Cambridge Quarterly of Healthcare Ethics* 8: 501-13.

Weiss Roberts, L., J. Battaglia, and R.S. Epstein. 1999. "Frontier Ethics: Mental Healthcare Needs and Ethical Dilemmas in Rural Communities." *Psychiatric Services* 50: 497-503.

Werhane, P.H. 1999. *Moral Imagination and Management Decision Making.* New York: Oxford University Press.

Willett, F., and A. Luloff. 1995. "Urban Residents' Views of Rurality and Contacts with Rural Places." *Rural Sociology* 60: 454-66.

Part 5: Rural Health Issues

Chapter 16   **"Beyond Tired of Driving that Far":**
HIV/AIDS Information Exchange in
Rural Canada

R. Harris, T. Veinot, L. Bella, and J. Krajnak

Key Points

- Insights from the field of library and information science provide a useful framework for understanding the exchange of HIV/AIDS-related information in rural communities.
- If members of rural communities hold stigmatizing beliefs about HIV/AIDS, are unaware that it exists among them, and/or have little knowledge of the disease, then rural people living with HIV/AIDS (PHAs) and their family members can be silenced, and little accurate, up-to-date information is likely to be exchanged through local networks.
- Because travelling long distances for care extracts a heavy toll from PHAs, interdisciplinary HIV health-care teams should offer regular, travelling clinics in rural areas, especially for routine care. These teams can also provide education, in collaboration with local AIDS service organizations (ASOs), to increase the capacity of community members, including local health and social service providers, improve prevention, and respond more effectively to those affected by the disease.

Canadians who live in rural, remote, and northern regions of the country face special challenges when it comes to maintaining their health (Mitura and Bollman 2003; Sutherns, McPhedran, and Haworth-Brockman 2004). In comparison with urban dwellers, they experience more accidents, poisonings, and incidents of violence; they face a higher prevalence of health risk factors, shorter life expectancies, and higher rates of disability (Chapters 2 and 3 of this volume); they are more likely to feel that their health-care needs are not being met (Mitura and Bollman 2003); and they can find it more difficult to gain access to immediate care (Sanmartin and Ross 2006). When seeking health care, rural residents commonly encounter barriers such as severe weather, inadequate transportation systems, limited local health and social services, few choices among service providers, and a lack of privacy (Harris and Wathen 2007). For those who are coping with complex, chronic, and/or stigmatized health conditions, such as people living with HIV/AIDS, life in a rural or remote community can be particularly difficult.

To manage their health effectively, PHAs and their caregivers require reliable, up-to-date information on HIV/AIDS and its treatment (Canadian AIDS Treatment Information Exchange 2003; Hogan and Palmer 2005). However, if they live in a geographically remote and possibly medically under-serviced area, then ready access to such information might be difficult. In this chapter, we explore the issues associated with the exchange of HIV/AIDS-related information in rural communities. Drawing on material gathered during more than 100 interviews with PHAs and their caregivers from British Columbia, Ontario, and Newfoundland, we describe how networks of HIV/AIDS-related information exchange operate in rural areas and how they can facilitate or block access to needed support.

HIV/AIDS

An estimated 58,000 PHAs live in Canada, and approximately 2,300 to 4,500 new infections occur each year (Boulos et al. 2006). The disease primarily affects men who have sex with men and injection drug users, although the rate of infection is rising among women and Aboriginal people (Public Health Agency of Canada 2007). Although new drug therapies have had a dramatic impact on the treatment of HIV/AIDS and reduced AIDS-associated morbidity and mortality (Schanzer 2003), these therapies are not a cure, and many PHAs face significant challenges in coping with complex medication regimes, medication side effects, and co-morbidities with conditions such as hepatitis C (Canadian AIDS Treatment Information Exchange 2003).

When managing their health, PHAs who live in rural areas are often at a disadvantage. For instance, although rural dwellers in general might have more difficulty finding a physician than urban dwellers (Statistics Canada 2004), the problem is exacerbated for PHAs. In the United States, many general practitioners have stopped providing HIV care (Lewis and Donohoe 2000), and in Ontario only about 100 of the approximately 13,000 family physicians routinely order HIV tests and provide HIV care (Ontario Advisory Committee on HIV/AIDS 2003). Indeed, the lack of HIV prevention, support, and treatment services has been identified as a serious weakness in the province's HIV/AIDS service infrastructure (Ontario Advisory Committee on HIV/AIDS 2003). PHAs are likely to receive better care from physicians with higher HIV caseloads (Golin, Smith, and Reif 2004), and physicians who practise in rural and remote settings often lack specific HIV/AIDS-related training. Most have limited experience providing HIV-related care. Therefore, it is not surprising that PHAs from rural areas often choose to, or have little choice but to, travel to urban centres for care. In fact, a US study revealed that "almost three quarters of rural residents with HIV/AIDS obtained their health care in urban areas" and that the majority of these PHAs "incurred significant inconvenience in obtaining care, had substantially longer mean travel times, and over 25 percent had put off obtaining care in the past 6 months because they did not have a way to get to their provider" (Schur et al. 2002, 337).

Apart from an important exploratory study based on a small sample of respondents (Groft and Vollman 2007), relatively little research has focused specifically on the experiences of PHAs who live in rural Canada. However, some reports suggest that the local presence of the disease in these areas is largely unacknowledged and that the conservative attitudes prevalent in some small communities can result in both isolation of members of at-risk populations (e.g., injection drug users and gay men) and limited attention to their needs in health-care and social service planning. In British Columbia, for example, Marchand (2001, 55) reported that "prejudice and discrimination against gay men and lesbians continue to be part of the culture, especially in smaller communities. Religious organizations and older generations of citizens are often the community gatekeepers. They influence local funding, access to schools and the development of community health programs."

The infrastructure that supports HIV/AIDS-related information exchange for PHAs and their caregivers is also unevenly distributed outside Canada's urban centres. Although AIDS service organizations, a diverse collection of resource and support groups, do exist in some rural areas, many small communities have no such groups (for a listing of Canadian ASOs, see the website of the Canadian AIDS Society, http://www.pwhce.ca). Even where they do exist, local ASOs are often staffed largely by volunteers who come and go. These ASOs might not always be welcoming to members of at-risk groups, and some lack connections with other relevant organizations. For instance, the linkages between gay community groups and ASOs in British Columbia have been described as "fragile" (Marchand 2001, 56). Given this fragmentation, how is HIV/AIDS-related information passed to and between rural-dwelling PHAs and the caregivers who support them?

Understanding Information Exchange

Understanding how people look for information and how their access to information can be facilitated or blocked is crucial to delivering relevant health and social services, yet this process is not always recognized or taken into account in the design of service delivery systems (Harris and Dewdney 1994). Research from the field of library and information science (LIS) provides useful insights into what is sometimes referred to as "everyday life information seeking" (Spink and Cole 2001). For instance, it is well documented that (1) information needs arise from personal contexts; (2) information seekers rely on sources that are readily accessible (often regardless of quality), especially interpersonal sources, particularly from others like themselves; and (3) information seekers expect emotional support to be wrapped into the delivery of information, regardless of the type of problem for which help is sought (Harris and Dewdney 1994). Common obstacles to successful information searches have also been identified. For example, the information necessary to resolve a problem might not exist, or the person looking for help might be unsure what information is needed to resolve a problem and where to locate the information. The help seeker might also be unaware that information relevant to the problem actually exists. Language and literacy issues (including the ability to navigate successfully using information technology) pose additional barriers, especially when information relevant to the searcher's problem is particularly complex or technical. The last challenge is discussed at length in Chapter 14 of this volume, where the authors describe the importance of "health literacy" in enabling people to use information to enhance their health.

Along with the various factors that influence successful information seeking, all of us live in information environments in which we are exposed to material incidentally, through conversation, reading, and popular media. This "incidental information" plays a significant role in everyday life decisions, including those related to health (Williamson 1998). Local gatekeepers or mediators who participate in the exchange of incidental information can influence the knowledge bases of communities by linking individuals, groups, and organizations, both inside and outside the immediate community, and by filtering information that is passed through these links or networks (Agada 1999). These networks can facilitate or constrain information exchange by affecting those with whom actors can make contact, which information their contacts can provide, and to which contacts actors can forward information (Haythornthwaite 1996). The positions of actors within the networks indicate who controls, inhibits, or facilitates the flow of information and the nature of the connections or ties between the actors. In other words, the structure of the network helps to reveal how information flows through the social environment.

In the study described here, we identify some of the barriers and facilitators that influence the exchange of HIV/AIDS–related information in rural communities and explore the nature and extent of the links that comprise the exchange networks through which the information flows.

Methods

This study was conducted in three large rural regions of Canada – the Kootenays area of British Columbia, the Counties of Huron and Perth in southwestern Ontario, and the island of Newfoundland – as part of a larger investigation funded by the Canadian Institutes of Health Research (Harris et al. 2005).

Participant Recruitment

PHAs were recruited to participate through local health and social service agencies in each region. Using a snowball sampling method to identify the wider network for HIV/AIDS information exchange, we asked participating PHAs to nominate the people most involved in their management of HIV infection. We then invited these individuals, including friends, family members, informal caregivers, and health-care and social service providers living or serving in the study regions (including GPs, infectious disease specialists, public health nurses, social workers, and ASO support workers) to participate in the interviews. Between May 2005 and August 2006, we conducted semi-structured, audiotaped interviews with 114 participants (34 PHAs, 28 of their friends and family members, and 52 health and service providers). We asked the interviewees questions about their experiences with HIV/ AIDS, how they locate and use HIV/AIDS information, and for their assessment of their communities' strengths and weaknesses with regard to HIV/AIDS information and support. The interviews were transcribed, and the rich textual base was analyzed using NVivo (qualitative analysis software). To explore the networks of information exchange, we also asked interviewees to identify individuals who provide them with HIV/AIDS information and support. This allowed us not only to identify the members of the broad information exchange network(s) in each of the three rural study areas but also to map the relational "ties" among them. For a detailed description of the study methods, see Veinot (2009).

Regional Differences in HIV/AIDS Care

The design and delivery of health care in Canada are provincial responsibilities. Because the three regions that are the focus of our research are in different provinces, it is not surprising that the HIV/AIDS care system in each region is arranged quite differently. In Newfoundland, a multidisciplinary HIV care team and community-based ASOs play important roles. A nurse practitioner is the key caregiver for all PHAs in the province, working with other team members, including specialist physicians, a pharmacist, and a social worker. This service design recognizes the challenge of geography and the need for interventions that overcome distance to facilitate interpersonal connections. For the HIV care team, this approach includes periodically taking travelling HIV clinics to people in various regions of the province as well as extensive use of toll-free telephone lines and email communication with rural-dwelling patients. As well, ASOs hold regular retreats that allow PHAs and their friends/family members to gather from across the province and connect with one another.

In the Counties of Huron and Perth in Ontario, an under-resourced, community-based system that includes public health units and local ASOs is complemented by a strong multidisciplinary HIV team (as well as a large ASO) in an urban centre, London. PHAs who need access to the specialized HIV team must travel to London for service.

The service system in the Kootenays region of British Columbia includes a visible and well-regarded regional ASO. However, the HIV/AIDS health-care system in the area does not employ the multidisciplinary care model found in Ontario and Newfoundland, and a lone infectious disease specialist in Kelowna serves a vast region, without support from allied health professionals who are part of the treatment teams in Ontario and Newfoundland.

Findings

Living with HIV/AIDS in a Rural Community

With regard to access to health-care services, the PHAs in our study face many of the same challenges experienced by other rural dwellers. One such challenge is the problem of maintaining confidentiality in a small community. A PHA observed that "the problem in rural areas is you're bound to know that, if you're going to the local hospital or the local clinic to draw blood, nine chances out of ten, whoever's working in the clinic may or may not be a relative of the individual who's getting the blood drawn." Because of the stigma associated with the disease, PHAs can pay a heavy price for the lack of confidentiality. One woman told us that, when her HIV/AIDS status was disclosed in the community by a family member, she felt "like I'm stripped naked, like I'm wandering around town with no clothes on, and everybody can see me." Another PHA described the social isolation that followed disclosure of her diagnosis: "I've got one friend in my life, and she's been really supportive, and I've got one sister who's been really supportive. Since the rest have found out, they've drifted away from me."

Like other rural residents, PHAs also experience difficulties arising from limited local services, long travel distances for medical care, and a lack of public transportation. However, these conditions can be particularly problematic for PHAs because of their ongoing need for access to specialized health-care services. As one PHA explained,

> We don't even have a network anymore ... That little answering machine
> is nothing to me. When I'm in distress, that means nothing to me, and
> I would like to be able to speak to a live person and not have to make a
> long-distance phone call to do so. But there's nobody in the community,
> not a knowledgeable [person] like somebody who's involved with it.
> There isn't anybody.

As a result of the lack of local services, rural PHAs' information and help networks tend to be widely dispersed geographically. Indeed, nearly 60 percent of the individuals identified by the PHAs as key sources of HIV/AIDS information/help (i.e., their help "ties") were located more than an hour's travel away by car.

The challenges experienced by rural dwellers as a result of lengthy travel times for care and support described in Chapter 9 of this volume are also very significant for PHAs who live in areas that, by Canadian standards, are not necessarily remote but certainly rural. The average (mean) amount of time that it takes PHAs in our study to travel by car to reach members of their help networks is 1 hour and 38 minutes for those living in the Counties of Huron and Perth in southern Ontario, 3 hours and 43 minutes for those living in the Kootenays area of British Columbia, and 5 hours and 13 minutes for those living in rural New-foundland. These times do not take into account weather delays, an important factor since, in all three regions, winter driving is often treacherous and roads close, sometimes for considerable periods, as a result of ice storms or blowing snow.

Comments by PHAs reflect the toll of travelling these long distances for help.

> *There's no funding for help with gas costs, and that's a big deal for us from here. It takes me almost two hours to get to London, that's a big deal.*

> *I know I'm tired of driving that far. I'm beyond tired of driving that far ... I feel kind of resentful that we don't have something closer because the people that are in the hospitals that are here, they have no training.*

Information and communication technologies (ICTs) can be helpful tools for overcoming barriers posed by geography. For instance, where available, toll-free telephone lines were identified as an important means for PHAs to communicate with workers in ASOs, with health service providers in distant urban areas, and with national HIV/AIDS organizations. Interestingly, given the generally high levels of use of the Internet for health information among the general population (Fox 2006; Harris, Wathen, and Fear 2006), most PHAs in our study made relatively little use of email or online chat forums to discuss HIV/AIDS-related issues with their network members. This low use rate cannot be attributed simply to a lack of computer literacy or limited Internet access. For instance, although only 50 percent of the PHAs from British Columbia had ever used email, 90 percent of those from Newfoundland and Ontario were email users. Relative to respondents in other regions, more PHAs from Newfoundland had used email to discuss HIV/AIDS, primarily in conversations with their St. John's-based health-care and service providers. However, an HIV/AIDS care provider pointed out that this opportunity is not available to all rural PHAs as a result of policies in some health-care settings that preclude communication with patients via email, even when PHAs are willing to accept the potential risks to privacy.

Support Networks

PHA Networks

We observed considerable variability in the size and nature of PHAs' HIV/AIDS-related information and support networks. For instance, some PHAs identified a large number of actors with whom they had "help" ties (as many as 62), whereas others named a very small number (as few as 2). Overall, the average number of help ties ranged from a median of 7 for PHAs living in the Kootenays, to 8.5 for PHAs in rural Newfoundland, to 10.5 for PHAs in the Counties of Huron and Perth in Ontario. Importantly, many of these ties were with actors outside the PHAs' home communities (for PHAs in the Kootenays, 50 percent of their HIV/AIDS information and help-giving ties were with individuals outside the area; for the Ontario PHAs, 46 percent of their ties were located outside their home region; and for the Newfoundland PHAs, 65 percent of their identified ties lived away from their local area).

For most PHAs, a significant proportion of their HIV/AIDS-related information and help ties are with formal health-care and social service providers (38 percent for the Ontario PHAs, 42 percent for the BC PHAs, and 63 percent for the Newfoundland PHAs). The PHAs whom we interviewed placed a high value on the expertise and caring of these individuals, and in each region certain prominent care providers emerged as key supporters and brokers of information in the respondents' networks. Indeed, for some PHAs, formal care providers were their *only* connections with other people concerning their HIV status. The intensity of PHAs' reliance on these central support figures is reflected in their anxiety about the pressing workloads faced by their care providers and the possibility that these individuals might leave, either because they burn out or because funding is discontinued. As one PHA said of a person who was repeatedly identified by our respondents as a key care provider in Newfoundland, "I think if [she] ever left to do something else we'd all be stricken with grief. Like there's nobody can replace her, you know?" Reflecting similar sentiments about another key regional care provider, a PHA from Ontario said that "she's amazing. Very compassionate. Very knowledgeable, and she was a big help ... It really eased me into being able to talk to somebody because I had nobody." Another PHA said of one of these individuals that, "when you have good people, you don't give them up, you cling to them." Unfortunately, as in the US study reported by Schur et al. (2002), the formal care providers who are so central to the support of rural PHAs in Canada are generally located in urban centres, often far from where the PHAs live. Moreover, participants' concerns about their intense reliance on a few key individuals proved warranted since, at the time of writing, seven of the twelve health-care and service providers identified by the PHAs as central figures had left the positions they held at the time of the interviews.

As well as access to HIV/AIDS-specific care, several respondents raised as a concern the social isolation of rural PHAs, especially gay men. A gay PHA explained,

> *In the city, it was different. There's [a] lot of availability. You can join different workshops [for PHAs], different groups ... You actually meet people because at my age you don't go to bars ... It's just not possible, any of that stuff, anymore. So there was ways to socially connect there and have friends who would introduce. Here I'm pretty much isolated.*

Religious conservatism in their communities was also identified by several participants as contributing to the isolation of PHAs. One care provider said that "a lot of people I suspect haven't disclosed [their HIV status] because it's just not safe to do so." Indeed, when asked to describe the HIV/AIDS landscape in the local community, one respondent said that "it's very underground. Supremely underground. Some people think it's non-existent." Another health-care provider from the same area explained, "because it's a conservative community, it's not as accepting as some communities. But this is the way it is, and we have to deal with it. Right?" As a result, one care provider suggested that it might be a good idea for PHAs to "manage their HIV privately, out of town."

Care Provider Networks

The health and social service providers who took part in the interviews rely heavily on professional colleagues in other organizations for help and information related to HIV/AIDS. The median number of support ties identified by these respondents ranged from 4.5 for those in Ontario to 6 for those in the Kootenays. These ties often reflect interorganizational collaboration, for instance between ASO staff and public health nurses within a region, between rural ASO staff and urban HIV specialists, or among cross-agency members on boards of HIV-related organizations. Some ties also reflect service providers' involvement in professional networks across regions, such as regional HIV-related networks of public health nurses or AIDS organizations. Non-HIV specialist providers, such as those involved in addictions or housing work, most often named representatives of ASOs as sources of information and help. A number of care providers, particularly those from the Kootenays region, also reported that their clients/patients are important sources of HIV/AIDS-related information.

Information Exchanged through Networks

The interview participants described a wide range of HIV/AIDS-related help and information that they both receive and pass along through their network ties. Some of this help is practical, such as information about HIV/AIDS treatment, referrals to other services, or how to obtain institutional resources such as financial assistance, disability benefits, or transportation funds. Along with this practical assistance, the connections with network members are a source of emotional support. As one PHA said of her HIV/AIDS specialist social worker, "I trust her. I trust her that she's going to have some kind of an answer and she's going to listen to me ... I think everybody needs that. Sometimes you don't need an answer, you don't need somebody to solve it. You just need somebody to listen to you. And she's really good at that." Another PHA explained that "the people I've dealt with have been very supportive, and there are people I can turn to if I need to. That helps me get through my days and helps me feel like this isn't going to get the better of me."

Interestingly, relatives and close friends are rarely sources of useful HIV/AIDS information for PHAs. Instead, the information tends to flow in the other direction. That is, PHAs often share HIV/AIDS information with their friends and family members, not only to update them about their conditions (e.g., by reporting their blood counts), but also to pass along general information (e.g., new developments in treatment).

PHAs are also important sources of information and help for one another, as the following comments suggest:

Nobody really understands what a PHA is living with and what they're going through, except for another PHA.

It's a very subtle kind of support ... You just have a connection that's different, that's deeper.

One PHA described the important mentoring role played by other PHAs: "I was newly diagnosed and had questions, and these people had the disease for many years and have the answers, and I asked my questions, and they gave me their answers." As mentors, PHAs also help others to anticipate their futures in living with the disease: "She's told me stuff about her illness and how it affects her ... I haven't reached that stage ... so it's kind of like she's getting me ready for something that could happen." PHAs also offer one another advice on self-care and managing treatment side effects:

When I'm having diarrhea, I discuss that with my friends because they have diarrhea, and "how do you deal with your diarrhea, because when I have diarrhea I can't leave my house?"

She gave me advice on herbal remedies. If I was nauseous or something. Ginger ... She told me to like boil it for fifteen or twenty minutes into a tea.

The Role of Organizations in Rural HIV/AIDS Information Networks

A number of the PHAs, their friends and family members, and health and social service providers mentioned that rural communities are largely silent when it comes to HIV/AIDS. As one PHA commented, "it's rarely talked about. Rarely. Just, you know, living up here I don't, I don't even hardly hear anybody talking about it." This silence reduces the likelihood of encountering potentially useful "incidental" information on HIV/AIDS because it is simply not part of the "everyday life" information that passes through community networks.

In the early 1990s, residents in the regions included in our study created local ASOs to raise awareness about the disease. Although they vary in size and organizational vitality, these ASOs continue to provide support for PHAs and their family members, produce locally relevant HIV/ AIDS information through workshops and publications, and provide various community education activities. Some of the PHAs whom we interviewed, many of whom were currently or had been affiliated with these ASOs, disclosed their status publicly to raise community awareness, resist stigma about the disease, and help other PHAs overcome isolation and fear. These "out" activists are very much aware of the need to create and sustain viable information and help networks. As one of them pointed out, "if we don't speak about it, no one else will."

The people whom we interviewed repeatedly identified local ASOs as important sources of support. One PHA told the interviewer, "[the local ASO] has helped me [to] no end. It's been fantastic and connected me with all the other relevant streams and created further community, thereby supplying new answers and greater strength." Similarly, a family member of a PHA said of the local ASO, "I feel quite connected to them. If I had questions, they would try and find out for me. I just think that's a really wonderful organization." Although the ASOs are highly valued, fear of stigmatization prevents some people from using them. As a care provider explained, "there's a huge fear with living in a rural community, the way information spreads around a rural community, that people will see you going into a place (like the local ASO) and automatically assume that you're positive." Several respondents expressed concern about the lack of support for local ASOs. For example, one of the Ontario PHAs said that "the AIDS network that's here used to have a lot of funding, it has hardly any now, and we have to fund-raise everything." Similarly, a health-care provider in British Columbia commented that, not only is there too little funding for the ASOs, but also they serve areas that are "too vast. If they're travelling to do education, then their offices are closed."

Beyond the particular individuals who play a role in ASOs, the organizations themselves are also part of a network structure. Often local ASOs were the most central local organizations in rural organizational networks, with overall networks possessing a broad geographical range of ties, with connections extending from the local to the international.

Implications of Findings for Rural HIV/AIDS-Related Services

The well-documented patterns of information behaviour described at the beginning of this chapter were clearly evident in the experiences and expectations reported by the PHAs and caregivers who took part in our interviews. For instance, the PHAs emphasized the importance of their connections with others like themselves, and along with their friends and family members they stressed the value of access to knowledgeable people in their networks who show concern and compassion while providing information and advice. In terms of barriers to HIV/AIDS-related information and support, few respondents reported problems arising from a lack of information or uncertainty where to locate the information. Instead, the barriers that they identified resulted primarily from the physical and social conditions associated with rural living. In particular, for many of the PHAs, the services and information sources that they need are not available locally, and as a result they are forced to travel, in some cases very long distances, to gain access to care providers who have specialized knowledge. Also, as reported elsewhere (Groft and Vollman 2007), stigma attached to HIV/AIDS has a negative impact on PHAs and their friends and family members. If members of rural communities hold stigmatizing beliefs about the disease, are unaware that it exists among them, and/or possess little knowledge about the disease, not only is little up-to-date or accurate information on HIV/AIDS likely to be passed through local networks (see Harris et al. 2008 for further details regarding the exchange of misinformation in rural networks), but also PHAs might understandably be reluctant to disclose their status and/or use local services.

Important regional differences emerged in our findings, most of which seem to be the result of variations in the configuration of HIV/AIDS-related care services. In the Counties of Huron and Perth in Ontario, community-based volunteers, particularly a few "out" PHAs and friends/family members, educate their communities and support others within the limits of their personal time, energy, and health. Few PHAs and friends/family members in this area use email or the telephone to contact their care providers, partly due to institutional policies, and lack of available services and participants' poverty and low information literacy skill levels. Although the London-based HIV care team and overstretched community volunteers are vital resources for the interviewees from this region, we found evidence of significant fragmentation of information access, misunderstanding, and exchange of misinformation.

In the Kootenays region of British Columbia, PHAs travel long distances for care, to Calgary, Vancouver, and Kelowna, and they appear to confront many difficulties in establishing ongoing, supportive, and informative relationships with health-care providers. They also rarely communicate with their caregivers via email, a fact that is linked in part to poverty among participants as well as under-resourcing of HIV specialist care. The local ASO is able to address some of the challenges of information access by providing helpful staff members who are accessible via a toll-free information line and through drop-in offices located in two small cities in the region. Nonetheless, interviewees described many problems in gaining access to and/or interpreting information about HIV/AIDS treatment and confronted considerable misinformation in their communities. In contrast, PHAs from Newfoundland generally described good access to HIV/AIDS information and strong connections with members of the province's multidisciplinary care team. They reported few misunderstandings or difficulties in gaining access to care, although they complained of limited access to information in their home communities.

Our findings suggest that several components are needed to achieve effective access to HIV/AIDS-related information and support in rural Canada. In particular, we recommend that, if they do not already exist, interdisciplinary HIV health-care teams should be created in each province and territory. We suggest that, based on the Newfoundland experience, rather than expecting PHAs to travel long distances, especially for routine care, these teams should provide, among other things, regular, travelling HIV health-care clinics that bring service (and education) to community members (including local health and social service providers), a model similar in many respects to what is recommended in Chapter 13 of this volume for the support of mental health needs in rural areas. This approach will not only lessen the emotional and financial burdens of travel experienced by many rural PHAs and their family members, but it will also build capacity among local providers.[1] We also recommend that provincial and territorial governments provide sufficient funding to enable regional ASOs to employ knowledgeable staff members rather than rely solely on volunteers to provide local support and community education. Again this is a matter of building and sustaining local capacity and encouraging the development of reliable networks of information exchange. Reasonably staffed ASOs are well placed to develop safe opportunities for PHAs to meet one another and, by so doing, foster and extend supportive interpersonal networks. Finally, we suggest that key service providers, HIV/AIDS specialist services, and ASOs collaborate with one another to provide email access and toll-free telephone lines to enable PHAs to maintain links with knowledgeable and supportive network members.

Acknowledgments

We thank our participants and community partners in the Counties of Huron and Perth, the Kootenays, and Newfoundland. We are grateful for the support received from the Canadian Institutes of Health Research for the Rural HIV/AIDS Information Networks Project, funded under the HIV/AIDS Community-Based Research Program (principal investigator: Roma Harris).

Note

1 It could be argued that travelling clinics pose risks to confidentiality for those who use their services. However, we suggest that the alternative – travelling long distances to urban centres for health care – is not only inconvenient and costly for PHAs but also often visible to others in PHAs' home communities. To address the problem of confidentiality, one option for travelling HIV health-care clinics is to combine their visits with those of other travelling health services.

References

Agada, J. 1999. "Inner-City Gatekeepers: An Exploratory Survey of Their Information Use Environment." *Journal of the American Association of Information Science* 50, 1: 74-85.

Boulos, D., P. Yan, D. Schanzer, R.S. Remis, and C.P. Archibald. 2006. "Estimates of HIV Prevalence and Incidence in Canada, 2005." *Canada Communicable Disease Report* 32, 15: 165-74.

Canadian AIDS Treatment Information Exchange. 2003. *Many Voices: Report on Stakeholder Consultations.* Toronto: Canadian AIDS Treatment Information Exchange.

Fox, S. 2006. *Online Health Search 2006.* Washington, DC: Pew Internet and American Life Project, http://www.pewtrusts.org/.

Golin, C.E., S.R. Smith, and S. Reif. 2004. "Adherence Counseling Practices of Generalist and Specialist Physicians Caring for People Living with HIV/AIDS in North Carolina." *Journal of General Internal Medicine* 19, 1: 16-27.

Groft, J.N., and A.R. Vollman. 2007. "Seeking Serenity: Living with HIV/AIDS in Rural Western Canada." *International Electronic Journal of Rural and Remote Health Research* 7: 677.

Harris, R.M., and P. Dewdney. 1994. *Barriers to Information: How Formal Help Systems Fail Battered Women.* Westport, CT: Greenwood Press.

Harris, R., T. Veinot, L. Bella, I. Rootman, and J. Krajnak. 2008. "Helpers, Gatekeepers, and the Well-Intentioned: The Mixed Blessings of HIV/AIDS Info(r)mediation in Rural Canada." In *Mediating Health Information: The Go-Betweens in a Changing Socio-Technical Landscape,* edited by C.N. Wathen, S. Wyatt, and R. Harris, 167-81. Basingstoke: Palgrave Macmillan.

Harris, R., T. Veinot, I. Rootman, and J. Krajnak. 2005. Rural HIV/AIDS Information Networks Project. Funded by the Canadian Institutes of Health Research under the HIV/AIDS Community-Based Research Program.

Harris, R., and N. Wathen. 2007. "'If My Mother Was Alive I'd Probably Have Called Her': Women's Search for Health Information in Rural Canada." *Reference and User Services Quarterly* 47, 1: 67-79.

Harris, R., C.N. Wathen, and J. Fear. 2006. "Searching for Health Information in Rural

Canada: Where Do Residents Look for Health Information and What Do They Do When They Find It?" Paper 274. *Information Research* 12, 1, http://informationr. net/.

Haythornthwaite, C. 1996. "Social Network Analysis: An Approach and Technique for the Study of Information Exchange." *Library and Information Science Research* 18, 4: 323-42.

Hogan, T.P., and C.L. Palmer. 2005. "Information Preferences and Practices among People Living with HIV/AIDS: Results from a Nationwide Survey." *Journal of the Medical Library Association* 93, 4: 431-39.

Lewis, C.E., and T.J. Donohoe. 2000. "Changing Sources of Care for HIV Infection in California." *AIDS Education and Prevention* 12, 1: 15-20.

Marchand, R. 2001. *Gay Men Building Local Knowledge: Community-Based Research in HIV Prevention and Health Promotion.* Vancouver: Community Based Research Centre.

Mitura, V., and R.D. Bollman. 2003. "The Health of Rural Canadians: A Rural-Urban Comparison of Health Indicators." *Rural and Small Town Canada Analysis Bulletin* 4, 6: 23. Statistics Canada Catalogue No. 21-006-XIE.

Ontario Advisory Committee on HIV/AIDS. 2003. *A Proposed HIV/AIDS Strategy for Ontario to 2008.* Toronto: Ontario Ministry of Health and Long-Term Care.

Public Health Agency of Canada. 2007. *HIV and AIDS in Canada: Selected Surveillance Tables to June 30, 2007.* Ottawa: Surveillance and Risk Assessment Division, Centre for Infectious Disease Prevention and Control, Public Health Agency of Canada, http://www.phac-aspc.gc.ca/.

Sanmartin, C., and N. Ross. 2006. "Experiencing Difficulties Accessing First-Contact Health Services in Canada." *Healthcare Policy* 1, 2: 103-19.

Schanzer, D. 2003. "HIV/AIDS Mortality Trends in Canada, 1987-1998." *Canadian Journal of Public Health* 94, 2: 135-39.

Schur, C.L., M.L. Berk, J.R. Dunbar, M.E. Shapiro, S.E. Cohn, and S.A. Bozzette. 2002. "Where to Seek Care: An Examination of People in Rural Areas with HIV/AIDS." *Journal of Rural Health* 18, 2: 337-74.

Spink, A., and C. Cole. 2001. "Introduction to the Special Issue: Everyday Life Information-Seeking Research." *Library and Information Science Research* 23, 4: 301-4.

Statistics Canada. 2004. "Canadian Community Health Survey 2003." *The Daily,* 14 June, p. 15.

Sutherns, R., M. McPhedran, and M. Haworth-Brockman. 2004. *Rural, Remote, and Northern Women's Health: Policy and Research Directions: Final Summary Report.* Winnipeg: Centres of Excellence for Women's Health, http://www.pwhce.ca/.

Veinot, T. 2009. "Social Capital and HIV/AIDS Information/Help Exchange Networks in Rural Canada." PhD diss., University of Western Ontario.

Williamson, K. 1998. "Discovered by Chance: The Role of Incidental Information Acquisition in an Ecological Model of Information Use." *Library and Information Science Research* 20, 1: 23-40.

Chapter 17   **Shifting the Burden: The Effects of Home-Based Palliative Care on Family Caregivers in Rural Areas**

R. Donovan and A. Williams

Key Points

- Family caregivers are highly motivated to provide care, yet they are poorly supported, especially in terms of informal support from other family members.
- A more "caregiver-centric" approach to providing palliative/end-of-life (P/EOL) care is needed that includes rural-based family caregivers (FCGs) as both a *partner in care* and the *unit of care*. This would help them to balance their roles better and reduce caregiver distress.
- Better integration between the spectrum of providers and services is needed in the provision of P/EOL care in rural areas so that FCGs receive the support that they need.

It is acknowledged that family caregivers are an essential component of the health-care system, providing immeasurable support for elderly, ill, or disabled family members in the home (Fast 2005; Romanow 2002). This reliance is an enduring feature of health-care system reform and particularly notable given the shift in the delivery of health care from formal settings (e.g., hospitals) to informal settings (e.g., the home). Such is the case for those receiving palliative/end-of-life P/EOL care, in which one of the goals is to support people suffering from a terminal illness to die at home (Stajduhar and Davies 1998). Indeed, the desire for a home death is increasing; however, to facilitate death at home, there *must* be someone in the home (typically a family member or friend) to provide care. Although often rewarding, providing P/EOL care in the home is exceedingly demanding for FCGs, both emotionally and physically, compromising their overall health and well-being. Access to formal (paid) and informal (unpaid) support is known to enhance caregiving and mediate negative outcomes (e.g., caregiver burden), although the degree to which it is available and utilized varies. In fact, it is suggested that less than 20 percent of the Canadian population has access to P/EOL care services (Carstairs 2005); this can be exacerbated for those living in rural areas, where issues in accessing health-care services in general persist (see also Chapter 12, this volume). We recognize that the provision of P/EOL care is not restricted to the elderly; however, given that rural areas tend to have higher proportions of elderly people, general trends suggest that they are the largest users of P/EOL care services.

P/EOL care in Canada is a relatively new phenomenon, and not much is known about the experiences of FCGs, especially those living in rural and remote areas (McRae et al. 2000). Most of the work that has been done on rural P/EOL care is international in scope (Aoun et al. 2005; Evans, Stone, and Elwyn 2003; Hughes et al. 2004) or specific to service provider perspectives (Kelley, Sellick, and Linkewich 2003). The objectives of this research were to understand and describe the P/EOL caregiving experiences of rural-dwelling FCGs and their effects on self-assessed health. We begin with an overview of issues implicated in rural health-care service provision, highlighting the gaps specific to P/EOL care. Following a discussion of the research methods, we present a summary of the cases and thematic results. We conclude the chapter with a discussion of the implications of the research and suggestions for improving support for FCGs.

Rural Service Provision: The Case of P/EOL

Geographical Context

Canada is the second largest country in the world, spanning an area of almost 10 million square kilometres. With a population of just over 33 million, population density is just 3.5 persons per square kilometre (Statistics Canada 2007a). Although the majority of Canada's population is concentrated in southern Ontario and Quebec, and along the southern border of Canada (Bone 2002), more than 20 percent reside in rural areas (du Plessis, Beshiri, and Bollman 2002). Ontario, where this study took place, is the second largest province in the country and home to more than 12 million people (Government of Ontario 2008). Northern Ontario encompasses almost 90 percent of the land area in the province yet contains just 6 percent of the population (Northern Development and Mines [NDM] 2007). Thirty-five percent of the population in northern Ontario reside in rural areas compared with just 11 percent in southern Ontario. Furthermore, rural areas are characterized as having larger elderly populations than urban areas. The process of "aging in place," common in rural areas due to the out-migration of youth (e.g., for education or employment opportunities) and in-migration of elderly (e.g., for retirement) (Bryant and Joseph 2001; see also Chapters 23 and 24, this volume), contributes to higher dependency ratios relative to urban areas, which can impact both the need for care and the availability of support networks to provide care.

Health-Care Services

Although the above-noted geographical and demographic factors present unique challenges for delivering and accessing health care in rural areas (see Chapter 25, this volume, for further discussion), these issues have been exacerbated by the impact of broader systemic reform. The desire to contain costs in light of the increased and anticipated demand on resources due to the aging population has been a major impetus for restructuring. However, given that health-care delivery is a provincial responsibility, the changes in Canada have not been uniform. In Ontario, decreased funding for health care has occurred alongside an overhaul of the long-term-care sector in general (see Cloutier-Fisher and Joseph 2000; Cloutier-Fisher and Skinner 2006; and Williams 1996, 2006). This has involved streamlining access to community-level services via district-level Community Care Access Centres (CCACs), implemented in Ontario in 1996. Forty-three centres were created to offer one-stop access to community-level health-care services. Efforts to regionalize health-care services were undertaken in 2007 with the creation of fourteen local health integration networks (LHINs) (Ministry of Health and Long-Term Care 2007). Under this system, CCACs were also reorganized to correspond with the LHINs. The health districts remain but now serve as boundaries in which CCAC branch offices are located. The seven districts located in northern Ontario were organized into two LHINs: the North East and North

West LHINs. The North East LHIN, where this study took place, comprises five of the seven health districts.

CCACs are responsible for the organization and delivery of community-level health-care services. Services are provided by various for-profit and not-for-profit agencies on a limited contractual basis. This format, designed to improve the quality of services, has in effect led to the reduction or elimination of services, including homecare, in rural areas. Furthermore, most efforts at reform have included shifting the responsibility for care onto families, either directly, through increased caregiving, or indirectly, through the purchase of services.

Due to the lack of a rural health services model in place in Ontario or anywhere in Canada, and P/EOL care services having little recognition as a stand-alone set of services, the latter are tacked onto the existing set of services, albeit inadequately. This translates into limited P/EOL care services being provided through homecare, long-term care, and hospital care, where available.

Provision of P/EOL Care in Rural Areas
P/EOL care services have typically been developed in urban areas and applied to the population at large (Evans, Stone, and Elwyn 2003; Williams 1996; see also Chapter 12, this volume, for further review). Issues of service provider recruitment and retention are problematic, and the high turnover of health-care professionals in these areas in general interrupts continuity of services and rapport with patients (Huttlinger et al. 2003). Although the physician shortage does not compare with the acute nursing shortage in rural Canada, the literature suggests that physicians generally take on P/EOL care as a specialty. Therefore, because of human health-care shortages – particularly those at the high end of the health-care hierarchy, other front-line practitioners such as registered nurses, social workers, and volunteers play larger roles in the delivery of P/EOL care (Evans, Stone, and Elwyn 2003; Kelley, Sellick, and Linkewich 2003). Given that many of these non-physician service providers are generalists rather than palliative care specialists (Community Care Access Centre for the Districts of Thunder Bay and Kenora/Rainy River [CCAC-TB/KRR] 2005; Kelley, Sellick, and Linkewich 2003; McRae et al. 2000), the quality of service is unknown. This is in contrast to large urban centres where patients and families are served by long-established palliative homecare teams composed of all types of providers specialized in providing P/EOL care

(Williams 1998). Additionally, service providers suggest that they lack training and experience specific to palliative care (Kelley, Habjan, and Aegard 2004). At the community level, there are fewer palliative care situations in which to develop knowledge and implement strategies to meet the needs of the dying and their families. Furthermore, organized volunteer programs designed to support patients and families at home are vulnerable, due in part to liability issues and the inability to remunerate volunteers adequately for travel expenses (CCAC-TB/KRR 2005). Barriers to service provision are known to exist; they include insufficient homecare support, inadequate funding for supplies and equipment, lack of access to specialized care facilities, and problems with continued communication and coordination of services (Kelley, Habjan, and Aegard 2004; MacLean and Kelley 2001). Numerous other gaps exist in services, including access to adequate respite services, dedicated palliative care beds, and specialized hospital services. It is thus impossible sometimes to keep people in their home communities to die.

Despite these known deficiencies in rural service provision, few studies have been undertaken to explore the experience of caregiving from the FCGs' perspective (Evans, Stone, and Elwyn 2003; Robinson et al. 2009; Wilson et al. 2006). Although limited, research suggests that caregiving experiences are similar across urban and rural locations and that rural-dwelling FCGs are, in general, satisfied with the services that they receive at the local level. They appear, however, to have higher unmet information needs and rely heavily on non-physician service providers, family members, and friends for support (Hughes et al. 2004; McRae et al. 2000). Furthermore, rural-dwelling FCGs often experience problems transporting patients to various appointments and accessing hospital care outside their communities (McRae et al. 2000; Thomas, Morris, and Harman 2002).

Methods

We used a multiple case study design (Yin 2003) to examine the caregiving experience over time. This method was chosen to facilitate the collection of data from multiple sources and for its efficacy in examining the experience longitudinally. Data were collected from FCGs via semi-structured interviews, surveys, and direct observations. The surveys included the Caregiver Reaction Assessment (Given et al. 1992) and the Self-Rated Burden Scale (van Exel et al. 2004) but are not central to the results presented herein. Information from various documents (e.g., websites, brochures, and newspaper articles), together with R. Donovan's field notes (e.g., physical characteristics of the home and study area), was also used in the interpretation. Various themes – including scope of the caregiver role, how FCGs were prepared for and supported throughout the process, experience of the caregiver burden, satisfaction with the experience, and self-assessed caregiver health – were explored in the interviews.

Sample

A combination of criterion and maximum variation sampling strategies was used to gather a heterogeneous sample (Patton 2002). Rather than the "Rural and Small Town" definition of rural (see Chapter 1, this volume), we used a macro-level conceptualization of rural in which the entire region was designated as rural based on its status as a medically under-serviced area (Williams and Cutchin 2002). Participants were recruited from the homecare caseloads of two district-level CCACs located in the North East LHIN. Ethics approval was obtained from the McMaster University Research Ethics Board prior to beginning the study. Five FCGs were recruited to the study; they were interviewed on average three times over the caregiving process at approximately six-week intervals. Through the informed consent process, FCGs were advised of their rights as participants; signed consent forms were obtained prior to each interview. With permission, all interviews were audiotaped.

Site Characteristics

The five FCG participants were drawn from four different communities situated within the North East LHIN. Two of the five participants came from the same urban centre (population < 55,000) within the largely rural LHIN, with the remaining three participants residing in communities with populations ranging from < 1,200 to < 85,000. The North East LHIN contains approximately 4.6 percent of Ontario's population, a number in steady decline since 1994 (Bains et al. n.d.). Much of the population is concentrated in the southeast quadrant of the region. Relative to Ontario as a whole, this LHIN contains a higher than average proportion of elderly people and is characterized by higher unemployment rates, lower labour force participation rates, and lower levels of education. Additionally, life expectancy rates are significantly lower for both men and women, and the population has higher than average rates of arthritis, rheumatism, high blood pressure, diabetes, and heart disease. Residents also have significantly less contact with physicians than the provincial average.

Data Analysis

All tapes were transcribed verbatim, and conventional content analysis (Hsieh and Shannon 2005) was used to analyze the data. This method is appropriate when there is little understanding of the phenomenon in question. The transcripts were read numerous times, both while listening to the tapes and without doing so, to capture any nuances, such as the tone used or pauses in speech. Coding involved the identification of words/phrases related to managing the caregiving experience, caregiver health, caregiver burden, and other significant ideas. These codes were then developed into themes. The cross-case analysis was completed in a similar fashion, with the categories clustered into four themes (one overarching principal theme and three sub-themes). A record of the exact sources for each of the categories generated during the coding process was kept. Multiple sources of data, including the thematic analysis, were used to develop case summaries, which provided an in-depth account of each unique caregiving experience.

Thematic Results

The FCGs in this study reflect a diverse set of individuals strongly committed to caring for their family members; FCG characteristics are summarized in Table 17.1. All names have been altered to protect identities.

As can be seen, each situation is unique, reflecting different family structures, disease trajectories, and lengths of time in the caregiver role. Individually, FCGs faced various challenges and had varying degrees of support, both through the health-care system and through informal networks. The results point to a high degree of personal satisfaction in fulfilling the caregiver role but with numerous challenges and many accommodations along the way – all of which had implications for the FCGs' health. The findings are arranged around one organizing principle, suspension of self and time, and three sub-themes relating to support, motivation, and health.

Table 17.1   Case summaries

	Family caregiver participants				
Characteristics	#1: Lisa	#2: Tom	#3: Angela	#4: Barb	#5: Maddie
Age	50	79	38	68	53
Marital status	Married	Married	Married	Married	Married
Relationship to patient	Daughter-in-law	Spouse	Daughter	Spouse	Daughter
Age of patient	75	79	71	78	79
Family structure in home	Spouse, no dependants	Spouse, no dependants	Spouse, 2 dependants	Spouse, no dependants	Spouse, 1 adult child
Working status	Quit work to provide care	Retired	Quit work to provide care	Retired	Self-employed
Residential location	Rural township (pop. <1,500)	Rural community (pop. <12,000)	Urban centre* (pop. <55,000)	Urban centre (pop. <75,000)	Urban centre* (pop. <55,000)
Duration of caregiving	16 months	>12 years	8 months	>4 months	8 months
Number of interviews					
C = during caregiving	C: 1	C: 4	C: 3	C: 2	C: 1
B = in bereavement	B: 2		B: 1		B: 1
Place of death	Home	n/a	Home	n/a	Home

*   Two of the family caregivers resided in the same urban centre within the NE LHIN.

Overarching Theme: Suspension of Self and Time

Suspension of self and time is an organizing theme that captures the temporal and spatial dimensions of caregiving. With the exception of one FCG, the caregiving role was assumed suddenly, with little previous experience or understanding of what lay ahead. Managing care required a great deal of self-sacrifice by the FCGs. Their ability to do so was directly related to the level of support that they had, their ability to accommodate to the role, and the patient's health status. Caregiving required considerable flexibility and patience. The extent of tasks associated with care was tremendous:

> *If someone is in the hospital, and they need medication, you're there as a family member, you're there to hold their hand ... you know, just be there*

*for them. So if they need medication, the nurses do that, you know?
You are "in between" the medical. But when you are at home, you are
responsible for everything. Nurses come, but I mean, when they're not
here, you're responsible for every need ... every need.*

The transition to care appeared somewhat easier for the retired FCGs,
but the role was just as restricting. Two of the adult children had to quit
work in order to provide care so that their parents would not be insti-
tutionalized, and one felt unable to cope without her work. All FCGs
sampled had to decrease significantly, if not practically eliminate, their
social activities, thus tying them in many ways to their home environments. Transformations to the home environment, through the addition of medical equipment, assistive devices, and/or reconfiguration of
space, were also necessary, although such transformations were not
perceived as problematic. The following sub-themes speak to the influences on caregiving arrangements, highlighting both aggravating and
mediating factors that contributed to the degree of suspension of self
and time experienced.

Support

Formal Support
Formal support refers to services, supplies, and human resources paid
for through the health-care system. Home-based palliative care was
delivered and administered through the CCAC palliative care programs, with case managers coordinating services that went into the
home. In general, the FCGs in the study expressed satisfaction with the
support available in their communities.

Geography explained how services differed *across* space as well as the
implications *of* space in accessing various resources. All FCGs had access to a family physician, and hospitals were located in all but one
community. Palliative homecare services were available to all FCGs,
although most service providers were not palliative care specialists.
Although the quantity of homecare services was similar, their provision
differed between the two CCACs located within this LHIN and across
caregiving situations. For example, only one CCAC appeared to provide flexibility in how the FCGs could use the time allotted, thereby
providing them with some degree of personal control. Accessing specialty services (e.g., specialists or oncology centres) was problematic
due to the centralization of these services in larger centres. FCGs

tended to normalize the distance involved in accessing them but expressed concern with the impact of travelling on the care recipients, especially when they were particularly ill. All communities lacked adequate transportation services for palliative patients. For example, though the larger communities had wheelchair-accessible transportation systems, there were no options for transferring bed-ridden patients in non-emergency situations. As a result, the ability to access services outside the home (e.g., physician's appointments or respite services) was virtually non-existent for both patients and FCGs.

Numerous challenges were experienced to a greater extent by the FCG living in the small rural community. They included increased travelling (to physician's appointments or the hospital when the patient was admitted), adverse travelling conditions (inclement weather, dirt roads), and having to pick up supplies and prescriptions as opposed to having them delivered.

The primary concern for the FCGs in this study was to obtain adequate information and services for the *patient*. In the aggregate, FCGs' needs were tremendous. For example, they needed to know which services were available in the community and how to access them. More importantly, they required information concerning the disease, its trajectory, and the process of dying. Not only did FCGs want some indication that death was imminent, but they also needed to know what to do once death occurred. FCGs also needed guidance in performing specific tasks (e.g., treating bed sores, monitoring patient status, and handling and administering medications) and relied on having the patient's condition monitored. FCGs had to be proactive in the search for information, or their needs could be left unmet. They believed that, as difficult as it might be to receive the necessary information, getting it was essential for them to cope.

> *They are not going to volunteer something that is, like you said, taboo. Unless you ask that question, they are not going to tell you things that are ... negative. Or negative to them, even though you have to go through it. And I'm not one to wait around to find out, so I'll ask, and you prepare yourself. I think that was one of my ways of preparing myself for what was going to happen. Knowing what she was going to go through.*

Knowing whom to approach was often problematic, as evidenced by the lack of a team approach. For the most part, case managers and registered nurses were used as sources of information. Registered nurses were highly trusted and proved most accessible given that they visited frequently with palliative patients. FCGs were pleased with homecare services, such as those provided by registered nurses and personal support workers; however, physicians, though relied on, were not overly supportive. This was reflected in a number of ways, including insensitivity to the patient's condition, failure to provide information as needed, failure to show up for home visits as promised, failure to renew prescriptions, and encouragement of hospitalization over homecare. Only one FCG expressed a high degree of satisfaction with the physician throughout the entire caregiving process. This was because the physician included the FCG in treatment decisions, made regular home visits and random telephone calls, and was available to the family day or night via cell phone. Other professionals, such as occupational and physiotherapists (O/PT), were utilized on an as-needed basis, which often involved prolonged wait times. The use of spiritual or religious support was very limited, and social workers and bereavement services were not used.

Informal Support

Informal support refers to those people who are not paid for the support that they provide; this includes family members, friends, and volunteers. Families were geographically divided, and this separation severely limited the type and amount of support that FCGs could expect to receive from them. As a result, much of the support that FCGs received was much-valued emotional support as opposed to task-related assistance or respite. Additionally, family dynamics played a role in how caregiving responsibilities were handled in general. Even when family members were dispersed, their inability to provide support was understood by FCGs when it was clear that an effort was being made. Family gatherings and special occasions were meaningful, even if entertaining visitors required extra effort. However, tensions were created, and the demands of caregiving were overwhelming when there was little or no effort put forth by other family members – physically or emotionally – to assist with care.

Access to visiting volunteer organizations specializing in P/EOL care was limited to just one community. These volunteers were available to sit with palliative clients, thereby offering respite opportunities to FCGs; however, the service was under-used. Several limitations affected access to the service, including the fact that arrangements had to be made several days in advance (the unpredictability of a loved one's status often precluded this) and some restrictions in terms of when the services were available (e.g., not overnight).

This theme illustrates the variation that FCGs had with respect to support. To some degree, albeit perceived as minimal in this study, FCGs are limited spatially to services. Structurally, there is a high degree of compassion among formal care providers, yet services are targeted more at the patient than the FCGs. Outside the health-care system, few informal networks of support exist, except for those of an emotional nature. In general, the lack of support contributed to the degree of suspension of self and time for the caregiver. If caregivers had enjoyed increased support, they could have maintained some aspects of their normal routines and/or activities and alleviated some of their burdens.

Motivations for Continuing the Role

This theme refers to how FCGs were motivated, both internally and externally, to care and continue caring when faced with adversity. FCGs were often motivated internally to care out of feelings of love and respect for their loved ones. FCGs were also motivated to care because they sensed that it was the right thing to do. These feelings contributed to a sense of pride, one that sustained FCGs in the bereavement period. More prevalent, however, were external motivators. All FCGs found that it was easier and more desirable to provide care at home. For example, they did not have to travel to an institution to spend time with their loved ones, and they were better able to balance their responsibilities and retain some semblance of routine in their lives. Furthermore, dissatisfaction with the type of care received in hospitals and long-term-care facilities (in terms of personal attention and general cleanliness) was prominent. As a result, FCGs were highly motivated to avoid institutionalizing their family members.

The most significant external motivator was the wish of the patient to be cared for and die at home. FCGs did not want their loved ones to be alone or receive less than optimal care (whether real or perceived) and were therefore the only option for care given family relationships and structures. This motivator reflected the sense of obligation that FCGs felt toward their loved ones – particularly when death was imminent. In these cases, FCGs understood the importance of dying at home to their loved ones and were therefore motivated to go to great lengths to make this happen. Often the pressure that they felt to manage care in the home was overwhelming. Again this was particularly so for the adult-children FCGs and was exacerbated by the deteriorating

condition of the care recipient and the loss of identity through prolonged engagement in caregiving.

> *She doesn't want the options, and I [have] to respect her wishes; where*
> *she wants to be is here. She knows she is dying, and she want[s] it to be*
> *with us. And that was the only decision that we could have made. Let*
> *me tell you, it was hard, because we thought last night about taking her*
> *to the hospital and at least being able to sleep at night.*

Clearly, staying committed to the caregiver role was a tough test for
the FCGs and a testament to the deep respect that they felt for their
loved ones; honouring their loved ones' wishes to be cared for and die
at home was a powerful influence on their decision to continue in the
caregiving role. Motivation therefore contributed to the suspension of
self and time by tying them to the caregiver role, despite a lack of support, both formally and informally.

Prioritizing Health Maintenance

We sought to understand the effects of caregiving on physical and emotional health and well-being; however, we also discovered just how
valuable maintaining health was to this sample of FCGs in order to
sustain them throughout the process. Given the household structures
and family dynamics, there was simply no one else readily available to
step in to provide care should they become incapacitated. Maintaining
health included efforts to get enough rest, eat properly, attend to personal health-care needs, stay active (exercise), and take breaks from the
situation. The lack of support and changing intensity of caregiving over
time made these strategies difficult, if not impossible, to achieve with
any degree of consistency.

Generally speaking, the physical health of the FCGs remained stable
over the caregiving process; however, self-assessed health was rated
lower during bereavement. Physical and emotional exhaustion were
prevalent, and FCGs suffered minor aches and pains due to the physical
demands of caregiving, personal health status, and age. Mental health
was impacted by the culmination of physical exhaustion, stress (e.g.,
family dynamics, witnessing the decline of their loved ones, and dealing with difficult personalities), and few opportunities for self-care.
FCGs did find the caregiving experience highly rewarding insofar as
they thought that they had provided improved quality and quantity of
life to their loved ones. The experience of health was highly contingent

on the degree to which FCGs engaged in caregiving, the type and quantity of support available, and their motivations for care. These contingent elements highlight the important link between the context of care and health outcomes for FCGs.

Limitations

The results of this research add to the evidence base for program improvement; however, it is a small sample and locally contingent and therefore might lack generalizability beyond this northern Ontario context. Furthermore, this sample might exclude the voices of those who were unable to overcome the challenges and could not therefore manage caregiving and/or the time to participate in the research process.

Discussion and Conclusion

Recognizing the importance of FCGs within the wider context of health-care planning and to the palliative process in particular is important and timely. This study has illustrated the importance of *place* – in this case, *home space* in medically under-serviced areas in a predominantly rural geography – to the palliative family caregiving experience. The results of this study suggest that there is a high degree of reliance on FCGs to provide care for their dying loved ones and that it is provided under extraordinary circumstances. Access to resources for caregiving in the home can reduce the burden of care, but such resources are disconnected and unevenly distributed across space. Furthermore, it is assumed that FCGs have access to informal networks of support, yet the results here suggest that families are unable to manage the physical tasks of care work together because they are geographically dispersed. FCGs with access to resources – formal and informal – have a greater advantage over other FCGs in providing care in the home, with fewer negative consequences to their overall well-being. The fact that the lack of services and support did not materialize as a greatly perceived problem is likely because FCGs had low expectations of the health-care system, because they were highly motivated to accommodate to the caregiving situation, and because of easier access to services given the mainly urban communities within which these FCGs lived. Despite this, the challenge still exists to provide services in a more overt and integrated fashion to ease FCGs' navigation of the system.

Two important ideas flow from research: first, a more "caregiver-centric" approach is needed in the provision of home-based palliative care; second, health must be treated as a resource to sustain FCGs in this role. A caregiver-centric approach would ensure that FCGs are included as part of the health-care team and as the unit of care so that they are better able to balance caregiving. This approach would acknowledge that FCGs' needs for support and information are in response to their role, albeit unpaid, as a partner in care. In this study, essential services appeared to be focused on patient status rather than caregiver well-being or distress, and there were few mechanisms that led to regular and consistent assessments of FCG functioning. Taking more opportunities to assess FCGs' status, for example by speaking with the FCG privately and routinely, would help formal providers to appreciate more fully how FCGs are feeling, help them to find solutions to deal with issues before they become too problematic, and help them to implement any necessary supports. In this way, recommendations would be FCG specific, based on the context of the caregiving situation, in addition to the status of the patient.

A caregiver-centric approach strongly supports the idea of FCG health as a resource that needs to be nourished in order for FCGs to manage the situation and avoid burnout. This is especially important to consider given the current context of the caregiving situation in rural areas (patient-focused care at end of life and health-care restructuring in medically under-serviced geographies) and is most applicable to the primary FCG who has taken on the responsibilities of care. Personal context is important: adult-children FCGs, referred to as the sandwich generation, might have other responsibilities within which the caregiving situation takes place (e.g., dependants, work obligations), and the elderly might work at a diminished capacity due to poor health and aging (Fast and Keating 2000; Wells and Kendig 1996). Furthermore, FCGs in rural areas might experience increased pressure in their caregiving role due to the lack of support from informal sources, such as family members.

As a strategy for P/EOL care moves forward in Canada, it is important to have evidence on which to base the decisions that guide the development of policy. More attention must be directed at the context of care and the importance of health as a resource for FCGs given their essential role in the homecare process. Looking at the experience within different spatial contexts and scales and over time reiterates that a "one size fits all" approach to supporting FCGs is ineffective. Although

FCGs often find the experience rewarding, research has consistently shown that they continue to experience high degrees of physical and emotional distress that negatively impact their health. Although there has been some form of redress, the development of policy and relevant practice issues specific to FCGs are still in their infancy. There is an immediate need to see the care work that FCGs perform in this context and to include their voices in developing appropriate supports and services.

Acknowledgments

We would like to extend our heartfelt appreciation to the FCGs who made this research possible by taking the time to participate in the study and share their experiences. This research was made possible through scholarships from the Social Sciences and Humanities Research Council of Canada and the Ontario Ministry of Colleges, Universities and Training.

References

Aoun, S.M., L.J. Kristjanson, D.C. Currow, and P.L. Hudson. 2005. "Caregiving for the Terminally Ill: At What Cost?" *Palliative Medicine* 19: 551-55.

Bains, N., K. Dall, C. Hay, M. Pacey, J. Sarkella, and M. Ward. N.d. "Population Health Profile: North East LHIN." Toronto: Government of Ontario, http://www.health.gov.on.ca/.

Bone, R.M. 2002. *The Regional Geography of Canada.* 2nd ed. Toronto: Oxford University Press.

Bryant, C., and A.E. Joseph. 2001. "Canada's Rural Population: Trends in Space and Implications in Place." *Canadian Geographer* 45, 1: 132-37.

Carstairs, S. 2005. *Still Not There, Quality End-of-Life Care: A Progress Report.* Ottawa: Senate of Canada, http://sen.parl.gc.ca/.

Cloutier-Fisher, D., and A.E. Joseph. 2000. "Long-Term Care Restructuring in Rural Ontario: Retrieving Community Service User and Provider Narratives." *Social Science and Medicine* 50: 1037-45.

Cloutier-Fisher, D., and M.W. Skinner. 2006. "Levelling the Playing Field? Exploring the Implications of Managed Competition for Voluntary Sector Providers of Long-Term Care in Small Town Ontario." *Health and Place* 12: 97-109.

Community Care Access Centres for the Districts of Thunder Bay and Kenora/Rainy River (CCAC-TB/KRR). 2005. *End-of-Life Care Service Delivery Model for Northwestern Ontario.* Districts of Thunder Bay and Kenora/Rainy River: Community Care Access Centres.

du Plessis, V., R. Beshiri, and R.D. Bollman. 2002. "Definitions of Rural." Agriculture and Rural Working Paper Series No. 61. Ottawa: Statistics Canada.

Evans, R., D. Stone, and G. Elwyn. 2003. "Organizing Palliative Care for Rural Populations: A Systematic Review of the Evidence." *Family Practice* 20: 304-10.

Fast, J. 2005. "Caregiving: A Fact of Life." *Transition Magazine* 35, 2: 4-9, http://www.vifamily.ca/.

Fast, J.E., and N.C. Keating. 2000. "Family Caregiving and Consequences for Carers: Toward a Policy Research Agenda." CPRN Discussion Paper #F/10. Ottawa: Canadian Policy Research Networks.

Given, C.W., B. Given, M. Stommel, C. Collins, S. King, and S. Franklin. 1992. "The Caregiver Reaction Assessment (CRA) for Caregivers to Persons with Chronic Physical and Mental Impairments." *Research in Nursing and Health* 15: 271-83.

Government of Ontario. 2008. *About Ontario: Geography.* Toronto: Government of Ontario, http://www.gov.on.ca/.

Hsieh, H., and S.E. Shannon. 2005. "Three Approaches to Qualitative Content Analysis." *Qualitative Health Research* 15, 9: 1277-88.

Hughes, P.M., C. Ingleton, B. Noble, and D. Clark. 2004. "Providing Cancer and Palliative Care in Rural Areas: A Review of Patient and Career Needs." *Journal of Palliative Care* 20, 1: 44-49.

Huttlinger, K., J. Schaller-Ayers, T. Lawson, and J. Ayers. 2003. "Suffering It Out: Meeting the Needs of Health Care Delivery in a Rural Area." *Online Journal of Rural Nursing and Health Care* 3, 2: 17-28, http://www.rno.org.libaccess.lib.mcmaster.ca/.

Kelley, M.L., S. Habjan, and J. Aegard. 2004. "Building Capacity to Provide Palliative Care in Rural and Remote Communities: Does Education Make a Difference?" *Journal of Palliative Care* 20, 4: 308-15.

Kelley, M.L., S. Sellick, and B. Linkewich. 2003. "Rural Nonphysician Providers' Perspectives on Palliative Care Services in Northwestern Ontario, Canada." *Journal of Rural Health* 19, 1: 55-62.

MacLean, M.J., and M.L. Kelley. 2001. "Palliative Care in Rural Canada." *Rural Social Work* 6, 3: 63-73.

McRae, S., S. Caty, M. Nelder, and L. Picard. 2000. "Palliative Care on Manitoulin Island: Views of Family Caregivers in Remote Communities." *Canadian Family Physician* 46: 1301-7.

Ministry of Health and Long-Term Care. 2007. *Local Health System Integration Act, 2006.* Toronto: Ministry of Health and Long-Term Care, http://health.gov.on.ca/.

Northern Development and Mines (NDM). 2007. *Northern Ontario Overview.* Toronto: Northern Development and Mines, http://www.mndm.gov.on.ca/.

Patton, M.Q. 2002. "Designing Qualitative Studies." In *Qualitative Research and Evaluation Methods,* 3rd ed., edited by M.Q. Patton, 230-47. Thousand Oaks, CA: Sage.

Robinson, C.A., B. Pesut, J.L. Bottorff, A. Mowry, S. Broughton, and G. Fyles. 2009. "Rural Palliative Care: A Comprehensive Review." *Journal of Palliative Medicine* 12, 3: 253-58.

Romanow, R.J. 2002. *Building on Values: The Future of Health Care in Canada.* Saskatoon: Commission on the Future of Health Care in Canada.

Stajduhar, K.I., and B. Davies. 1998. "Death at Home: Challenges for Families and Directions for the Future." *Journal of Palliative Care* 14, 3: 8-15.

Statistics Canada. 2007a. *Population and Dwelling Counts, for Canada, Provinces, and Territories, 2006 and 2001 Censuses.* Ottawa: Statistics Canada, http://www12.statcan.ca/.

—. 2007b. *Local Health Integration Networks.* Ottawa: Statistics Canada, http://www.statcan.ca/.

Thomas, C., S.M. Morris, and J.C. Harman. 2002. "Companions through Cancer: The Care Given by Informal Carers in Cancer Contexts." *Social Science and Medicine* 54: 529-44.

van Exel, N.J.A., W.J.M. Scholte op Reimer, W.B.F. Brouwer, B. van den Berg, M.A. Koopmanschap, and G.A.M. van den Bos. 2004. "Instruments for Assessing the Burden of Informal Caregiving for Stroke Patients in Clinical Practice: A Comparison of CSI, CRA, SCQ, and Self-Rated Burden." *Clinical Rehabilitation* 18: 203-14.

Wells, Y.C., and H.L. Kendig. 1996. "Changes in Carers' Capacity and Motivation to Provide Care." *Journal of Family Studies* 2, 4: 15-28.

Williams, A.M. 1996. "The Development of Ontario's Home Care Program: A Critical Geographical Analysis." *Social Science and Medicine* 42, 6: 937-48.

–. 1998. "An Assessment of Community Palliative Care Needs: The Case of Niagara." *Palliative Care* 15, 2: 45-52.

–. 2006. "Restructuring Home Care in the 1990s: Geographical Differentiation in Ontario, Canada." *Health and Place* 12: 222-38.

Williams, A.M., and M.P. Cutchin. 2002. "The Rural Context of Health Care Provision." *Journal of Interprofessional Care* 16, 2: 107-15.

Wilson, D.M., C. Justice, S. Sheps, R. Thomas, P. Reid, and K. Leibovici. 2006. "Planning and Providing End-of-Life Care in Rural Areas." *Journal of Rural Health* 22, 2: 174-81.

Yin, R.K. 2003. *Case Study Research: Design and Methods*. 3rd ed. Thousand Oaks, CA: Sage.

Chapter 18   **Pain and Palliative Care with Seniors
in Canada's Northern Territories**

N. Novik and M. MacLean

Key Points

- The provision of palliative care services to seniors in Canada's northern territories must recognize the differences among regions, communities, and cultures.
- The factors identified as being most important in ensuring the quality of palliative care received by northern seniors include good communication, consistency, and the acknowledgment of and respect for
  the impact of culture.
- Culture and ethnic background have a direct impact on pain recognition, assessment, and management.

The nature of pain management and palliative care support for seniors
in each of Canada's three northern territories is as unique as each territory itself. Palliative care services for seniors in northern Canada appear to be driven by the specific needs of respective populations, the
intricacies of unique cultures, and the impacts and pressures of economic realities and development. This chapter explores the realities
and issues surrounding pain and palliative care with seniors in northern Canada from the perspectives of over fifty health and social work
practitioners, volunteers, and family members of former palliative care
patients from the Yukon, Northwest Territories (NWT), and Nunavut.
Information and data discussed have been gathered through a qualitative

study during which these individuals described their experiences in providing care to seniors who are/were palliative.

Northern Canada

Canada's three northern territories are situated across a large land mass but support a relatively low population base. The 2006 census reports a total Canadian population of 31,612,897, and the population of the Yukon is reported to be 30,392, the population of Nunavut is 29,474, and the population of the Northwest Territories is 41,464 (Government of the Northwest Territories 2008). In Canada, the three distinct groups of Aboriginals – North American Indian, Inuit, and Métis – make up approximately 1.2 million people (Statistics Canada 2006). However, the overall population of northern Canada is composed largely of individuals of Aboriginal descent. Approximately 19.1 percent of the population in the Yukon identify as Aboriginal, and 62.5 percent in the Northwest Territories and 88.7 percent of the population in Nunavut identify themselves as Aboriginal (Statistics Canada 2006). Aboriginal identity is defined as those individuals who identify with at least one Aboriginal group (North American Indian, Métis, or Inuit), who are treaty or registered Indian, and/or who are members of an Indian band or First Nation (Government of the Northwest Territories 2008). Each of Canada's three northern territories is unique and distinct. It is therefore necessary to explore briefly facts relevant to each territory.

As the youngest of the three territories, Nunavut was created on 1 April 1999 (Government of Nunavut 2008). When the Nunavut Land Claims Agreement was signed by federal, territorial, and Tungavik Federation of Nunavut (TFN) representatives in 1993, the decision was finalized to divide the Northwest Territories according to the unofficial borders that had divided the single territory into what was known at the time as the Western Arctic and the Eastern Arctic (Indian and Northern Affairs Canada [INAC] 1994). Prior to division of the territory, residents of the Eastern Arctic – now Nunavut – had followed a more traditional lifestyle. The Nunavut Land Claims Agreement, and the creation of a distinct territory, sought to ensure that this traditional lifestyle, language, and culture would be protected (INAC 1994). In addition to English and French, Inuktitut is one of the three official languages in the territory and is considered to be the working language. There are twenty-six communities in Nunavut, the largest being Iqaluit, with a population of 6,184. There is only one government-maintained road (twenty-one kilometres) in the entire territory (Government of Nunavut 2008). Other than that, communities are accessible by air year round or by ship and barge during the short summer months. The population of Nunavut is considered to be relatively young, with 60 percent of the current population under the age of twenty-five (Government of Nunavut 2008). The economic activities of the territory include mining, tourism, fishing, hunting and trapping, and arts and crafts production (Government of Nunavut 2008). Immigrants account for only 1.6 percent of the total population of Nunavut (Government of the Yukon 2008).

In the Northwest Territories, the most frequently reported ethnic origin is Aboriginal. In fact, there are eight distinct Aboriginal groups that reside throughout the territory, including the Dogrib, Yellowknives, Chipewyan, South Slavey, North Slavey, Gwichin', Inuvialuit, and Métis. However, the 2006 census report indicates that the immigrant population increased by 50 percent since 1996 (Government of the Northwest Territories 2008). Overall, immigrants account for 6.9 percent of the population of the Northwest Territories (Government of the Yukon 2008). There are thirty-three communities in the territory, the majority of which are accessible by road year round. The more remote communities, such as Tuktoyaktuk, are accessible by air and water or by ice road during the winter months. Yellowknife is the capital city, with a population of 18,510. This territory primarily has a resource-based economy. Recent development has focused on mining and natural gas exploration (Government of the Northwest Territories 2008).

The Yukon Territory was created in 1898, two years after gold was first discovered and the Yukon Gold Rush began. Today mining still accounts for 30 percent of industry in the Yukon, with tourism having emerged as a close second. In recent years, there has also been development in the forestry industry and commercial fishing. There are seventeen communities in the Yukon, the majority of which are accessible by all-weather roads. Whitehorse is the capital city, with a population of 24,473. There are six distinct Aboriginal groups in the Yukon, including the Kutchin, Han, Tutchone, Tlingit, Kaska, and Tagish. As of 2006, there were 3,005 immigrants residing in the Yukon. In fact, immigrants make up 10 percent of the total population (Government of the Yukon 2008).

Palliative Care and an Aging Population

The population of Canada is aging. As a result of low fertility rates and a longer life expectancy overall, the number of seniors aged sixty-five and older has increased by 68 percent over the past two decades (Turcotte and Schellenberg 2007). A medium growth scenario estimates that by 2056 seniors will represent over a quarter of the total Canadian population (Statistics Canada 2006). The number of Aboriginal people in Canada over the age of sixty-five has also increased by 43 percent since 2001 (Statistics Canada 2006). These figures suggest that, like non-Aboriginal people, the number of seniors in the Aboriginal population will represent a much higher percentage of their total population in less than twenty years (Lemchuck-Favel and Jock 2004; Parrack and Joseph 2007).

According to the Canadian Hospice Palliative Care Association (CHPCA), palliative care is a special service that provides health care to both individuals and families who are living with a life-threatening illness that is usually at an advanced stage (CHPCA 1997). Additional definitions of palliative care are found in Chapter 12 of this book.

The goal of palliative care is to provide comfort and dignity for the person living with the illness as well as to ensure the best quality of life for both the individual and his or her family. Relief of pain and other symptoms is an important objective, along with meeting not only physical needs but also the psychological, social, cultural, emotional, and spiritual needs of each person and his or her family (CHPCA 1997). Because family members and friends are often the primary caregivers, the palliative care team can provide respite not only to the patient but also to the caregiver. There has been significant research evidence demonstrating differences in accessibility to health care and social services in rural settings as opposed to urban settings (Kelley 2007; MacLean and Kelley 2001). Palliative care is an aspect of health services seen to be particularly important in rural and remote areas partly because most people would prefer to die in their home communities (Hotson, Macdonald, and Martin 2004; Kelley, Habjan, and Aegard 2004; MacLean and Kelley 2001; Wilson 2007). However, though differences in the palliative care experience between urban and rural settings are significant, the literature does acknowledge some similarities among the issues impacting these two diverse settings (McKee, Kelley, and Guirguis-Younger 2007).

Method

Focus groups and individual interviews were conducted with social service and health-care practitioners and volunteers who work specifically with seniors receiving palliative care in the Yukon, Northwest Territories, and Nunavut. However, before data collection could proceed, we conducted extensive ethics reviews specific to each territory. This process included in-depth written application and research explanation as well as participation in various stakeholder meetings. N. Novik participated in each of these meetings via conference call. Following this process of rigorous review, a research licence was granted by each territory. From beginning to end, the ethics review process spanned a period of five months. Partially due to the varying research guidelines in place within each territory, we decided to exclude current palliative care patients in this study. Instead, the research would include family members of *former* palliative care patients.

Individuals interviewed for this study included a number of registered nurses and social workers, four physicians, a number of homecare staff, two First Nations liaison staff, two pharmacists, one recreational therapist, three hospice staff, and one language interpreter. In addition, family members of seniors who were former palliative patients – representing one family from each of the three territories – were interviewed. Over half of those interviewed identified themselves as Aboriginal, Métis, or Inuit. A total of fifty-three individuals participated in this research study. Of this number, twenty-four were interviewed individually face to face, and the remainder participated in one of seven focus groups. Due to geographical restrictions, interviews were conducted during a one-month period in each territory's capital city – Whitehorse, Yellowknife, and Iqaluit. Participants were identified primarily through health and social service agencies as well as through word of mouth. The process of identifying individuals willing to participate in this study, and the scheduling of interviews, began approximately three months prior to Novik's arrival in the first location and continued throughout the one-month study period. The research participants were asked questions that focused on the types of services and supports available to seniors who are palliative in each community, the manner in which pain is assessed and the pain assessment tools most frequently utilized, the ways in which seniors express or demonstrate pain, how pain is treated and managed, and the impact of pain on seniors' quality of life. One limitation is that palliative patient perspectives were not included in the study; however, given the lack of information about palliative care among northern populations, this study generates more than sufficient information on a topic that warrants further investigation.

Interviewing is one of the most frequently used qualitative methods of data collection (Lincoln and Guba 1985). Typically, this approach results in significant masses of data (Grinnell and Unrau 2005). For this study, both focus groups and individual interviews followed the same general format. During data collection, extensive reflective process notes were also compiled.

Once the interviews and focus groups were completed, they were transcribed by an independent contractor. Novik then analyzed the transcriptions using a thematic analysis based upon the four main areas explored during the interviews. The process notes further informed data analysis since they recorded impressions of body language, facial expression, and dynamics evident during the focus groups. The data analysis was completed using a regular word-processing program that allowed for the sorting of data into emergent categories. As meaning units were identified during first-level coding, categories were established, and codes were subsequently assigned to each category. This intensive approach to data analysis allows one to become completely involved in the data and presents an opportunity to view the information holistically (Grinnell and Unrau 2005). The resultant findings are discussed in the next section.

Findings

Overall, across the three territories, there is recognition that culture and ethnic background have impacts on pain recognition, assessment, and management. Respondents highlighted this point as follows: "They [different cultures] each have their own belief system, and cultural backgrounds determine how they will deal with pain and the role in that of pain medication. Different cultures experience pain in different ways. Some have a lower tolerance for pain."

The significant differences between the three territories were evident in the results of this research study. The unique physical, social, cultural, and historical factors of each territory have resulted in unique circumstances and services for seniors receiving palliative care support. The findings from each territory are discussed later in the chapter, but there were also a number of general themes that arose out of this research. Provision of end-of-life care requires skill and knowledge in a variety of domains, including collaborative decision making, communication, and psycho-social factors that can impact a terminal patient's care preferences (Carter et al. 2006). These areas of skill and knowledge were highlighted as being important in ensuring the quality of palliative care received by seniors in all three territories. Specifically, respondents discussed the importance of good *communication*, the importance of *consistency* in terms of both assessment and care provision, and the importance of acknowledging and respecting the impact of *culture*.

Communication

Across all three jurisdictions, respondents spoke about how critical communication is between the palliative care providers, the patient, and the family members. One care provider offered her thoughts on the importance of good communication and the challenges that can arise when communication falters: "You and [the] relative you're caring for know exactly what the information is and exactly what's happened and what you want to happen – ideally – if you can control it. Whereas here [in the hospital] you have got all these different players and different shifts. The communication may not be as good as it should be."

A number of care providers also discussed other impacts of poor communication, especially between the individuals working with seniors in palliative care and a patient's family members:

> So if someone's experiencing pain, or any other issues, and a family
> are feeling that they are only being half heard or half listened to or half
> understood or half responded to, then that is huge. It's huge in the short
> term in terms of frustration and security and comfort level. And it's
> huge in the long term in terms of the emotional trauma.

One social worker discussed the experience of working with a family using a collaborative team approach in which communication was clear and followed appropriately:

> I said, "what about communication? How do you want to communicate
> with the staff? We're going to do this for pain management." We went
> through all the different domains. The daughter, who was living here,
> was present, and the son, who was visiting, was present, and it went so
> smoothly. Even the therapists, they were in the meeting. And, "okay,

you're going to give them the air mattress, you're going to do the gel pad
for the chair, you're going to monitor and evaluate the positioning every
two days and the skin integrity every few days." Like it was a real team
effort – and the family were involved – and it was really lovely, actually,
how it unfolded.

Difficulty in communication will impact the palliative health-care team's propensity to care for those with a terminal illness (Ingleton 2000). Although this issue is common between both rural and urban settings, in northern Canada these difficulties can be heightened by differences in the language spoken, the cultural background, or the ensuing relationship between patient and health-care provider.

Consistency

Across northern Canada, health and social service regions continue to experience difficulty in recruiting and retaining health-care and social service professionals (Government of the Northwest Territories 2002, 2008; Government of Nunavut 2008; Government of the Yukon 2008). This difficulty has resulted in chronic shortages of physicians, registered nurses, social workers, and pharmacists. Health-care professionals who do choose to practise in northern locations will often seek opportunities over shorter, albeit more intense, periods of time. In essence, this creates a revolving door approach to filling vacant positions. The interviews for this research study revealed that it is especially difficult to recruit professionals with experience and training in palliative care. Of particular concern is a perceived shortage of physicians: "It used to be you could come to town and get a doctor. You can't come to town and get a doctor now."

Many of those interviewed talked about the importance of the relationships between the palliative senior and his or her health-care providers and how consistency in care comes from that relationship: "As you build a relationship with folks and trust, they begin to disclose things like that, not only related to medications, but to certain family situations, to all those multi-factorial things that relate to pain, that contribute to pain."

Related to issues of recruitment and retention are opportunities for professional education. The registered nurses and social workers interviewed for this research study all spoke about the importance of educational opportunities specific to palliative care. Although they spoke about financial constraints and limitations currently placed on educational opportunities, all expressed an interest in accessing professional education through any means available to them. This would include opportunities for on-site, in-service training and training via some form of distance or telehealth technology.

The issue of consistency within the health-care team itself was also discussed by respondents, especially as it related to pain assessment. Individuals interviewed from all three territories talked about the lack of a universal pain scale that incorporates aspects of different cultures. One registered nurse spoke at length about the fact that many of her colleagues do not use any pain scale when working with seniors in palliative care:

> *I feel strongly that it's time to get some issues in place, and facts and protocols and scales, and some structure in providing good palliative care and management of pain, because it's been way too loosey-goosey, depending on staffing and experience and structure. There's no continuity, and we need the – structure, continuity – in how we are going to be providing palliative care and standards of care and standards of practice and protocols and all of that. Right now pain assessment depends too much on the person doing the assessing.*

Consistency of care creates a level of comfort and a sense of safety and security for the palliative patient, his or her caregiver(s), and his or her family. Providing health and social service professionals with educational opportunities is one approach to improving recruitment and retention. Education also improves skill levels and increases feelings of professional competency. All of these factors can vastly improve the senior's quality of life at the end of life.

Culture

All of the individuals interviewed for this research study talked about the impact of culture on both pain assessment and pain management with seniors in palliative care. Obviously, given the large Aboriginal and Inuit populations across the North, much attention was paid to the importance of recognizing these cultures in particular. In fact, the necessity of cultural awareness was the most prominent theme that evolved from the interviews. Other themes included the impact of culture on decision-making processes related to end-of-life care, the impact of family involvement in the process, and, more generally, the impact of culture on communication among everyone involved. One health professional spoke about some of the ways that she has learned to remain cognizant of culture and the importance of doing so:

> *I'm very mindful of the different traditions of the people here, different customs. I'm always, forever, learning different rituals and ceremonies around the dying, around the life celebrations or potlatches. There's a lot of different groups, so – and even working in a facility such as this – I have to really be mindful of the role I take and how I walk with people, support people. Some elders will simply look at me to walk them through. Other elders will boss me around. So it's like I kind of walk with what's happening. Sometimes what we find is that there's a real clash of cultures within mainstream and the traditional practices of the people. And so sometimes you feel like you're caught in the middle – it's very interesting.*

A registered nurse described her experiences in working with Aboriginal seniors:

> *I find that First Nations clients tend to be less verbal about their pain, especially elderly people. I don't know if stoic is the right word, but they are, they don't express pain. Even the word pain has different implications for different people. Well, some people, if you ask them if they have pain, they'll say "no, oh, no, I'm okay." But I'll say, "does your body feel the same as it did when you were twenty, or before you got sick," and they'll be like, "well, no." "Okay, can you tell me more about that?" Because they don't want to say it's pain, because pain sounds like it would be really unbearable.*

Palliative care is often influenced by the values and beliefs found in Aboriginal and Inuit cultures. Of particular importance, decision-making processes are strongly influenced by culture. One of the most important decisions for a physician is how or when to provide palliative care, which requires a high degree of physician discretion (Fetters, Churchill, and Danis 2001). It is accepted in Western societies that the physician will tell the patient his or her prognosis directly. As Kelly and Minty (2007) point out, compared with their non-Aboriginal counterparts, Aboriginal cultures often have different approaches to telling bad news to and maintaining hope for patients. Some Aboriginal cultures believe that positive thinking has an essential role in fighting disease and maintaining good health. As such, the discussion of death related to a terminal illness can be seen as causing the patient to die more quickly. For this reason, some Aboriginal families choose not to disclose prognoses to family members. The use of interpreters can create more confusion. Physicians have found that the use of trained non-family interpreters is the best approach in that it is then possible to avoid potential complications due to differences in values and beliefs related to medical care.

Physicians aim to diagnose a disorder, whereas patients attempt to find meaning and understand their illness (McKechnie and MacLeod 2007). Therefore, how patients choose to live their last days is often a reflection of how they have lived their lives, and such decisions might be the most important ones that they ever make. In Aboriginal populations, the involvement of family and community members in decision making on end-of-life issues is common and tends to complicate palliative care planning (Kelly and Minty 2007).

One registered nurse talked about the importance of enabling family and community members to be present with the senior in palliative care. Not only does their presence improve the overall quality of life for the senior, but also the added comfort and security of a traditional dying process can reduce the senior's anxiety:

> *The Aboriginals are very unique in their own ways, and so if they have someone dying all of the family and the community wants to participate. It's not unusual to have most of the community come in when someone is dying – maybe 50, 100 family and friends from the community would come in. We try to keep the bulk of it contained near to the resident, because it's traditional that they stay until the person passes away. They all come, and they have to pay their respects to the elder.*

The same nurse talked about the challenges of effectively addressing pain experienced by Aboriginal seniors in palliative care:

> *There are those cues that, all of a sudden they become quiet, and then they were fine for a few days, and then they're not responding as much, or they're wanting to talk. We'll sit down, because pain – a lot of elderly people want the pain. I think some of them see taking medication as a weakness, right? Because, out in the community, especially the Aboriginals,*

they're tough, they're very tough individuals. Maybe they're afraid to be there, because they all know. So often it helps if you sit down with them and talk to them. And I usually try to do that pre, before we get into more difficult pain.

As demonstrated, the significant impact of culture on palliative care as experienced by seniors in northern Canada was discussed by respondents from all three territories. Of particular importance is the impact of culture on decision-making processes, the level of family involvement, and the nature of communication.

This section highlighted the importance of communication, consistency, and culture as expressed by individuals interviewed from the territories. However, there were also issues specific to each territory. The next two sections examine issues related to palliative care services available to seniors within each territory.

Nunavut

Given the relatively young population of Nunavut, the number of seniors requiring palliative care support appears to be very low. Whenever possible, most seniors prefer to remain in their own communities to die. However, those who live in Iqaluit most often prefer to die in the hospital. It has been speculated that these seniors view this option as potentially creating less of a burden for their families. As well, a stay in the hospital actually increases the amount of company and community support that they receive, and this support is perceived to have a positive impact on the death experience. Health-care staff spoke openly about the limited resources available to seniors requiring palliative care in Nunavut:

I think we fail them. I really do, truly, not even just here but trying to get a patient back to their home community who wants to die in their home community. The resources are so limited. There's so many vacant positions. We're short on staffing, and even in the new hospital we have only one palliative care bed.

According to all accounts, pain management with this population appears to be straightforward, and oral pain medication often meets the needs of seniors who are palliative:

*Looking at the people that we have got, pain control has not been a big
issue. I don't know if this has anything to do with it at all. There's also
some documentation, and they – with First Nations and whomever – had
noticed that this population doesn't respond to medications like other populations do. And I don't know if that has anything to do with pain control
[for] Inuit or not, I don't know. Typically, we have not had – I'm trying
to think, but I can't think of anyone that we have actually had to admit in
the hospital because their pain has not been controlled at home. But, typically,
we have never had to use like a pain pump at home or anything like that.*

Although there appears to be some suggestion that members of Inuit
populations have a higher tolerance for pain, there is no doubt the Inuit
culture impacts on the expression of pain that does exist:

*The Inuit are a very quiet, very passive people. They're not aggressive
people at all. They will sit, the majority of them will sit, and they'll wait
to ring the bell. Some will just lie there, and you have to notice the very
subtle things ... if they are in pain, like the laboured breathing, the
shuffling in the bed, or the little bit of agitation. Usually, it's us asking
a family member, who will ask them.*

Given the traditional lifestyle, and the lower numbers of seniors who
linger in palliative care, the majority of Inuit involved in this research
study were not aware of the word *palliative* and still view it as a foreign
concept: "But I had never used or heard about it [palliative care] before,
but now, in the last few years, they have been using it. So I had to look
it up in the dictionary to find out what it meant."

Although the traditional lifestyles of the Inuit are beginning to
change, some changes are slower than others. There is only one small
care facility for seniors in Nunavut, and that facility, located in Iqaluit,
is not staffed by registered nurses or professionals with medical backgrounds. Some staff members have received minimal training similar to
that of a home health aide. Currently, there is no specifically defined
palliative care team available in the territory, and there are no hospice
services. Yet Inuit do recognize the changes to their traditional com-
munity- and family-oriented lifestyles:

*The Inuit are starting to take the elders to group homes. You know,
that's something new to us. To take elders – they lose contact with their
families. It's not the same, it's not like leaving for a month. I'm just glad*

in a way that both of my parents died among us when they died. Because
we had a job to do. I don't know about other families. I see people taking
their elders to group homes now because they can't look after them.

Finally, the individuals from Nunavut who were interviewed for
this research study did not report dementia as a common factor for
seniors who are palliative. In fact, dementia appears to be virtually non-
existent among the Inuit. Although this absence might be related to
genetics, to lower rates of mortality, or to the traditional lifestyles of
Inuit seniors, we could not locate any research specific to this topic.
Clearly, this issue requires further investigation.

Northwest Territories and Yukon

Although both the Northwest Territories and Yukon maintain distinct
cultures and related traditional lifestyles, they have been more impacted
perhaps by outside influences than has Nunavut. Consequently, both
territories offer a wider range of palliative care services and supports to
seniors. The Yukon offers hospice services as well as palliative care coordination. Many of the registered nurses and physicians in the Yukon
have received palliative care training through the Victoria Hospice
Program. Although the Northwest Territories does not offer hospice
services, it does have a palliative care working group. Both territories
currently have physicians with an interest, and some specific training, in
palliative care.

Although the differences between the Northwest Territories and
Yukon are many, a number of factors related to palliative care and pain
management with seniors were consistently identified between the two
territories. Consequently, these issues will be discussed jointly in relation
to both the Northwest Territories and the Yukon. In particular, three
themes consistently came out of the interviews with individuals from
these territories: the impact of former and current patient *addictions* on
pain management; the impact of *soul pain* on pain management; and the
recognition of *alternative and traditional approaches* to pain management.

Addictions

In the interviews, a number of individuals talked about the impact that
addictions have on the assessment and management of pain with seniors
in palliative care. It appears that this issue is twofold. First, there is the

belief that there are health practitioners who will not administer pain medication to palliative patients because they fear that the individuals will become addicted to the medication. Second, there are family members who have concerns about pain medications and fear that their loved ones will become addicted to them. The literature suggests that these are common beliefs and concerns and are not unique to northern and remote locations (Aranda et al. 2004; Ward, Emery Berry, and Misiewicz 1996). The following excerpts describe these two situations.

I think there's a challenge there, there's still a lot of stigma out there with the older nurses in regards to addictions and giving too much of medications, you know, or dealing with that also.

If they're in pain, there's things we can do. And a lot of education with the families too. A lot of family members will not understand and say, "wow, she's taking an awful lot of morphine. I don't want her to get addicted to that." And we say, "because of the pain, we've increased the morphine." There are times with the families, when they're giving these meds, so you want to make sure that they have a really good understanding of that.

All individuals who spoke about the impact of addiction during their interviews acknowledged that communication and education are key to improving the situation, including developing and implementing an appropriate pain management plan.

Soul Pain

Many of the individuals interviewed from the Northwest Territories and Yukon spoke about the impact of "soul pain." Essentially, the term was used by respondents to describe lingering emotional and spiritual issues that the patient might have. Although many people referred to soul pain, and expressed their belief that soul pain increases physical pain and impacts the manageability of physical pain, there appeared to be hesitancy to explain or discuss the concept in detail. One of the First Nations liaison workers described her understanding of soul pain as follows: "[Soul pain is] just that deep pain at the core of you, it's that anguish of unresolved issues or emotional stuff or spiritual stuff."

One of the social workers described her experience with the impact of soul pain. In particular, she discussed how soul pain was the only explanation that she could offer in cases where all physical reasons for pain had been addressed and/or ruled out:

> *Now, if there's no reason for physical pain and they're still sort of, there's a closed door there to get anywhere else with them, then my belief is that then there's an incredible amount of soul pain at that point. And it's so painful, what they're going through, and because of life stuff, that they can't go there. We have to deal with both – the soul pain and the physical pain. I think that's just a very, very important part of the diagnosis.*

The practitioners who spoke about soul pain also spoke about the importance of a holistic approach to treatment and pain management. Holistic approaches, as described by the respondents, also include alternative and traditional approaches.

Alternative and Traditional Approaches

Many of the health and social service practitioners from both the Yukon and the Northwest Territories spoke about the incorporation of alternative and traditional approaches into their own professional practices. As well, they spoke about the interest and willingness of seniors in palliative care to incorporate alternative and traditional approaches into their own pain management plans. The approaches that they discussed included acupuncture, therapeutic touch, massage, and the use of traditional medicines. One homecare nurse mentioned that "I've seen, I had a couple of elders, First Nations elders, who opted for all three – naturopathic and homeopathic, herbal approaches, as well as traditional [Indian medicine]."

There is a general understanding that many of the traditional medicines are not talked about or shared openly with outsiders. However, the hospital in Whitehorse does have staff who make available both traditional foods and traditional herbs and medicines. They have also worked to develop a database that lists possible drug interactions related to traditional herbs and medicines.

Implications for Practice

Parrack and Joseph (2007) remind us that national policies based upon the assumption that all communities face the same caregiving challenges fail to recognize important regional, economic, social, and cultural distinctions. This fact resonates through most rural and northern Canadian populations and particularly among Aboriginal seniors and their family caregivers. This research study serves to highlight the importance of recognizing the differences among regions, communities, and cultures. Each of Canada's three northern territories offers very different services to seniors in palliative care, and seniors from each territory have their own distinct needs. Health and social service practitioners who work with seniors in palliative care must work to ensure that these differences are acknowledged and respected.

Acknowledgment

Preparation of this chapter was supported by a Canadian Institutes of Health Research New Emerging Team grant.

References

Aranda, S., P. Yates, H. Edwards, R. Nash, H. Skerman, and A. McCarthy. 2004. "Barriers to Effective Cancer Pain Management: A Survey of Australian Family Caregivers." *European Journal of Cancer Care* 13: 336-43.

Canadian Hospice Palliative Care Association (CHPCA). 1997. *Frequently Asked Questions, Extracted from "Palliative Care: A Fact Sheet for Seniors."* Ottawa: CHPCA, http://www.chpca.net/.

Carter, C.L., J.G. Zapka, S. O'Neill, S. DesHarnais, W. Hennessy, J. Kurent, and R. Carter. 2006. "Physician Perspectives on End-of-Life Care: Factors of Race, Specialty, and Geography." *Palliative and Supportive Care* 4: 257-71.

Fetters, M.D., L. Churchill, and M. Danis. 2001. "Conflict Resolution at the End of Life." *Critical Care Medicine* 29: 921-25.

Government of the Northwest Territories. 2002. *HSS Recruitment and Retention Plan.* Yellowknife: Government of the Northwest Territories, http://pubs.aina.ucalgary.ca/.

—. 2008. *Newstats: Bureau of Statistics.* Yellowknife: Government of the Northwest Territories, http://www.stats.gov.nt.ca/.

Government of Nunavut. 2008. *Nunavut Fact Sheets.* Iqaluit: Government of Nunavut, http://www.gov.nu.ca/.

Government of the Yukon. 2008. *Yukon.* Whitehorse: Government of the Yukon, http://www.gov.yk.ca/.

Grinnell, R.M. Jr., and Y.A. Unrau, eds. 2005. *Social Work Research and Evaluation: Quantitative and Qualitative Approaches.* 7th ed. New York: Oxford University Press.

Hotson, K.E., S.M. Macdonald, and B.D. Martin. 2004. "Understanding Death and Dying in Select First Nations Communities in Northern Manitoba: Issues of Culture and Remote Service Delivery in Palliative Care." *International Journal of Circumpolar Health* 63, 1: 25-38.

Indian and Northern Affairs Canada (INAC). 1994. *Tungavik Federation of Nunavut (TFN) Comprehensive Claim: Northwest Territories.* Ottawa: INAC, http://www.ainc-inac.gc.ca/.

Ingleton, C. 2000. "Reactions of General Practitioners, District Nurses, and Specialist Providers to the Development of a Community Palliative Care Service." *Primary Health Care Research and Development* 1: 15-27.

Kelley, M.L. 2007. "Developing Rural Communities' Capacity for Palliative Care: A Conceptual Model." *Journal of Palliative Care* 23, 3: 143-53.

Kelley, M.L., S. Habjan, and J. Aegard. 2004. "Building Capacity to Provide Palliative Care in Rural and Remote Communities: Does Education Make a Difference?" *Journal of Palliative Care* 20, 4: 308-15.

Kelly, L., and A. Minty. 2007. "End-of-Life Issues for Aboriginal Patients: A Literature Review." *Canadian Family Physician* 53: 1459-65.

Lemchuck-Favel, L., and R. Jock. 2004. "Aboriginal Health Systems in Canada: Nine Case Studies." *Journal of Aboriginal Health* 1: 28-51.

Lincoln, Y.S., and E.G. Guba. 1985. *Naturalistic Inquiry.* Beverly Hills: Sage.

MacLean, M.J., and M.L. Kelley. 2001. "Palliative Care in Rural Canada." *Rural Social Work* 6, 3: 63-73.

McKechnie, R., and R. MacLeod. 2007. "Facing Uncertainty: The Lived Experience of Palliative Care." *Palliative and Supportive Care* 5: 255-64.

McKee, M., M.L. Kelley, and M. Guirguis-Younger. 2007. "So No One Dies Alone: A Study of Hospice Volunteering with Rural Seniors." *Journal of Palliative Care* 23, 3: 163-72.

Parrack, S., and G.M. Joseph. 2007. "The Informal Caregivers of Aboriginal Seniors: Perspectives and Issues." *Journal on Innovation and Best Practices in Aboriginal Child Welfare* 3, 4: 106-13.

Statistics Canada. 2006. *Aboriginal Identity Population by Age Groups, Median Age, and Sex, 2006 Counts, for Canada, Provinces, and Territories – 20% Sample.* Ottawa: Statistics Canada, http://www.statcan.ca/.

Turcotte, M., and G. Schellenberg. 2007. *A Portrait of Seniors in Canada.* Ottawa: Statistics Canada, http://www.statcan.ca/.

Ward, S.E., P. Emery Berry, and H. Misiewicz. 1996. "Concerns about Analgesics among Patients and Family Caregivers in a Hospice Setting." *Research in Nursing and Health* 19: 205-11.

Wilson, D.M. 2007. *An Ethnographic Study to Define the "Good" Rural Death in Alberta: Executive Summary.* Edmonton: Faculty of Nursing, University of Alberta, http://www.nursing.ualberta.ca/.

Chapter 19   Reflections on the Socio-Economic
and Psycho-Social Impacts of
BSE on Rural and Farm Families
in Canada

V. Pletsch, C. Amaratunga, W. Corneil,
S. Crowe, and D. Krewski

Key Points

- Canadian rural and farm families still harboured feelings of bitterness, worthlessness, hopelessness, and uncertainty four years after the announcement of the first BSE case in a Canadian herd.
- "Nobody gave a damn!" captures the sentiment echoed in rural and remote communities. "Nobody" included the government, farm organizations, the media, local and urban communities, and fellow producers; each faltered, to some degree, in giving social and economic support to distressed families, during and following the BSE crisis.
- Meeting the mental health needs of rural communities is challenging, laden with barriers. Crises such as BSE have an extensive socio-economic impact on rural families. Inevitably, this is followed by psycho-social distress.
- BSE is only one crisis in a string of events in recent years to hit Canadian agricultural communities. Farmers are resilient and protective. Many are determined to take extra precautions in their operations and are demanding the same of the industry.
- Farmers are more realistic about the future of the "family farm." Many of their children, after witnessing a string of crises, agree that, without outside financial support, family farmers will exist only as "a family centre where we can raise a cow or have a garden."

The 1989 Canada-US Free Trade Agreement removed any remaining limitations on the transfer of cattle between the two countries and placed Canadian beef farmers in a position to expand their herds and take advantage of this new financial opportunity. However, the situation changed abruptly in May 2003 when one cow in northern Alberta tested positive for bovine spongiform encephalopathy (BSE), and approximately forty countries immediately closed their borders to live ruminants, meat products, and animal by-products from Canada (Lewis, Krewski, and Tyshenko 2010). Some relief came four months later when the United States opened its border to slaughtered "boneless meat from cattle less than 30 months old" (Leblanc 2007, 1). The border remained closed to live cattle less than thirty months old until July 2005 and to older cattle until November 2007 (Canadian Food Inspection Agency [CFIA] 2005, 2007, 2008a). It is estimated that Canada's soaring cattle and beef exporting industry suffered losses exceeding $6.3 billion and affected 90,000 producers nationwide (Broadway 2008; Emilson 2005; Mitura and Di Piétro 2004). As other chapters in this volume have shown, meeting the mental health needs of rural communities has many challenges and barriers. With the added element of the BSE crisis, rural communities are increasingly vulnerable to growing socio-economic concerns and their inevitable psycho-social impacts.

A review of the scientific and grey literature on BSE, both in Canada and internationally, reveals that, although the significant financial losses to farmers are well recognized, the subsequent psycho-social stresses experienced by rural and farm families are largely excluded (McCallum and Sutherns 2006; Sutherns and Amaratunga 2007; Wellmann and Thurston 2006).

This chapter contributes to the rural health literature by examining the impacts of circumstances such as BSE on rural peoples and examining aging in rural contexts as well as cultural and spatial barriers to accessing mental health services (e.g., pride of farmers). We review the results from focus groups conducted with farm family members in five provinces across Canada in 2007, four years after the announcement of the first indigenous case of BSE in Canada.[1] Table 19.1 describes the focus group sample, and Table 19.2 describes the research and analysis process. The forty-eight participants (averaging fifty years of age) represented farmers involved in animal and mixed farming, agricultural students, producers' associations, and agricultural organizations. The recruitment strategy, which included mail-outs to 800 rural and agricultural organizations, and advertisements through the news media,

Table 19.1   Description of focus groups

Province	City	Women	Men	Total participants
Ontario	Kemptville	4	6	10
Quebec	Ste-Hyacinthe	4	8	12
Manitoba	Brandon	5	3	8
Saskatchewan	Moose Jaw	0	12	12
Alberta	Lethbridge	0	6	6

might explain the gender bias in the focus groups, because participation was voluntary. In addition, a number of male participants noted that their partners/spouses were unable to participate due to their off-farm work schedules. Both male and female participants suggested that subsequent focus groups on this subject, centring on women, are needed to understand better the different experiences of the BSE crisis between men and women on the farm.

Although a number of farms have always been located close to urban centres, most of the participants were from rural and remote communities. The definition of rural is outlined in Chapter 1 of this book. As shown in Chapter 13, however, the term "rural" is not well defined and is often based on the researcher's purpose (Bosak and Perlman 1982; Deavers 1992; du Plessis et al. 2002; Halfacree 1993, 1995). For the purposes of this chapter, it is important to understand that significant distinctions exist within rural contexts and especially between agricultural and non-agricultural communities (Judd et al. 2006; Lobley et al. 2004; Mitra et al. 2009). From the focus group discussions, farmers who participated self-identified as a distinct culture (i.e., distinct from "rural non-farming communities"), and they thought that their experience of the BSE crisis was different from that of their rural neighbours. "Nobody gave a damn!" captures the sentiment echoed during the dialogue with participants in the five focus groups. As much as possible, the original statements from the participants are used to capture their responses regarding the impacts of BSE on their families, their communities, and their health and well-being. In retrospect, the inadequate financial and emotional support and the subsequent unrecoverable losses left families harbouring feelings of bitterness, worthlessness, hopelessness, and uncertainty. In essence, the socio-economic impact

Table 19.2 Research process and analysis

Structure and analysis	Description
Structure	• Semi-structured interview guides • Structured Interview Matrix methodology (Chartier 2002); participants interview each other in pairs, followed by small group and larger group discussions • Total of 8 questions per focus group • Running time: 5 hours • Approved by University of Ottawa Research Ethics Board
Analysis	• Results thematically analyzed • Qualitative research software: QSR NVivo 7 • Summary reports circulated to participants and recruiting organizations through regular mail
Participants	• Livestock and mixed-farming producers; agricultural students; members of producers' associations; agricultural organizations • 48 in total • Average age: 50 and above (some younger participants included)

of BSE is further shaping rural and remote situations under changing and increasingly strained circumstances.

Emotional and Social Stress

When the discovery of BSE in Canada in May 2003 was announced, many farmers instantly experienced feelings of devastation and emotional stress. For example, one participant reported that "I was baling, listening to CBC Radio. I literally shook for the rest of the day." What is clear from the findings of the focus groups, and consistent across all five provinces surveyed, is the sustained high level of stress caused by the discovery of BSE in the Canadian cattle herd. The source of this stress was multi-layered; however, from the participants' point of view, the financial losses, particularly the sudden loss in equity (anywhere from 20 percent to 80 percent in annual income), continued to be the main stressor.

The majority of participants agreed that the lack of export markets for cattle left cow-calf producers shouldering the costs, resenting the fact that packers and processors benefited, first by buying cheap cattle, then by profiting inequitably from government assistance programs. In particular, confusion and frustration ensued from the fact that the price of their cattle was greatly lower while the price of beef in grocery stores remained the same. One participant reported that "farmers don't feel appreciated. They lose money and can't pass the costs on to the middle-men because they [farmers] are at the bottom of the food chain. Who am I to have to work for free to feed the population?"

Most participants shared the perception that even during good times farmers are less likely to visit a physician than non-farmers. However, with the added stress of false promises, off-farm jobs, and burnout ex-perienced during the BSE crisis, farm families reported that "colds turn into pneumonia, sore knees turn into arthritis, and sleep deprivation leads to injuries – often ignored and untreated, all because farmers can't 'call in sick.'" Moreover, for some participants, the physical impact of the stress related to BSE has been persistent. One man reported, "I still don't sleep at night, still disoriented, and have constant headaches." The health of the animals often circumvents a farmer's well-being. The rationalization of one farmer follows: "There are so many low blows in agriculture that we end up developing thick skin, which prevents us from properly evaluating the impact it has on our health, physically as well as psychologically, and it eventually surfaces in the form of illness or depression."

Although difficult to measure, some participants believed that de-layed health problems such as high blood pressure, strokes, and heart attacks were directly related to the BSE crisis, and many agreed that the "independent nature of farmers may have a lot to do with these illnesses," describing themselves as having "short fuses" and being "angry in general" because of the disaster. Many people chose farming not only as an occupation but also as a way of life for their families. Under extreme economic pressure, family relationships, including par-ents and partners, became disconnected. Over time, as farm families increasingly had to manage uncertainty and economic decline, the stresses on relationships and marriages increased. One participant ex-plained: "Feelings toward family members turn to bitterness. We went from a vivacious loving family to this [anger and isolation]."

Participants affirmed that women were especially vulnerable as they attempted to add more responsibilities to their usual tasks. The extra workload created additional isolation and separation among family members. One husband, for example, stated that "we take our stress out on our wives. What about the wife's problems? Everything now takes money, and she has to deal with it." Not only did the women of the family take off-farm jobs when things got tough financially, but they also continued to be the rural community volunteers.

Endeavouring to shelter the family from the distress of social isolation has been a major challenge. Try as they might, parents cannot shield children, even young ones, from worrisome family concerns such as the lack of money to support sports, community events, or further education. In some cases, participants reported that children left school to help their parents on the farm. One participant explained: "It's hard to watch and hear the children talking at school – children can't participate in social events or go on in school."

With little cash to purchase or enjoy the extras, combined with the shame of unpaid bills, farmers began to withdraw from their neighbours. "In your own community, you can't pay your bills, so you don't want to meet the dealership owner or the banker at the mailbox or in church. Your pride is hurt because you feel that your reputation is tarnished." A number of participants discussed their experiences of finger pointing and negative attitudes toward farmers in general, causing some to withdraw from community workshops and other functions – "even the free ones." Others explained that the most humbling experience was the loss of prestige and social standing within their communities, but the "ultimate shame" for any farmer "comes when a farmer, whose job it is to produce food, has to make a stop at the food bank."

From the participants' point of view, a sense of upheaval and isolation struck rural and remote agricultural communities on multiple fronts. Many discouraged producers have given up on farming and have left the industry only to be followed by farm support service operators and labourers. For example, machine dealerships have been unable to pay their investment costs, and local grocery stores often fold as farming communities shrink and farmers find ways to cut costs. In the worst-case scenarios, especially in the western provinces, where farmers and rural people are already isolated by geographical distance, participants thought that BSE has had a devastating effect on local commercial centres. One farmer stated: "We watched the town close down, and it won't reopen. It's a ghost town, even the rink stands empty." Others told of the demise of trucking businesses and the closure of schools and churches. Whether warranted or not, the fallout from BSE has caused many farm families to feel estranged from the mainstream of life, leaving them with little or no incentive to seek psychological and social supports – services that they believe they need.

Who Can We Trust?

Most participants claimed to have a fair to above-average knowledge of BSE. One producer explained: "I have a slight overview – not a vet's or doctor's knowledge, but a layman's." Obviously, many know what is reported but suspect that much more is to be learned and reported. Following announcement of the discovery of BSE in Canada, most farmers continued to trust veterinarians to deal with animal health. One participant stated: "Vets are probably the best source of information about BSE. They have ethics, and they are paid by us. They were also affected by BSE. They lost business." Rural families also trusted their physicians (especially rural physicians) to seek out the latest information on BSE and to deal with their patients' physical and psychological issues related to it. However, according to one participant, veterinarians and physicians were receiving the same information (often through the media, by facsimile, or by email) at the same time as everyone else. As an example of the confusion at the time, one farmer explained: "One doctor asked [me] what he should be looking for, and I said, 'Don't worry about the physical side, expect stress and depression.'"

Documented research available through university websites and government news releases was accepted as trustworthy information. Farm, veterinarian, and medical journals were also seen to be credible, but, as the participants explained, many of these publications did not reach the general public, resulting in a lack of local and urban support. Information provided by agricultural organizations was available to farmers but reported by the participants to be accepted with more enthusiasm if the association's leaders were perceived to have training and experience in agriculture – a vested interest in the producers' overall welfare. Participants explained that they are more likely to trust professionals with farming experience, since they would be better positioned to understand the daily issues that farmers face, and respect and appreciate a farmer's method of business and way of life, which they perceived as unique.

Farm and rural families do not always trust the mainstream media to provide truthful facts, and most of the participants thought that the press, radio, and television frequently used "sensational, scary tactics." Media reports, participants maintained, did not put farming in a positive light or explain the short- and long-term economic, emotional, and social impacts of BSE on the farming community. Nor did news updates attempt to clarify government-announced assistance programs, leaving the public with the idea that the money was simply a handout to farmers. One farmer stated that "media people have little knowledge of the industry, so how can they describe the plight of the farm community? They can't educate the public." Much of the anger was directed toward inaccurate, shocking accounts of BSE and the need for someone to step up in defence of the positive steps being taken by producers to supply safe, quality food for Canadians. One participant stated: "The media has denigrated us – alarmists that provoke mistrust of our products. You feel very small in their depiction."

Coping

When BSE hit, most farmers "waited out the storm" for a few months; however, when the reopening of export borders appeared to be hopeless and government assistance programs proved to be more of an "insult than help," families, determined to hang on to their farms and their animals, relied on their own ingenuity. Off-farm employment, for one or more family members, became the main coping mechanism. Farm women, usually responsible for the household budget – and in many cases for the farm books – took on full-time off-farm jobs and found creative ways to cope. "Women were car-pooling to bigger centres to save gas and buy cheaper milk, etc."

Farm families seem to have coped less successfully with their emotional and psycho-social stresses. One reason might be the fact that, as a number of participants affirmed, farmers are "an independent and tough lot" when it comes to seeking outside help. However, under the circumstances, many learned to cope emotionally by keeping a positive attitude, taking advantage of any support services that did not cost money, and by learning to laugh. One woman explained that she had decided, very early, to laugh: "The alternative," she said, "was to go behind the barn and bury myself in the manure pit."

Less costly events that included close friends and family prevented many families from isolating themselves socially. For one participant, it meant taking extension courses, at no cost, to keep his "mind and soul together." For another, it was frequent visits to the local coffee shop or a rotating coffee-and-muffins routine among friends. "I was in a rut," reported one woman, "so I suggested we get friends together to watch a movie or a hockey game. Have a potluck – anything that doesn't cost. Then give each other a break; don't talk about agricultural issues." Many agreed with her strategy. And many, especially women, agreed that they could handle giving up the annual vacation but were determined to make time for their children and grandchildren even as they struggled with off-farm jobs.

Nevertheless, many participants knew of someone whose marriage had ended in divorce because of the ramifications of BSE, and a surprising number reported suicide cases that were perceived as being directly related. One simply stated: "I sold the farm and divorced."

For many, "there was a huge financial impact." Unfortunately, declaring bankruptcy has been the only alternative for a number of Canadian farmers. One former farmer described how "we used up all the kids' university money and savings. I am using my RSPs and still had to get out of it in the end." Another explained: "You can only tighten so far – life gets sapped out."

Amazingly, many have managed to maintain a positive attitude. "It's very discouraging but not hopeless yet. We have to be the most optimistic crowd, us farmers," stated one participant. Another used the following analogy: "The impact of BSE, it's similar to a death. Eventually, you get to the point of accepting that death. Everyone has to come to his own conclusion about how and when this acceptance will take place."

Support

Over the past two or three decades, farming practices in Canada and globally have changed dramatically. Farms are big business operations involving larger land areas (especially in the western provinces), huge machinery, and a greater concentration of animals – a far cry from the days of mixed farming, when neighbours knew each other, worked together, and relied on businesses in nearby villages and towns. One farmer explained: "There's a tremendous shift in the mentality of farming as the farms get bigger and not operated by family anymore. It's impersonal, competitive."

In rare cases, where that sense of community still exists, participants reported receiving support during the BSE crisis; for example, a few local dealerships cut prices. One producer explained: "There was little money changing hands. People paid by bartering services. There was more of that going on than paying off debts to each other, because everyone's tight for cash." The response of rural non-farmers was somewhat similar to that of urban dwellers. They attended local beef barbecues, believing that they were offering their support, and it was reported that "they bought even more beef because it was cheap." Local physicians and veterinarians continued their support; however, in communities depleted of people who moved out to seek jobs, remaining members became financially strapped, and rural churches, traditionally recognized as community centres of concern, tended to have fewer resources to offer.

Nonetheless, the majority told of the total lack of community support. Even fellow producers competed for the best prices, taking advantage of another's loss. The following statement portrays this sense of disappointment and betrayal: "The community will mobilize only in the face of a major event, like a suicide (always support in death) or a fire, but afterwards their support vanishes. If a farmer has a mental breakdown, you don't see the neighbours coming over."

This deficiency in support for mental health issues might not be unique to rural communities since mental health has a stigma no matter where people live. However, as discussed in Chapter 13 of this volume, there is growing debate over the role that cultural characteristics of rural, remote, and agricultural communities (e.g., stoicism, isolation) play in stigma concerning mental health problems and help-seeking behaviour (Canadian Agricultural Safety Association [CASA] 2005; Fuller et al. 2000; Judd et al. 2006; Mitra et al. 2009; Parry et al. 2005; Peck et al. 2002).

The lack of community support might be explained by the fact that farmers tend to communicate with and support those who are in the same type of production. Their connections are through the commodity groups of which they are members. "People today don't realize. We've all been isolated into our own industry. So nobody sees the big picture. Farmers are so individualized." Moreover, participants felt further constrained by the impact of the processors and packers on the smaller producers: "Feedlots are like businesses, made up of independent businesspeople. So they took it out on cow-calf guys by offering to pay less for cows and forcing the industry prices down. There was no trickle down to cow-calf producers."

Reviews varied among the focus groups concerning the amount of support offered by agricultural organizations. The issue of trust lies in the fact that these decision makers are elected or government appointed to paid positions and do not "represent the grassroots producer." Dairy farmers attending the focus groups reported feeling particularly neglected – they did not qualify for assistance because they operated under a quota-regulated system of supply management.

The federal government announced a Cull Animal Program in 2003 ($120 million) and both a Transitional Industry Support Program ($930 million) and a Repositioning the Livestock Industry Strategy ($458 million) in 2004. As well, the Canadian Agricultural Income Stabilization Program (CAIS), which has been replaced by AgriStability and AgriInvest (Agriculture and Agri-Food Canada 2008), was available. In addition, the provinces implemented their own support and compensation programs. Despite these supports, Canadian cattle sales declined drastically during the same years (Broadway 2008). The participants in all focus groups were consistent in their criticism of government support at all stages of the BSE crisis – the lack of a prevention plan, the complete breakdown of communications that included broken promises, and the inadequate, inequitable financial assistance programs that followed. This injustice they attributed to the dearth of understanding about farming by government officials at all levels, the desire to turn farming into big business, and a politician's preoccupation with being re-elected. Again the general feeling from a majority of participants was that "nobody gave a damn."

One positive support was supplied in the form of rural and farm stress lines, and in some cases agricultural associations provided not only farming advice but also stress counselling. One participant explained: "I was on the cattlemen's board, and it was easy to let them scream and curse. They didn't want answers, just wanted to be mad. They couldn't get away from it. I was on the phone three or four hours every day, and it was extremely stressful." However, a number of participants stated that the private, proud nature of farmers and the "stigma of having to reach out" often resulted in avoidance, causing the withdrawal of government support. One participant emphasized the fact that "farmers are so independent, they won't use crisis call lines; they would rather deal with things internally – between husband and wife."

With few exceptions, the greatest immediate and long-term moral and financial support was provided by the immediate family. One farmer stated: "Our family is pulling together to make ends meet," and another credited his wife, a nurse, for being "the only reason we kept any sanity around the house" after the family declared bankruptcy. In general, communications among family members were highly appreciated and recommended.

Future of the Family Farm

For a number of years, the future of the Canadian family farm has been a topic of debate among academics, politicians, farm organizations, and individual farmers. When the focus groups were conducted, recent disasters, such as the drought in the west and the high value of the Canadian dollar (Baxter and Stoneman 2008), added to the discussion, and the focus group participants agreed that the immediate and lasting effects of BSE have contributed to the possible demise of the family farm, large or small. Although measuring the reach of these perceived impacts is challenging and beyond the scope of this chapter, concerns from a majority of the participants raise questions about the viability and sustainability of the family farm in Canada. Particularly since farming and rural communities are aging (as shown in Chapter 25 of this book), exacerbating the challenges for rural and remote communities to meet the health-care needs of the older members of their populations. For example, one young participant pointed out that "the young have struggled, trying to get into the beef industry. Many are selling the cows and getting out. Why are they giving up? They're running out of money." Another young farmer stated:

> I went to work in the oil fields and sent money home to keep the farm running. It changes the dynamics of the farm when you have to work to keep it going. I will not go into farming, and I want you to tell that to the general public and to the government. Our family knows they will not earn a living. Get rid of that dream. If you don't have that quarter section to take over and produce, you're not going to do it.

Many parents who have used their savings and their retirement reserves to survive the BSE crisis are discouraging young people from taking up farming as a means of supporting a family. One producer offered the following explanation: "My dad retired at my age (sixty-two) and wrote himself a cheque from the farm to buy a house in town. I couldn't do that now, no way. And I'm the same age that he was then." To demonstrate further the challenges faced by farm families, one participant asked: "Do I want to pass on this frustration, risk, and lack of social support investment?" Participants explained that traditionally their farms had been in their families for several generations, with children usually taking over the farms after their parents retired.

However, the participants reported that they now found themselves discouraging their children from farming and inheriting the financial burden. This sentiment was in contradiction to the pride and strong attachment that participants expressed in regard to the way of life of farming. This contradiction appeared to cause some stress among a number of the participants.

In five focus groups, with an average age of at least fifty years, the older generation was well represented. Many older farmers tried to stay on to save the family farms, but they reported that "accidents are up because of long hours and poor eyesight." Moreover, they were further challenged by the changing business of farming: "Some farmers are just too old to learn computers or to catch and tag their cattle." Because of BSE, many could not afford to retire. "My health is okay," reported one. "I'm retired, but part of my retirement fund went down the tube, and that's common." Another retiree explained the inheritance dilemma: "After BSE, people couldn't make payments, and the problem is that the intergenerational transfer of land isn't done traditionally anymore. So someone has to sell the land at top dollar, and this takes away from financing on debt money. No one can get out of debt." Traditionally a son or daughter remained on the farm, sharing the responsibilities with elderly parents. In many cases, BSE depleted the cash flow, requiring immediate sale of the farm, limiting possibilities for continuing operations, because siblings expected to receive their inherited shares.

All of these dilemmas impact rural and remote communities; families leave the land, and farms are left without replacements to continue farm operations or fill community positions traditionally taken up by the younger generation of farmers. "There aren't enough people to provide leadership for the organizations," explained one participant, who had contributed many volunteer hours in his community. "We all have a burnout period – we'd love to see the twenty-five year olds step up, but they won't get involved." Many agreed with the explanation that, "as rural communities disappear, kids go to the city for education and sports. They are being exposed to city ethos and are losing the farming/ rural life attitude."

Recommendations

In all five focus groups, participants offered recommendations both to other producers and to governments. Their hope was that their suggestions would assist in dealing with the current impacts of the BSE crisis and help to mitigate future crises. The summary of these recommendations is discussed below.

To Other Producers

Reflecting on their experiences during the crisis, participants wanted to remind other producers that "knowledge is power." "Study the impact of the disease on your product," advised one farmer. "Be aware of the financial and psychological repercussions and know the regulations." Some participants thought that looking beyond government, with the exception of grants, and developing a long-term plan for sustainability could be a useful strategy. In other cases, participants shared a loss of hope for the industry, offering what they thought was a more realistic solution: "Ditch the dream if there's no hope, get another job, or bite the bullet. Exit the business and educate your children not to go into farming."

Operating a closed herd rated a top position on the list of suggestions. "Label, record, and be able to trace every animal from the gate to the plate," cautioned one farmer: "It will also lower your vet costs." Building alliances by bartering within the community was also promoted as a means of saving money and offering support. "Support your agricultural associations. They need a quorum to operate. Time is money to a farmer, so keep your meetings short and meaningful."

Equally important, farmers must present themselves and their products in a more positive light. Participants suggested direct involvement – at least communication – with the media, farm organizations, members of Parliament, and international trading partners. "Invite the media and demonstrate positive steps that are taking place in your locality or province."

Even though these suggestions might seem out of the question for a busy and independent farmer, participants emphasized the urgency of putting agriculture back in "its rightful place in society," and they called on the industry to "stay honest" in its dealings. "'Made in Canada' is misleading," one farmer warned. "Industry must live up to its part of the deal." This comment refers to the discussion regarding the frustration that a number of participants felt concerning misleading labels permitted on imported products. For example, the term "Made in Canada" on agricultural products sold to consumers can mean that only a small percentage of the finished product (e.g., the packaging) is actually made in Canada.[2]

To Governments

Angered by the social and economic injustices that BSE bestowed on them, a number of participants viewed the focus groups as a forum to voice their concerns and make recommendations to governments. When the next disaster hits, they want to see a risk management plan, with a trellis life line in place, that will allow everyone to survive – even small farmers. "Government must anticipate the problem before it happens," insisted one man. "What's the protocol? These are the steps to take. Outline them." Being prepared, they say, will require the involvement of those trained to handle rural problems. This further supports the postulation in Chapter 13 of this volume for community-based approaches in designing mental health and social care supports and interventions for rural and remote communities and farmers in particular.

Producers also called for a much more aggressive attempt to educate the general public, including farmers, about farming practices. When giving advice on soliciting the support of the general public, one farmer insisted that "the Federation of Agriculture, and the media, must give more useful, accurate information to farmers," and the "government must step up to defend the farming community against false accusations by the media." Other recommendations involved financial safeguards to protect the industry from future disasters, for example "using crop insurance as a prototype, develop[ing] a program to cover livestock." Another participant added: "Put some safeguard money aside, perhaps in the hands of an agricultural organization, to be invested for farmers – not just on an emergency basis. Farmers could pay a monthly pre-mium, to be matched by the government, to create a pension fund."

Farmers fear that they alone will bear the expense of implementing government specified risk materials (SRM) regulations,[3] and they im-plore the present government to develop a means whereby all stake-holders can share the costs: "Sensitize the public on specified risk materials and the feasibility of the proposed laws and policies," warned an apprehensive producer. "They need to be aware of constant changes regarding food safety and health risks." Another participant echoed the concerns of many by suggesting that agriculture should be returned to the school curriculum.

The majority of participants voiced their approval of testing all Canadian cattle – "Every cow should be tested at the slaughter house" – and a "tightening of regulations regarding the traceability of each animal from birth to consumption is absolutely necessary." As well, they encouraged the government to seek access to diversified markets.

The hesitancy among rural families to seek physical, psychological, and social assistance during the BSE disaster can be associated with the lack of time and money. Their recommendations to governments were straightforward: "First identify the tension. Then find ways to provide financial and emotional support." More specifically, one suggested that the government "provide mental health counsellors, similar to those who go into schools following a tragedy. Do the same with legal and therapeutic help – only medical is free."

Conclusion

The sentiment "nobody gave a damn" was voiced by participants in virtually each of the focus groups and is indicative of the feelings of bitterness, worthlessness, hopelessness, and uncertainty harboured by rural and farm families four years after the announcement of the first BSE case in the Canadian herd. The "nobody" included not only governments but also a wide range of people and organizations that, consciously or not, failed to offer adequate social and economic supports to the distressed families. Farm organizations, the media, local and urban communities, and even fellow producers all faltered in their support to some degree.

The BSE experience demonstrated one more time that "farmers have the resiliency to 'bounce back' during adversity." Yes, some good things have resulted from the struggle: many farmers are determined to take extra precautions in their operations, and they are demanding similar action from the industry. More than ever, they are anxious to promote safe and healthy products and are willing to face the media and government to defend their cause. One woman declared: "We won't let this happen again!" As well, current farmers have become more realistic about the future of the family farm, and many of their children, regardless of age, have experienced the financial, emotional, and social anxieties that can plague a career in farming.

BSE is only one crisis in a string of events in recent years to "deliver a blow" to Canadian agricultural communities and one among many stressors affecting rural (i.e., farming) communities. For many, the unremitting "big hurt" that followed BSE extended well beyond a monetary crisis. It cut into the soul and threatened the very existence of the farm family as a Canadian institution. If the family farm continues to exist, it will require outside financial supports and networks, or it will become what one young participant called merely "a family centre where we can raise a cow or have a garden."

During the summer of 2006, the Blyth Festival's production of *Another Season's Harvest* skilfully portrayed the story of farmers coping – in their own ways – with the BSE disaster. In reflection, one farmer said, "I thought I could handle it; I knew my non-farming friends were enjoying the humour, but it got me right in the pit of my stomach. Only those who experienced it will ever understand."

Acknowledgments

The research team would like to thank the staff, research assistants, and students from the Women's Health Research Unit who helped to prepare and successfully hold the five focus groups across the country. We are especially grateful to the agricultural organizations and farmers across the country that helped to recruit participants and for their on-going support of our work. Finally, we would like to thank all the participants who took part in the focus groups. The funding of PrioNet Canada, a National Centre of Excellence, is gratefully acknowledged. The views contained in this chapter are those of the authors and do not represent the views of PrioNet Canada.

Notes

1   This study is one component of a national program of research led by researchers at the University of Ottawa who are developing an integrated risk management framework for prion diseases, including BSE (Leiss et al. 2010; Mitra et al. 2009).
2   In January 2009, the government of Canada announced that it intended to implement tougher laws on labelling, including stricter rules for "Product of Canada" labels. Prior to this announcement, "Made in Canada" labels only needed to contain 51 percent of production costs spent in Canada (Davis 2009).
3   On 12 July 2007, the government of Canada implemented an enhanced regulation on SRMs, materials in which BSE proteins are concentrated (e.g., brain, eyes, and spinal cord). In 1997, they were banned from bovine animal feed, and in 2007 SRMs were banned from all animal feeds, including pet foods and fertilizers. In addition, stricter regulations and paper trails regarding the transportation of SRMs were implemented (CFIA 2008b).

References

Agriculture and Agri-Food Canada. 2008. *The Canadian Agricultural Income Stabilization (CAIS) Program*. Ottawa: Agriculture and Agri-Food Canada, http://www4.agr.gc.ca/.

Baxter, M., and D. Stoneman. 2008. "Managing the Wavering Loonie." *Better Farming* 10, 1: 12-24, http://www.betterfarming.com/.

Bosak, J., and B. Pearlman. 1982. "A Review of the Definition of Rural." *Journal of Rural Community Psychology* 3, 1: 3-34.

Broadway, M. 2008. "BSE's 'Devastating' Impact on Rural Alberta: A Preliminary Analysis." *Prairie Forum* 33, 1: 123-45.

Canadian Agricultural Safety Association (CASA). 2005. *National Stress and Mental Survey.* Winnipeg: CASA, http://www.casa-acsa.ca/.

Canadian Food Inspection Agency (CFIA). 2005. *Canadian Livestock Shipments Moving across United States Border.* Ottawa: CFIA, http://www.inspection.gc.ca/.

–. 2007. *Exporting Cattle, Bison, and Their Products under USDA Final Rule on BSE Risk.* Ottawa: CFIA, http://www.inspection.gc.ca/.

–. 2008a. *Bovine Spongiform Encephalopathy (BSE) in North America.* Ottawa: CFIA, http://www.inspection.gc.ca/.

–. 2008b. *Enhanced Animal Health Protection from BSE.* Ottawa: CFIA, http://www.inspection.gc.ca/.

Chartier, R. 2002. *Tools for Leadership and Learning: Building a Learning Organization.* 3rd ed. Ottawa: Public Works and Government Services Canada, http://www.managers-gestionnaires.gc.ca/.

Davis, J. 2009. "Tougher 'Made in Canada' Regs Kick In." *Embassy,* 7 January, 1-15, http://www.embassymag.ca/.

Deavers, K. 1992. "What Is Rural?" *Policy Studies Journal* 20, 2: 184-89.

du Plessis, V., R. Beshiri, R.D. Bollman, and H. Clemenson. 2002. "Definitions of 'Rural.'" Agricultural and Rural Working Paper Series No. 61. Ottawa: Statistics Canada.

Emilson, K. 2005. *Just a Matter of Time.* Vogar, MB: Nordheim Books.

Fuller, J., J. Edwards, N. Procter, and J. Moss. 2000. "How Definition of Mental Health Problems Can Influence Help Seeking in Rural and Remote Communities." *Australian Journal of Rural Health* 8: 148-53.

Halfacree, K.H. 1993. "Locality and Social Representation: Space, Discourse, and Alternative Definitions of the Rural." *Journal of Rural Studies* 9, 1: 23-37.

–. 1995. "Talking about Rurality: Social Representations of the Rural as Expressed by Residents of Six English Parishes." *Journal of Rural Studies* 11, 1: 1-20.

Judd, F., H. Jackson, A. Komiti, G. Murray, C. Fraser, A. Grieve, and R. Gomez. 2006. "Help-Seeking by Rural Residents for Mental Health Problems: The Importance of Agrarian Values." *Australian and New Zealand Journal of Psychiatry* 40: 769-76.

Leblanc, M. 2007. "Chronology of BSE-Related Events and Government Initiatives (PRB 04-12E)." *In Brief,* Issue PRB 04-12E, revised 20 June 2007, 1-8. Ottawa: Parliamentary Information and Research Services, Library of Parliament, http://www.parl.gc.ca/.

Leiss, W., M.G. Tyshenko, D. Krewski, N. Cashman, L. Lemyre, M. Al-Zoughool, and C. Amaratunga. 2010. "Managing the Risk of Bovine Spongiform Encephalopathy: A Canadian Perspective." *International Journal of Risk Assessment and Management* 14, 5: 381-435.

Lewis, R., D. Krewski, and M.G. Tyshenko. 2010. "A Review of Bovine Spongiform Encephalopathy and Its Management in Canada and the USA." *International Journal of Risk Assessment and Risk Management* 14, 1-2: 32-49.

Lobley, M., G. Johnson, M. Reed, M. Winter, and J. Little. 2004. "Rural Stress Review: Final Report." Exeter: Centre for Rural Policy Research, University of Exeter, http://www.centres.exeter.ac.uk/.

McCallum, M., and R. Sutherns. 2006. "Bovine Spongiform Encephalopathy: An Annotated Review of International Literature." Calgary: Prairie Women's Health Centre of Excellence, University of Calgary, http://www.webapps2.ucalgary.ca/.

Mitra, D., C. Amaratunga, R. Sutherns, V. Pletsch, W. Corneil, S. Crowe, and D. Krewski. 2009. "The Psychosocial and Socio-Economic Consequences of BSE: A Community Impact Study." *Journal of Toxicology and Environmental Health, Part A: Current Issues* 72, 17: 1106-12.

Mitura, V., and L. Di Piétro. 2004. "Canada's Beef Cattle Sector and the Impact of BSE on Farm Family Income 2000-2003." Agriculture and Rural Working Paper Series No. 69. Ottawa: Statistics Canada.

Parry, J., H. Barnes, R. Lindsey, and R.F. Taylor. 2005. "Farmers, Farm Workers, and Work-Related Stress." Research Report 362. Sudbury, UK: HSE Books.

Peck, D.F., S. Grant, W. McArthur, and D. Godden. 2002. "Psychological Impact of Foot-and-Mouth Disease on Farmers." *Journal of Mental Health* 11, 5: 523-31.

Sutherns, R., and C. Amaratunga. 2007. "Canadian Farmers in the Wake of BSE: Resilience amidst Uncertainty." Unpublished technical report, University of Ottawa.

Wellmann, L., and W.E. Thurston. 2006. *Canadian BSE Annotated Literature Review.* Calgary: University of Calgary, http://www.webapps2.ucalgary.ca/.

Part 6: First Nations in Rural Settings

Chapter 20   Decolonizing First Nations Health

K. Jacklin and W. Warry

Key Points

- Colonialism is a major determinant of health for Aboriginal peoples in Canada.
- Self-determination, community control, and capacity building are necessary ingredients in the decolonization of Aboriginal health care and improved health status for Aboriginal peoples in Canada.
- Approaches to Aboriginal health care that include an understanding of historical and contemporary relations between Aboriginal and non-Aboriginal people in Canada can facilitate culturally safe and competent care of Aboriginal peoples.
- Decolonizing Aboriginal health care requires the application of an Indigenous social determinants of health model to policy and practice at the federal, provincial, and community levels.

This chapter views First Nations health and health services through a historical and critical lens. The history of relations between Aboriginal peoples and the Canadian government provides a foundational backdrop to the health of First Nations people today and the rationale for current health policy.[1] We contend that Aboriginal health status and policy have evolved from, and are part of, colonial systems, and we conclude with the suggestion that the decolonization of First Nations health care is a necessary step toward the equality of health care for

Aboriginal peoples in Canada. Our perspective has grown from decades of community-based research with community representatives, leaders, and elders who have suggested that an appropriate way to conceptualize Aboriginal peoples' health is through a historical lens. Aboriginal health researchers (Duran and Duran 1995; McCormick 2000; Yellow-Horse Braveheart 2003) as well as Aboriginal organizations (e.g., the Aboriginal Healing Foundation [AHF] and the National Aboriginal Health Organization [NAHO]) have also endorsed the necessity of understanding Aboriginal health from this perspective.

There are many reasons why Aboriginal health requires special attention from health-care practitioners. They include (1) the unique status of Aboriginal peoples, entrenched in the Constitution and in treaty agreements, entitling them to specific health-care rights and benefits; (2) poorer overall health status compared with the non-Aboriginal population; (3) socio-economic and political circumstances that are unique to being Aboriginal; (4) cultural differences from mainstream society and cultural heterogeneity within the Aboriginal population; and (5) unique demographic structures and trends. Despite the need for special attention to Aboriginal people's health, it is poorly understood by mainstream health-care providers. This lack of understanding is due to the complexity of Aboriginal health-care policies and services and to the lack of attention paid to Aboriginal health in health education. Some health disciplines, notably nursing, have sought better knowledge of and education on Aboriginal health in the past decade. Physician education on Aboriginal health is improving; national organizations such as the Indigenous Physician Association of Canada-Association of Faculties of Medicine of Canada (IPAC-AFMC) are providing leadership concerning learning objectives and content (IPAC 2008), and select medical schools are pursuing Aboriginal-specific curriculum as an elective (Silversides 2008) and as a core curriculum (Northern Ontario School of Medicine).

Rural health in Canada cannot be understood in isolation from the Aboriginal populations living off reserve or within First Nation communities. This chapter focuses on registered/status Indians governed under the Indian Act, commonly referred to as First Nations. There are 615 First Nation reserves in Canada and 748,371 registered Indians representing 52 cultural groups and over 50 languages (Indian and Northern Affairs Canada [INAC] 2007). Most reserves are either rural or remote, isolated from major cities. Remote First Nation communities are generally thought of as those with seasonal and/or fly-in access;

they include communities that are dependent on winter ice roads, summer boat transportation, and air service. We believe that all reserves that are not remote can be considered rural (see Chapter 1 of this volume for the definition of rural). For example, on reserves such as Six Nations near Brantford, Ontario, which have large populations and are located close to urban centres, the invisible walls of federal policy create communities with differing social, economic, and health opportunities that more closely approximate remote reserve communities than the urban community only steps away. Larger First Nations often experience degrees of rurality within the reserve; for example, reserves such as the Wikwemikong Unceded Indian Reserve on Manitoulin Island, Ontario, and the Six Nations Reserve are often comprised of one larger, fully serviced settlement (e.g., municipal water and sewer) and several other "rural" villages.

Aboriginal population density varies considerably among provinces with the highest densities in the northern territories followed by the prairie provinces. Intraprovincially, higher densities occur in the northern portions of the provinces; for example, in some northern Ontario municipalities, Aboriginal people represent up to 24.5 percent of the population, while provincially they represent 2 percent. Fifty-four percent of Aboriginal people live in urban centres compared with 81 percent of the non–Aboriginal population (Statistics Canada 2006). Despite the trend of movement to urban centres, the 2001 census revealed that more Aboriginal people moved onto reserves (mostly from rural communities) than off reserves (Statistics Canada 2001).

First Nations health has improved over the past century but remains much poorer than the health of the non-Aboriginal population. Life expectancy has increased while infant mortality and rates of infectious disease have decreased. However, life expectancy for First Nations women remains 5.2 years less, and for Aboriginal men 7.4 years less, than for non-Aboriginal Canadians. Infant mortality rates are 16 percent higher for First Nations people (Health Canada 2000). On average, one in five Aboriginal adults (20 percent) has diabetes (First Nations and Inuit Regional Health Survey [FNIRHS] 2002). First Nations people have higher levels of all infectious diseases compared with other Canadians, higher rates of vaccine-preventable diseases, higher rates of hospitalization, and higher levels of smoking (62 percent). Some of the greatest disparities in health status between Aboriginal people and other Canadians occur in rates of suicide (three to five times higher), tuberculosis (on average six times higher), and accidental death (three and a half times higher) (Health Canada 2000). Chapter 21 of this book offers a more detailed discussion of health status.

In presenting these data, we do not wish to perpetuate images of the "pathologized" Aboriginal population (Kelm 1998; O'Neil, Reading, and Leader 1998). Health surveillance of Aboriginal communities contributes to popular views of Aboriginal peoples as "sick" and serves to justify continuing policies of paternalism. This portrayal also creates feelings of hopelessness when it comes to Aboriginal health issues (Kelm 1998, xvi). Thus, despite challenges, it is important to realize that community-based models of care have led to improvements in health and that there is reason to hope that current actions to enhance Aboriginal self-determination in health will lead to a decrease in disease burden in the future (Warry 2007, 151-63).

Our work places the relationship between the federal government and Aboriginal peoples at the root of current health status. Specific explanations for current health status, such as historical and intergenerational trauma, are part of this framework. There are two caveats to this perspective. First, occasionally it is necessary to generalize about the effects of colonization on health status; in no way should this generalization mask Aboriginal cultural diversity. Second, we do not wish to convey an image of Aboriginal people as passive to colonialism.[2] One of the most inspiring aspects of working with First Nations is having knowledge of the adversity that they have faced and seeing how their culture has survived and even strengthened (see Jacklin 2007). Throughout this difficult history, there have been many accounts of resistance to assimilation. We hear about resistance from residential school survivors, and we read about it in mission diaries. And today we see it in the advocacy of national associations such as the Assembly of First Nations (AFN).

Colonialism as a Determinant of First Nations Health

Colonial processes and policies have had a major impact on First Nations health. Arguably, colonialism influences all other determinants of health under the social determinants of health model (Jacklin 2009). Warry (1998, 215-16) argues that it is only through increased awareness of the colonial process that community healing will be realized. This argument echoes an earlier statement by the AFN (1994, cited in FNIRHS 1999, 30): "First Nations need to know their history. History provides a context for understanding individuals' present circumstances, and is an essential part of the healing process."

The idea that health and health care today are intimately linked to colonialism should not be difficult to accept, yet in our experience few health-care providers even comprehend the notion of colonialism.[3] The colonial process brought with it new economies, political structures, religions, languages, values, technologies, and diseases. Over the past 100 years, forced relocation of reserves and individuals, ineffective and inappropriate health policies and practices, residential schools, the criminal justice system, welfare, the Indian Act, and more have continued the assault on the life ways of Aboriginal peoples. State actions placed health care in the hands of the colonizers and undermined culturally based conceptions of disease, illness, and treatment rooted in Indigenous knowledge. As this medical paradigm shift occurred, authority over Aboriginal life was increasingly placed in the hands of the colonial government, which sought to abolish Aboriginal culture and identity.

Aboriginal health status rapidly declined following contact with Europeans. Virgin soil epidemics occurred where new pathogens were brought to North America by Europeans and introduced to Aboriginal people, who had no immunity. These epidemics, which continued well into the twentieth century, reduced regional populations between 53 percent and 89 percent (Waldram, Herring, and Young 2006, 54-55). The adoption of bio-medicine and the impact of disease were closely associated. Whenever virgin soil epidemics occurred, they were sufficiently devastating that they began to undermine Aboriginal healing systems and beliefs and left communities vulnerable to encroaching Christian values and Western medical beliefs (Young 1988, 96). Christian missions, aided by federal laws, principally the Indian Act, led the assault on important spiritual practices and ceremonies, such as the Midewin among the Ojibwa (Hallowell 1992) and the Potlatch among the cultures of the northwest coast (Steckley and Cummins 2008, 172-77), that contained important healing rituals at the individual and community levels. European belief in the superiority of bio-medicine was also integral to the cultural blindness that led to other colonial actions aimed at supplanting Indigenous medical science. The Wikwemikong Community Health Plan (WCHP 1989) substantiates this: "As many illnesses were unknown to the Indian people, they increasingly had to turn towards western medicine for affective [sic] cures. Slowly, *confidence* in the traditional healing practices ... eroded and [was] replaced by western medicine."

Over time, many Aboriginal people questioned their Indigenous medical beliefs, and a false dichotomy or rift between Indigenous and

Western health practices occurred. Yet we now know that Indigenous knowledge and medicine went underground, where they were protected and not lost. Today many First Nations are actively pursuing the revitalization of Indigenous medicine despite a lack of support for these practices by the federal government (Martin-Hill 2003). Research into Indigenous knowledge and medicine is also currently a major emphasis of the Institutes of Aboriginal Peoples Health, as are newfound collaborations between Western and Indigenous practitioners.

History has shaped Aboriginal perceptions of the health-care system and has influenced patients' trust of services provided by non-Aboriginal providers. Negative experiences at residential schools with those in positions of authority, including physicians, have caused many people to avoid bio-medical services. It is incorrect to think of residential schools and policies of assimilation as belonging in the distant past and thus worthy of being forgotten. Traumatizing colonial processes continued well into the "postcolonial" period. The last residential school continued to operate into the 1990s in Yellowknife, Northwest Territories (Aboriginal Healing Foundation [AHF] 2005, A19-A20). Residential school experiences existed within a backdrop of social, economic, and health policies aimed at the assimilation of Aboriginal peoples. During the 1960s, Child and Welfare Services was responsible for the removal of Aboriginal children from their families during what came to be known as the "60s Scoop" (AHF 2005, A20). Prior to 1960, about 1 percent of children who were legal wards of the state were Aboriginal; by the late 1960s, this had increased to between 30 percent and 40 percent (Kirmayer, Brass, and Tait 2000). Although the number of First Nations children being placed in care has decreased nationally, it was still five times higher than the number for non-First Nation communities in 1989 (Armitage 1995).

Such experiences create mistrust between Aboriginal peoples and mainstream institutions, and this mistrust influences where they seek care, from whom, and other aspects of health-seeking behaviour. For example, a recent evaluation of the community-based Canadian Prenatal and Nutrition Program among Wikwemikong people in Ontario found that the requirement of nurses to report any child welfare issues to the Children's Aid Society produced low participation rates by this community (Jacklin 2007). To take another example, during an Aboriginal cancer-care training session, we were told by one Aboriginal partner that her grandmother still warned the family not to accept blankets from nurses when in hospital. This caution had been handed down through oral tradition recounting the "gift" of smallpox blankets to Aboriginal peoples by the British (see Steckley and Cummins 2008, 180). Furthermore, colonial health practices included the removal of Aboriginal tuberculosis patients to sanatoriums, the removal of Aboriginal women from their communities to give birth, and the coerced sterilization of women (Warry 2007, 65n10). Today Aboriginal patients are reminded of these times as they continue to be removed from their communities to seek cancer treatment or other hospital-based care, a practice that separates patients from their families, often for weeks at a time, and forces Aboriginal people to make difficult decisions about treatment and long-term care.

Thus, although health-care practitioners are apt to assume that the role of medicine in relation to Aboriginal communities has been benign, if not positive, it is important to recognize that bio-medicine is one of the many state systems that are part of the colonial legacy.

Such examples point to the continuing historical impacts of colonial actions on contemporary health behaviours. Although not yet fully understood or documented, it is clear, for example, that some Aboriginal peoples have a fear, mistrust, or suspicion of bio-medical institutions and practitioners (Cancer Care Ontario [CCO] 2002) and that cultural beliefs influence many aspects of health and illness throughout the life course – from parental decisions to immunize infants (Tarrant and Gregory 2003) to end-of-life care (Hampton 2010). Much remains to be understood about the impacts of colonialism and culture on health-seeking behaviours, perceptions of specific illnesses, and treatment decisions. It is within this context that we must strive to understand health and health care of First Nations. We must remember that colonialism is an ongoing process. First Nations continue to be viewed as "in the way of development" by the dominant society, and Aboriginal peoples continue to suffer the negative health effects of major resource industries, including oil and gas development, mining, and hydro-electric projects (Blaser, Feit, and McRae 2004; Martin-Hill 2008). The Aboriginal Healing Foundation (2005, 41) writes that "Aboriginal people in Canada continue to be trapped by social, political and economic policies that promote dependency by preventing self-determination." Current government policies, from land claims to economic development, must be understood as part of the social determinants of Aboriginal health.

First Nations Health Policy and Health Care

The level of health service provided by the federal government for Aboriginal people has a history of inadequacy (Waldram, Herring, and Young 1995, 156-61). Bio-medical health care was introduced as treaties were signed. Aboriginal people were granted access to physicians, usually annually on "treaty days." Aboriginal people attempted to have medical care formally included as a treaty provision in several cases but were successful only in the case of Treaty Six (Waldram, Herring, and Young 2006). This treaty contains the "Medicine Chest Clause," interpreted by First Nations to mean that the federal government has a legal obligation and responsibility to provide health services to First Nations: that is, an entitlement to universal health care. The federal government denies this interpretation and argues that the provision of health care was not the intent of this clause and that services are provided as a matter of policy, not due to a legal obligation (Waldram, Herring, and Young 1995, 141, 149). In reality, the government has federal legislative authority under the Indian Act (section 73) to provide health services to status Indians; however, this represents not a responsibility to provide services but the right to provide services *at its discretion.* The government has always maintained that it provides such services on humanitarian grounds rather than due to any legal obligation.

There have been several bureaucratic changes in Aboriginal health services; the most significant came in 1945 when health services were transferred from Indian Affairs to Health and Welfare. In 1962, the Medical Services Branch (MSB) was established, later renamed the First Nations Inuit Health Branch (FNIHB) in 1999 and First Nations and Inuit Health (FNIH) in 2007 (see Chapter 21, this volume, for discussion). The move to Health and Welfare was important since it separated health from broader Indian Affairs policies concerned with housing, water, and sanitation, thereby denying a more holistic understanding of health. Today the determinants of the health model embraced by Health Canada recognize the significance of the relationship between health and social environment. But bureaucratic structures leading to compartmentalized policy making remain, so that Aboriginal health policy making is isolated from the broader socio-political and environmental concerns seen as part of the mandate of Indian Affairs.

During the 1970s, health-care policy around the world began to move toward models of participation and health promotion. In 1979, the Indian Health Policy was formed, and, like the 1978 World Health

Organization (WHO) Alma Ata statements, it recognized the broad determinants of health. This policy also stressed the need for socio-economic, cultural, and spiritual development and the importance of Aboriginal people's participation in their health-care system (Young 1984, 263). However, this period saw only limited participation of Aboriginal people in their own health care. In the 1980s, steps were taken toward improved primary health-care services (Waldram, Herring, and Young 1995, 235). This improvement was to be achieved primarily through Health Transfer. In 1986, the Indian Health Transfer Policy was announced. This policy proposed the transfer of health funding and administrative responsibilities to First Nations. It allowed First Nations to determine community health needs and respond with appropriate programming using their own governance and administrative structures within the accountability guidelines set out by FNIH, as long as mandatory programs (as defined by FNIH) continued to be provided. Since its inception, the Health Transfer Policy has been evaluated three times and has been modified to provide greater flexibility to communities that wish to pursue varying degrees of authority over the provision of health services. Now referred to as consolidated contribution agreements, "transfer" is offered in three forms: "general," which does not give communities authority to reprioritize or redirect health resources; "transfer/targeted," previously known as Health Transfer, which allows First Nations to design and deliver health programs based on local needs provided that FNIH "mandatory programs" continue to be delivered; and "integrated/targeted," which shares responsibility with FNIH to administer health programs. Communities are now also eligible for self-government models (Health Canada 2007). Currently, 46 percent of First Nations have opted to participate in the Health Transfer process transfer/targeted, 33 percent in integrated/targeted, and 4 percent in self-government agreements (FNIH 2008). Other First Nations remain under FNIH control.

The Health Transfer Policy reflects national and international calls for Aboriginal participation in and control over health services; however, the motives of the policy have been called into question. Aboriginal leadership groups such as the Assembly of First Nations and the Union of Ontario Indians have criticized the policy as assimilationist, and researchers examining evolution of the policy since its inception have concluded that it has become one of cost containment rather than self-determination (Jacklin and Warry 2004). Despite the restrictions and reduced emphasis on self-determination, Health Transfer remains the best option for communities seeking greater control over local health care.

Programs and services outside Health Transfer are funded through separate initiatives by federal and/or provincial governments. Commonly, these funds must be spent in a specific area within a limited time period. Programs and positions funded through the Canadian Prenatal and Nutrition Program, the Fetal Alcohol Syndrome Strategy, and the Diabetes Initiative are examples of such specific funding. In one First Nation in northern Ontario, we found that Health Transfer funding makes up only 40 percent of the global budget for health, 60 percent of the funding coming from a multitude of small sums for individual programs or projects. Although these other funding agencies do provide important services for the communities, they also present great administrative challenges.

Provincial responsibility for health in First Nations contexts is contentious because, according to many chiefs and advocates, it can undermine the federal government's fiduciary and treaty-based responsibilities. The reality, however, is that federal financial contributions to health care are woefully inadequate, and provinces can play a key role in health delivery. In Ontario, off-reserve health centres funded by the Aboriginal Healing and Wellness Strategy (AHWS) provide specialized services in the form of nurse practitioners, dieticians, and researchers. AHWS is co-managed by representatives from provincial ministries and Aboriginal organizations. It funds both urban and reserve programs and has been essential in funding crisis intervention and traditional healing programs that the federal government has refused to fund.

Our experience evaluating First Nations programs over the past twenty years suggests that enhanced community control has improved the quality and effectiveness of services and, from a client perspective, has led to services regarded as accessible and culturally appropriate (Jacklin and Warry 2000, 2005; Warry 2007, 151-63; Warry and Jacklin 2004). We have found that First Nations health systems, though complex, are well integrated into referral networks within regional systems of care. It is still the case that Aboriginal clients can choose to go "outside" their own health system for specific stigmatized health issues such as mental health or sexual health, but generally First Nations health services have decreased reliance on mainstream services (and associated health-care costs) while providing cost-effective and culturally appropriate care, often in the patient's own language (Jacklin and Warry 2005).

Community-based systems of care that have emerged within this policy context can be diverse and unique yet effective in responding to the needs of particular First Nations. For example, a northern Ontario tribal authority for several smaller First Nations has consolidated Health Transfer funding under one governance structure with representatives from each of the communities on the board of directors. This approach has reduced the amount of funding allocated to governance and increased the total amount of funding available for direct health services. We have also found that communities have been responsive to the need for diabetes programming by combining various funding sources (Health Transfer/FNIH, Northern Diabetes Network, Ministry of Health and Long-Term Care, and Aboriginal Diabetes Initiative) to create programs responsive to community needs. In one community, this approach resulted in the creation of a diabetes program that utilized traditional medicine, and in another it resulted in hiring a lay educator to work with a diabetes nurse educator to translate information and material into the local language.

Mental health programming is another area that has required community-based solutions. Completely devoid of a mental health strategy, FNIH does not provide funding for mental health programming. Communities access funding and resources through various means: the AHF; provincial funders; partnering with other programs, such as the federal Native Alcohol and Drug Addiction and Building Healthy Communities and Brighter Futures programs; and (in Ontario) partnerships with AHWS health centres. Community-based mental health programming often includes a combination of the following: case management, counselling, traditional medicine, wilderness camps, talking circles, youth programs, workshops, and health promotion. We have found that, when local mental health services are available, most community members access these services locally, and referrals "out" are largely made due to a lack of specialist services or long waiting lists.

For the health-care professional, this community-based approach means that programming and administration will be different in each First Nation. This variation often leads to frustration among health-care providers who service multiple First Nations, but this frustration usually results from a lack of knowledge of or respect for the self-determined process that created the service. This process blends the availability of funding with community needs and priorities to create the most appropriate program possible. Having conducted several Health Transfer evaluations for First Nations, we have found that, despite the underlying and often invisible administrative challenges associated with this approach, client satisfaction with these services is high, and in one case we were able to detect a decrease in hospital admissions related to community-based diabetes programming (Jacklin and Warry 2005).

These examples confirm what other research suggests – that increased Aboriginal control over health care leads to improved health care: that is, there is a relationship between self-determination and community health (Warry 1998). Work by Chandler and Lalonde (1998), for example, demonstrates that communities that exercise greater degrees of control over community life also experience the lowest suicide rates. It is in the direction of Aboriginal self-determination, the promotion of Indigenous medicine, and the search for culturally appropriate health care that the solutions to the ill health of First Nations are to be found.

Decolonizing Aboriginal Health Care

Given the relationship between colonialism and the ill health of First Nations, it is easy to suggest that improvement in Aboriginal health care will come only through a process of decolonization – literally, by ending colonial processes and policies and by reconstructing health-care practices in keeping with the aim of Aboriginal self-determination. Although it is difficult to glimpse the future, and though pointing to "solutions" in the Aboriginal context can be naively idealistic, this brief review is sufficient to suggest a number of key elements in the process of decolonization.

The solutions to Aboriginal ill health are complex and lie outside what is arbitrarily labelled the health sector. To take one example, behaviours associated with youth mental health are as easily linked to inadequacies in housing or educational policy as they are to access to mainstream services or lack of Aboriginal counsellors or psychiatrists. Mounting evidence suggests that the continuing disparities between mainstream and Aboriginal health will be addressed only through the application of an Indigenous social determinants of health model to policy and practice at the federal, provincial, and community levels. In addition, there is a need for greater appreciation of, and direct monetary support for, self-determination to enhance Aboriginal-controlled health programs and institutions where culturally appropriate health practices can take root. Unfortunately, there is little indication that such an understanding exists, at least among government policy makers. The AFN's report card on the federal government's implementation, or lack thereof, of recommendations of the Royal Commission on Aboriginal Peoples (RCAP) over a decade ago (AFN 2007) notes the government's abject failure to address RCAP's health recommendations. They include, for example, failure to expand Health Transfer Agreements to provide for a true degree of self-control over services; failure to implement a network of healing centres and lodges (i.e., to recognize and fund Indigenous healing practices); and failure to implement a national Aboriginal health and human resources strategy. Concrete action by the federal government in all these areas – and many others – is essential to create the structural change necessary to improve the health of First Nations. Likewise, action by provincial governments, through tripartite negotiations, cost-sharing and other agreements, and, as in Ontario, the development of Aboriginal-specific health policies, is needed to ensure adequate funding of First Nations services.

Perhaps the first step toward decolonization is enhanced awareness of cultural diversity and of Indigenous medical science in health curricula at all levels. There is a dearth of Aboriginal health professionals of all kinds – from health administration to psychiatry. Recruiting, training, and retraining Aboriginal health professionals and paraprofessionals are part of the solution to the challenges facing First Nations. Providing culturally relevant information to all health professionals is also essential to improve care and to develop policies that are respectful of Aboriginal culture at local and regional levels (Warry 2007, 151-63).[4]

Recognizing cultural diversity means that there is no single way to improve Aboriginal health, but improving Anishinabe, Carrier, or Dene health is indeed possible. Different cultures and local histories require regional health systems that interface with provincial and territorial health systems in a relatively seamless fashion. However idealistic, a decolonized health-care system would respect the integrity of local Aboriginal primary care systems, including traditional systems of care, while ensuring that these systems are linked to mainstream health institutions where Aboriginal patients can receive culturally competent and culturally safe[5] specialized or tertiary care. This system would require greater understanding and cooperation between health-care providers and Aboriginal providers and healers.

Similarly, improving health promotion is dependent on a better understanding of Aboriginal health beliefs, so as to ensure that health promotion messages are locally and culturally effective. Perhaps the classic example of this is the work being done by CCO on traditional versus contemporary use of tobacco to address the dramatically higher incidences of smoking (in some cases as high as 75 percent of youth) on reserves. Decolonizing regional health-care systems will also require structural and legislative change, for example to recognize traditional systems of midwifery and to ensure that Indigenous healers can work within mainstream hospitals or clinics while remaining outside current legal definitions of medical liability. Likewise, funding and policy development are needed to ensure the protection, promotion, and distribution of traditional medicinal plants.

For individual health professionals, decolonizing health care begins with the honest effort to understand the culture and everyday experience of Aboriginal patients. We can hope that, as health education changes, the next generation of health professionals will receive specific training in Aboriginal health. But for current and future practitioners, cross-cultural awareness can be found in local engagement with First Nations and by participation in Aboriginal cultural activities. For physicians and other health-care professionals, decolonizing health care means, first and foremost, understanding that Aboriginal patients have choices that are different and often attenuated or restricted compared with those of mainstream Canadians. Aboriginal patients can choose between Western and Indigenous medicine or pursue treatment that combines these approaches. Aboriginal patients, faced with the choice of relocating to urban centres for long-term care or specialized treatment, might choose instead to manage chronic diseases at home, where the support of family and Aboriginal primary care professionals is assured. Patient communication, patient perception, and patient "compliance" are then all influenced by colonial history, by local cultural contexts, and by the accessibility of specific medical interventions.

In the end, health-care delivery for Aboriginal peoples will be improved by deconstructing the jurisdictional and geographical barriers that surround First Nations – barriers that are the products of history and colonialism. The challenge will be to remove the invisible walls that divide Aboriginal and mainstream Canadians while allowing ourselves to see and honour the uniqueness of the cultural spaces within First Nations health environments.

Notes

1 Throughout this chapter, we use the terms "Aboriginal" and "First Nation(s)." The former term refers to the descendants of the original inhabitants of North America, including Indian, Métis, and Inuit, as defined in the Constitution Act, 1982. Aboriginal

peoples represent approximately 4.4 percent of the population; 53 percent identify as registered Indians, 30 percent as Métis, 11 percent as non-registered Indians, and 4 percent as Inuit (Statistics Canada 2006). Following the National Aboriginal Health Organization (NAHO) terminology guide (2003), we use "Aboriginal" when making general comments that apply to or include all original inhabitants of North America. "First Nation" is used to refer to reserve communities/bands and "First Nations" to refer to registered Indians. See also Chapters 21 and 22 of this book.

2 Similarly, although colonialism is a determinant of health, Aboriginal agency in health continues, and Aboriginal peoples recognize that individual and community responsibility for health is an important aspect of health-care reform. The idea of community responsibility is examined more closely in our discussion of Health Transfer and in Chapter 21 of this volume.

3 Colonialism is defined as the forms of exploitation that followed European expansion over the past 400 years. The ideologies of capitalism, racism (and the "crude application of Social Darwinism"), and paternalism were all implicit to the process (Ashcroft, Griffiths, and Tiffin 1998, 45-47). The AHF (2005, A19) describes colonialism as "the process of taking control over and assimilating Aboriginal people through formal government policies. From an Aboriginal perspective, it refers to the theft of ancestral homelands and resources, as well as attempts to destroy Indigenous languages and cultures."

4 The Aboriginal Health Human Resources Initiative (AHHRI) has begun to respond to these issues. Announced in 2004, the AHHRI currently funds work concerned with increasing the number of Aboriginal people working in health careers, improving retention of health workers in Aboriginal communities, and creating and improving health-care education curricula to improve cultural competence (AHHRI 2006).

5 There are no universally accepted definitions of cultural competence or cultural safety. In our view, cultural competence implies care that incorporates knowledge of a people's culture and history accompanied by a change in attitude and honing of clinical skills in response to this knowledge; cultural safety stresses the need to address power inequalities in health-care delivery and patients' ability to express themselves in an environment that is conducive to communication and understanding.

References

Aboriginal Healing Foundation (AHF). 2005. *Reclaiming Connections: Understanding Residential School Trauma among Aboriginal People: A Resource Manual.* Ottawa: AHF Research Series.

Aboriginal Health Human Resources Initiative (AHHRI). 2006. *Program Framework: Aboriginal Health Human Resources Initiative (AHHRI),* http://www.fnhealthmanagers.ca/.

Armitage, A. 1995. *Comparing the Policy of Aboriginal Assimilation: Australia, Canada, and New Zealand.* Vancouver: UBC Press.

Ashcroft, B., G. Griffiths, and H. Tiffin. 1998. *Key Concepts in Post-Colonial Studies.* London: Routledge.

Assembly of First Nations (AFN). 2007. *Assembly of First Nations, Royal Commission on Aboriginal Peoples at 10 Years: A Report Card,* http://www.afn.ca/.

Blaser, M., H.A. Feit, and G. McRae. 2004. *In the Way of Development: Indigenous Peoples, Life Projects, and Globalization.* London: Zed Books.

Cancer Care Ontario (CCO). 2002. *Aboriginal Cancer Care Needs Assessment: It's Our Responsibility.* Toronto: CCO, http://www.cancercare.on.ca/.

388   *First Nations in Rural Settings*

Chandler, M.J., and C.E. Lalonde. 1998. "Cultural Continuity as a Hedge against Suicide in Canada's First Nations." *Transcultural Psychiatry* 35, 2: 191-219.

Duran, E., and B. Duran. 1995. *Native American Postcolonial Psychology.* New York: SUNY Press.

First Nations and Inuit Health (FNIH). 2008. *Transfer Status as of March 2008.* Ottawa: FNIH, http://www.hc-sc.gc.ca/.

First Nations and Inuit Regional Health Survey (FNIRHS). 1999. *First Nations and Inuit Regional Health Survey, National Report.* Ottawa: FNIRHS National Steering Committee.

–. 2002. *Regional Health Survey Selected Results 2002-2003.* Ottawa: AFN, http://www.rhs-ers.ca/.

Hallowell, A.I. 1992. *The Ojibwa of Berens River, Manitoba: Ethnohistory in History.* Edited by J.S.H. Brown. Fort Worth: Harcourt Brace Jovanovich College Publishers.

Health Canada. 2000. *A Statistical Profile on the Health of First Nations in Canada.* Ottawa: Minister of Supply and Services Canada.

–. 2007. *First Nations and Inuit Health Program Compendium.* Catalogue H34-178/2007 E-PDF. Ottawa: Health Canada, http://www.hc-sc.gc.ca/.

Indian and Northern Affairs Canada (INAC). 2007. *Registered Indian Population by Sex and Residence.* Ottawa: INAC, http://www.ainc-inac.gc.ca/.

Indigenous Physician Association of Canada (IPAC). 2008. *Newsletter,* winter, http://www.ipac-amic.org/.

Jacklin, K. 2007. "Strength in Adversity: Community Health and Healing in Wikwemikong." PhD diss., McMaster University, Hamilton.

–. 2009. "Diversity Within: Deconstructing Aboriginal Community Health in Wikwemikong Unceded Indian Reserve." *Social Science and Medicine* 68, 5: 980-89.

Jacklin, K., and W. Warry. 2000. "Wikwemikong Unceded First Nation Health Transfer Evaluation Report." Prepared by Northwind Consultants for the Wikwemikong Health Board. Document held at the Wikwemikong Health Centre.

–. 2004. "The Indian Health Transfer Policy: Toward Cost Containment or Self-Determination?" In *Unhealthy Health Policy: A Critical Anthropological Examination,* edited by M. Singer and A. Castro, 215-34. Walnut Creek, CA: Altamira Press.

–. 2005. "Mnaamodzawin Health Services Health Transfer Evaluation Report, September 2005." Prepared for Mnaamodzawin Health Services Health Board. Document held at Mnaamodzawin Health Services.

Kelm, M. 1998. *Colonizing Bodies: Aboriginal Health and Healing in British Columbia 1900-50.* Vancouver: UBC Press.

Kirmayer, L.J., G.M. Brass, and C.L. Tait. 2000. "The Mental Health of Aboriginal Peoples: Transformations of Identity and Community." *Canadian Journal of Psychiatry* 45, 7: 607-16.

Martin-Hill, D. 2003. *Traditional Medicine in Contemporary Contexts: Protecting and Respecting Indigenous Knowledge and Medicine.* Ottawa: NAHO, http://www.naho.ca/.

–. 2008. *The Lubicon Lake Nation: Indigenous Knowledge and Power.* Toronto: University of Toronto Press.

McCormick, R.M. 2000. "Aboriginal Traditions in the Treatment of Substance Abuse." *Canadian Journal of Counselling* 34, 1: 25-32.

National Aboriginal Health Organization (NAHO). 2003. *Terminology Guide.* Ottawa: NAHO, http://www.naho.ca/.

O'Neil, J.D., J.R. Reading, and A. Leader. 1998. "Changing the Relations of Surveillance: The Development of a Discourse of Resistance in Aboriginal Epidemiology." *Human Organization* 57, 2: 230-37.

Silversides, A. 2008. "Aboriginal Curriculum Framework Developed." *Canadian Medical Association Journal* 178, 13: 1650.

Statistics Canada. 2001. *North American Indians.* Ottawa: Statistics Canada, http://www12.statcan.ca/.

–. 2006. *Aboriginal Peoples in Canada in 2006: Inuit, Métis, and First Nations, 2006 Census.* Catalogue No. 97-558-XIE. Ottawa: Statistics Canada, http://www12.statcan.ca/.

Steckley, J.L., and B.D. Cummins. 2008. *Full Circle: Canada's First Nations.* 2nd ed. Toronto: Pearson, Prentice-Hall.

Tarrant, M., and D. Gregory. 2003. "Exploring Childhood Immunization Uptake with First Nations Mothers in North-Western Ontario, Canada." *Journal of Advanced Nursing* 41, 1: 63-72.

Waldram, J.B., D.A. Herring, and K. Young. 1995. *Aboriginal Health in Canada: Historical, Cultural, and Epidemiological Perspectives.* Toronto: University of Toronto Press.

–. 2006. *Aboriginal Health in Canada: Historical, Cultural, and Epidemiological Perspectives.* 2nd ed. Toronto: University of Toronto Press.

Warry, W. 1998. *Unfinished Dreams: Community Healing and the Reality of Aboriginal Self-Government.* Toronto: University of Toronto Press.

–. 2007. *Ending Denial: Understanding Aboriginal Issues.* Peterborough, ON: Broadview Press.

Warry, W., and K. Jacklin. 2004. "Wikwemikong Unceded First Nation Health Transfer Evaluation Report." Prepared by Northwind Consultants for the Wikwemikong Health Board. Document held at the Wikwemikong Health Centre.

Wikwemikong Community Health Plan (WCHP). 1989. "Wikwemikong Community Health Plan." Document held at the Nahndahweh Tchigehgamig – Wikwemikong Health Centre.

Yellow-Horse Braveheart, M. 2003. "The Historical Trauma Response among Natives and Its Relationship with Substance Abuse: A Lakota Illustration." *Journal of Psychoactive Drugs* 35, 1: 7-13.

Young, T.K. 1984. "Indian Health Services in Canada: A Sociohistorical Perspective." *Social Science and Medicine* 18, 3: 257-64.

–. 1988. *Health Care and Cultural Change: The Indian Experience in the Central Subarctic.* Toronto: University of Toronto Press.

Chapter 21   **Access to Primary Health Care in Rural and Remote Aboriginal Communities: Progress, Challenges, and Policy Directions**

J.G. Lavoie and L. Gervais

Key Points

- In the past twenty years, policies have created opportunities for improved access to appropriate and Aboriginal community-driven primary health-care services.
- Innovations that build on the idea that *the community is the constant,* and that strengthen community capacity, mitigate the impact of nursing staff turnover and improve continuity of care.
- The impact of these innovations is constrained, however, by jurisdictional confusion. Although some provinces and territories have embedded provisions in legislation and policies to address and clarify roles and responsibilities, these responses have been partial and fail to add up to a comprehensive approach.
- A national Aboriginal health policy framework must be created to guide current and emerging initiatives while entrenching common minimal standards.

Reports continue to show that Aboriginal peoples bear a disproportionate burden of physical and emotional illness (Adelson 2005; Canadian Institute for Health Information [CIHI] 2004; First Nations and Inuit Regional Health Survey [FNIRHS] National Steering Committee 1999; First Nations Regional Health Survey [FNRHS] National Committee 2005; Health Canada 2002, 2003; Health Council of Canada 2005). As discussed in the previous chapter, many of the social issues reported by Aboriginal peoples are related to involuntary and rapid cultural changes imposed by colonization, multi-generational trauma related to the legacy of oppressive policies, and the systematic removal of children to residential schools (Archibald 2006; Bartlett 2003; Wesley-Esquimaux and Smolewski 2004).

A number of studies have demonstrated that access to appropriate health-care services remains a challenge for Aboriginal peoples. Some have reported that jurisdictional barriers can lead to increased reliance on otherwise avoidable hospitalization (FNRHS National Committee 2005; Lavoie and Forget 2006; Lavoie et al. 2008; Martens et al. 2002; Shah, Gunraj, and Hux 2003). Others have focused on institutional violence and racism (Browne 2007; Browne, Fiske, and Thomas 2000). Although acknowledging these realities, this chapter will also highlight the progress made in ensuring access to appropriate and responsive primary health care.

Methods

This chapter brings together three different sources of data. The demographic data were garnered from the 2006 census. It is the most complete source of demographic data on Aboriginal peoples and the only source that reliably distinguishes between Aboriginal, First Nations, Inuit, and Métis.

In contrast, health statistics and information on access to care remain remarkably patchy. More information is available for First Nations, particularly those living on-reserve. Some information is available for Inuit. For other individuals of Aboriginal ancestry, the Métis, and those who do not qualify for registration under the Indian Act, invisibility is the norm. The information reported here was garnered from the most current sources, including the Canadian Institute for Health Information, Health Canada, the 2005 First Nations Regional Longitudinal Health Survey (FNRLHS), and the published literature.

Finally, information on Aboriginal health policies and self-government activities is based partly on a study of Aboriginal health policies and legislation in Canada conducted on behalf of the National Collaborating Centre for Aboriginal Health in 2007-8 (Lavoie et al. 2011). The overall objective was to develop a comparative inventory of public/community health policies and legislation impacting on/relevant to Aboriginal health in Canada, from the late 1960s on (Waldram, Herring, and Young 2006). For each jurisdiction (Aboriginal, federal, provincial, and territorial), Internet searches were used to locate primary documents (legislation, policies, regulations) produced by ministries or departments of health.

Terminology

In this section, we define key concepts used in this chapter. The collective term "Aboriginal peoples" encompasses First Nations, Inuit, and Métis and is entrenched in the Constitution Act, 1982. However, the term glosses over cultural, legislative, and administrative complexities. The collective term "First Nations" is the preferred self-referent used by the peoples of Canada historically known as "Indians." This term veils a multiplicity of nations, including Nisga'a, Cree, Ojibway, Salish, Mohawk, Mi'kmaq, and Innu, to name a few. In administrative terms, there are currently 615 First Nations recognized by the federal government (Indian and Northern Affairs Canada [INAC] 2002).

An increasing number of individuals of First Nations ancestry who descend from treaty signatories do not qualify for registration as Indians under the Indian Act and find themselves in jurisdictional limbo. Some of them are born on reserves. This is a growing yet largely invisible group in Canada facing specific challenges (Lavoie and Forget 2006).

Inuit is also a collective self-referent that refers to the arctic peoples historically known as Eskimos. Inuit themselves recognize local groups with different names (Pallurmiut, Inuvialuit, etc.), reflecting the complexity of arctic history and subtlety in cultural differences glossed over by outsiders. Four Inuit regions are recognized in Canada: Inuvialuit in the Northwest Territories, Nunavut, Nunavik in Quebec, and Nunatsiavut in Newfoundland and Labrador.

Finally, and as discussed in more detail in the next chapter, Métis refers to the descendants of French or Scottish traders and Cree or Ojibway women who settled in the Red River area, north of what is now Winnipeg, Manitoba, developing their own blended culture and their own language, Michif. For the purposes of this chapter, the term "Aboriginal" will be used only when statements apply to First Nations living on- and off-reserve, Inuit, Métis, and non-status[1] individuals of First Nations ancestry. In other cases, preferred self-referents will be used. The term "Indian" will only be used when quoting historical documents or when speaking of the Indian Act's legal term "Indians," which defines access to certain federal programs and benefits.

The World Health Organization (WHO 2008) defines primary health care as

> the principal vehicle for the delivery of health care at the most local level of a country's health system. It is essential health care made accessible at a cost the country and community can afford with methods that are practical, scientifically sound and socially acceptable. Everyone in the community should have access to it, and everyone should be involved in it.

Community engagement has been recognized as a cornerstone of primary health care for at least thirty years (WHO 1978) and continues to be promoted in current debates on social and indigenous determinants of health as a key to addressing health inequities. The link between participation and improved gains was recently articulated by Solar and Irwin (2006, 183):

> The success of national efforts to reduce health inequities through action on social determinants ... will depend heavily on the extent to which these processes: (1) engage civil society and communities as committed yet autonomous partners; (2) empower civil society and community groups for knowledge and leadership on [social determinants of health, SDH]; (3) empower and support civil society for ongoing social monitoring for SDH conditions and policy responses.

In the Canadian Aboriginal context, where inequities continue to be reported, the right to some level of engagement has been entrenched in the Constitution Act, 1982, which recognizes Aboriginal peoples' right to self-government. Community engagement has been promoted through a variety of contractual arrangements promoting primarily local control over primary health-care services.

In this chapter, primary, secondary, and tertiary prevention activities will be included under the umbrella term "primary health care." Primary prevention activities refer to early interventions designed to prevent the onset of chronic conditions. Secondary prevention activities focus on assisting in the management of chronic illness to avoid or delay the development of complications. Tertiary prevention activities are designed to assist in the management of complications once they manifest themselves to ensure that optimal autonomy is retained (Last 1983).

Table 21.1   Type and number of services available in First Nations and Inuit
communities in Canada, based on community type

Community type	Type of facility and services			
	Health office (prevention services, <5 days a week)	Health station (screening and prevention, <5 days a week)	Health centre (emergency, screening, and prevention, 5 days a week)	Nursing station (treatment and prevention, 24/7 services)
Non-isolated: good telephone service, road access to physician services located within 90 km	46	12	2	1
Semi-isolated: access to scheduled flights, good telephone service, road access to physician services exceeding 90 km	90	26	13	7
Isolated: access to scheduled flights, good telephone service, but no road access	171	22	7	3
Remote-isolated: do not have scheduled flights, minimal access to telephone and radio, no road access	0	6	66	3
Resident nursing staff	No	No	Yes	Yes
Total	*307*	*66*	*88*	*14*

Source: Health Canada (2004).

Socio-Demographic Profile of First Nations, Inuit, Métis, and Other Aboriginal Peoples

According to the 2006 census, the Aboriginal population now totals
1,172,790 or 3.8 percent of the Canadian population. Although enumeration remains somewhat incomplete, Statistics Canada reported having

been able to secure the participation of the largest number of reserves to date. As shown in Table 21.2, nearly half of the Aboriginal population live either on reserves or in rural areas. Generally speaking, First Nations communities, reported here as North American Indians, are found across the country, with the exception of Nunavut. Inuit are mostly found in the northern parts of Newfoundland and Labrador, Quebec, the Northwest Territories, and Nunavut. The Métis are mostly found in Ontario and in provinces and territories west of it.

Health Status

This section presents an overview of the health status of Aboriginal peoples in Canada. Important variations exist between Aboriginal groups and across communities. Despite the recent flurry of activities in creating national health indicators that also capture progress in Aboriginal health (CIHI 2006), data on Métis, off-reserve First Nations, and non-status individuals of First Nations ancestry remain sketchy or simply non-existent (see Chapter 22, this volume). The reasons are partly historical, partly methodological, and partly conceptual (Smylie and Anderson 2006). Furthermore, where available, data on First Nations and Inuit tend to gloss over local and regional differences, rurality, and remoteness.

As shown in Figure 21.1, the life expectancy at birth for all Aboriginal groups is increasing. The gap in life expectancy that exists between Aboriginal peoples and non-Aboriginal Canadians is slowly narrowing. For Inuit, the gap remains wider. The available data suggest that in 2000 the remaining gap in life expectancy can be partly explained by higher rates of infant mortality among registered First Nations peoples living on reserves (8.0 per 1,000) and Inuit (15.0 per 1,000) compared with other Canadians (5.3 per 1,000) (CIHI 2004).

The rate of injury and accidental death for First Nations on reserves is four times the rate for all of Canada (CIHI 2004). According to the 2000-1 and 2003 Canadian Community Health Surveys, about 20 percent of Aboriginal persons between the ages of twelve and sixty-four living off-reserve reported having had an injury serious enough to limit their activities in the year prior to the study compared with 14 percent for other provincial residents (Tjepkema 2005). Aboriginal children also have much higher rates of death from injuries than all children in Canada. In 2002-3, 49.5 percent of First Nations youth (aged twelve to

Table 21.2 Aboriginal identity according to area of residence, 2006

Aboriginal identity	Total area of residence[1]	Area of residence			% living on reserve	% living in rural environments
		On reserve[2]	Rural	Total urban		
Total Aboriginal and non-Aboriginal identity population	31,241,030	342,865	5,926,685	24,971,480	1.1	19.0
Total Aboriginal identity population[3]	1,172,790	308,490	240,825	623,470	26.3	20.5
North American Indian single response	698,025	300,755	85,210	312,055	43.1	12.2
Métis single response	389,780	4,320	114,905	270,555	1.1	29.5
Inuit single response	50,480	435	31,065	18,980	0.9	61.5
Multiple Aboriginal identity responses	7,740	160	1,835	5,745	2.1	23.7
Aboriginal responses not included elsewhere	26,760	2,825	7,810	16,135	10.6	29.2
Non-Aboriginal identity population	30,068,240	34,375	5,685,855	24,348,005	0.1	18.9

1 "Area of residence" refers to the following geographical areas: on reserve, urban Census Metropolitan Area, urban non-Census Metropolitan Area, and rural area.

2 Statistics Canada warns that the counts for this item are more affected than most by the incomplete enumeration of certain Indian reserves and Indian settlements. In 2006, a total of 22 Indian reserves and Indian settlements were incompletely enumerated by the census. The populations of these 22 communities are not included in the census counts.

3 Statistics Canada uses its own identification categories that include North American Indian, single responses, and multiple responses. Specifically, the Aboriginal identity population is composed of those persons who reported "identifying with at least one Aboriginal group (i.e., 'North American Indian,' 'Métis' or 'Inuit (Eskimo),' Amérindien), and/or who report being a Treaty Indian or a Registered Indian as defined by the Indian Act of Canada, and/or who were members of an Indian Band or First Nation" (Statistics Canada 2004).

Source: Statistics Canada (2008a).

Figure 21.1   Life expectancy at birth, by sex, Canada, 1991 and 2001

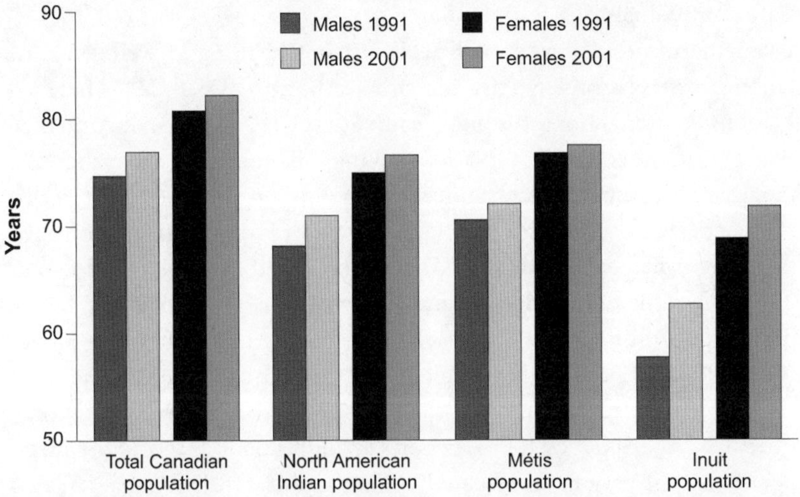

Source: Statistics Canada (2004).

seventeen) reported an injury requiring treatment compared with 13.6 percent for all of Canada (FNRHS National Committee 2005). The rate of death by suicide is 28 per 100,000 for First Nations living on-reserve compared with 79 per 100,000 for Inuit and 13 per 100,000 for Canada (CIHI 2004).

Canada's Aboriginal peoples continue to report being at an increased risk for infectious diseases. The rate of infection from tuberculosis is much higher among First Nations living on- and off-reserve and considerably higher for Inuit than among other Aboriginal groups and non-Aboriginal Canadians. For chlamydia, the rate of infection is seven times that of other Canadians for First Nations living on- and off-reserve and over fifteen times that of other Canadians for Inuit. HIV infection and AIDS are also of major concern to Aboriginal peoples (Public Health Agency of Canada 2003), especially in northern and remote communities, where HIV testing and AIDS treatment are limited or unavailable.

Chronic conditions, particularly diabetes mellitus, respiratory disorders such as asthma, cardiovascular diseases (including heart problems and high blood pressure), cancer, and digestive disorders are significant factors in Aboriginal illness and death (CIHI 2004). Important differences exist among Aboriginal groups. It appears that the prevalence of chronic diseases is highest among First Nations, with the notable exception of arthritis and rheumatism, which are highest among non-status individuals of Aboriginal ancestry.

Furthermore, diabetes mellitus is a major health and wellness issue among First Nations, Métis, and other Aboriginal peoples. The First Nations Regional Longitudinal Health Survey (FNRLHS) documented that the number of First Nations living on-reserve with diabetes is rapidly rising, especially among men. The survey also documented that the age of diagnosis is dropping: 1.5 percent of First Nations youth aged twelve to nineteen already have diabetes (FNRHS National Committee 2005). Cardiovascular disease and hypertension are also major health problems, with First Nations again experiencing the highest prevalence (CIHI 2004). These health problems also appear to be on the rise.

Aboriginal peoples suffer more end-stage renal disease (ESRD) than other Canadians. Dyck (2001) reports an eightfold increase in the number of dialysis patients between 1980 and 2000. Of 954 Canadian Aboriginal people with ESRD studied, 395 (41.3 percent) had diabetic ESRD.

Lung cancer is an emerging health concern among Aboriginal peoples due to the non-traditional use of tobacco products. The FNRLHS indicated that 58.8 percent of First Nations adults on reserves smoked either daily or occasionally (FNRHS National Committee 2005). The study documented that 37.8 percent of youth (aged thirteen to seventeen) already smoked on a regular basis. Among thirteen year olds, 9.4 percent of boys and 18.2 percent of girls smoked. In 1997, the First Nations and Inuit Regional Health Survey (FNIRHS) documented that 78 percent of First Nations adults living on-reserve and Inuit adults smoked (Reading 1999). Trends in the non-traditional use of tobacco have not been documented. Data for other Aboriginal groups are not available.

The picture of health conditions that emerges shows that Aboriginal Canadians are increasingly living with chronic conditions requiring access to primary health care. The next section summarizes the available data on access to health services.

Access to Primary Health Care

To some extent, before the advent of Medicare, access to health care for at least some Aboriginal peoples living in rural and remote communities was somewhat better than that of their national counterparts. For example, the federal government began to offer health services in First Nations and Inuit communities in the 1920s to address the spread of tuberculosis.[2] By the late 1960s, most communities had access to some level of primary health-care services, delivered by registered nurses (RNs) assisted by translators and community health representatives (CHRs). In remote areas, RNs offered treatment, provided midwifery, performed X-rays, and dealt with broken limbs (Waldram, Herring, and Young 2006).[3] These services were provided free of charge.

Access to health services for Métis, however, remained a matter of provincial responsibility. Provincial engagement in the provision of health services began later than that for First Nations and Inuit and co-incided with the spread of tuberculosis and syphilis. Waldram, Herring, and Young (2006) note that in Alberta, despite reports of periodic star-vation and extremely poor health, Métis communities had access to only irregular screening and services. Access to services likely varied across the country, at least until the advent of Medicare in the late 1960s. As for other Canadians, access was dependent on the presence of a physician, an unlikely occurrence in many rural and remote com-munities (Heeney 1995).

What services were accessible to Aboriginal communities, however, were largely delivered *to* them rather than *in partnership with* them (Lavoie 2001; Waldram, Herring, and Young 2006). As well, services reflected the practices of the time and focused on infectious disease screening, immunization, and treatment (Booz, Allen and Hamilton Canada 1969). Since 1989, First Nations and Inuit living south of the sixtieth parallel have had opportunities to plan and deliver on-reserve primary health-care services spanning prevention, health promotion, public health, and treatment services (in communities served by a nurs-ing station). The Health Transfer Policy provides communities ranging from a few hundred to 15,000 members with the option to deliver services previously offered by First Nations and Inuit Health (FNIH). New programs have been introduced over the years (e.g., the Aboriginal Diabetes Initiative, the First Nations Home and Community Care Program). As discussed in Chapter 20 of this volume, the Health Transfer Policy and other Aboriginal self-government activities have created opportunities for communities to experiment with different models of service delivery that acknowledge *community is the constant.* Innovations have included expansion of para-professional roles in health promotion and prevention activities, proactive care, inclusion of elders in program planning and delivery, local capacity development, and integration of other health professionals and providers into a web of community-based relationships of care that focuses on continuity at the community level (Lavoie et al. 2005). These providers can be urban based (visiting general practitioners and in some cases specialists or professionals accessed via telehealth), or they might be prepared to commit to community-based practice for a relatively short period of time (the average stay of RNs in First Nations communities is two years; Aboriginal Nurses Association of Canada 2002).

Strengthening the local health-care system through use and expansion of local capacity can mitigate the transience and scarcity of northern health-care professionals. O'Donnell and Tait's (2003) analysis of the 2001 Aboriginal Peoples Survey (see Table 21.3) showed that, whereas urban and rural residents are more likely to access primary care services from family physicians or general practitioners, Aboriginal people living on reserves and in arctic regions are much more likely to see a nurse. This is partly due to the documented lack of health service providers in Canada (RNs, general practitioners, and specialists), which creates barriers to and delays in accessing health care (Romanow 2002). The problem is compounded in many rural and remote Aboriginal communities, where RNs provide community-based public health and primary care services (Health Council of Canada 2005). When some positions become vacant, the nurse's role in prevention and health promotion activities becomes secondary as treatment takes precedence.

Recent efforts in the development of indigenous determinants of health frameworks (FNRHS National Committee 2005; Reading, Kmetic, and Gideon 2007) reflect approaches that have emerged in Aboriginal communities. Although every Aboriginal group has its own definition of health, these definitions are generally broader and more holistic and invariably include individual and community self-determination as a key component. For example, land claim and self-government discussions have resulted in new models of governance. The Nunavut Land Claim Agreement resulted in the creation of the territory of Nunavut. In the Inuvialuit and Nunatsiaq regions, Inuit have signed self-government agreements. In Nunavik, the James Bay and Northern Quebec Agreement gave rise to a unique model whereby Inuit-managed structures were seen as extensions of the provincial government's own structures. An agreement signed between Quebec, Canada, and Makivik in 2007 proposed the creation of the regional government of Nunavik. According to the proposal, this new order of government would answer directly to the National Assembly of Quebec.

Table 21.3   Contacts with health professionals within twelve months of the survey, Aboriginal identity non-reserve population, fifteen years and over, 2001

	Urban	Rural	Arctic regions
Family physician[1] or general practitioner	75%	69%	43%
Dentist or orthodontist	55%	47%	43%
Eye doctor (ophthalmologist, optometrist)	37%	37%	31%
Other medical doctor (surgeon, allergist, orthopedist)	23%	21%	15%
Registered nurse[2]	23%	27%	58%
Traditional healer	7%	6%	2%
Traditional medicine	34%	26%	14%

1 O'Donnell and Tait (2003) used the expression "family doctor and general practitioners."
2 O'Donnell and Tait (2003) used the term "nurses" only. We assume that they referred specifically to registered nurses.
Source: O'Donnell and Tait (2003).

The proposal was rejected, however, by Nunavik voters in the April 2011 referendum.

Self-government activities have also resulted in the restructuring and rationalization of local health services previously managed by multiple authorities. The community of Norway House in Manitoba is located approximately 800 kilometres north of Winnipeg by road. The overall community includes approximately 5,500 members of the Norway House Cree Nation (NHCN) and 1,000 Métis residents. For many years, the community had been studying options to improve residents' access to health care, which was remarkably fragmented. Local health services included (1) the Norway House hospital, funded and administered by FNIH; (2) the Pinaow Wachi Personal Care Home, funded by INAC and Manitoba Health and managed by NHCN; and (3) a complement of community-based health services, funded by FNIH and delivered by NHCN. Physician services were provided by the Northern Medical Unit of the University of Manitoba. Additional, albeit limited, services were provided by the Burntwood Regional Health Authority. Of these services, only homecare was delivered at the community level. The community recently created a single health authority tasked to administer, manage, and deliver all health services to all residents of Norway House, thereby bringing nine government and community stakeholders into a single integrated health-care plan (Lavoie 2006). This is an important initiative that will lead to better resource utilization, coordinated planning, and improved local access to care.

In spite of these innovations, recent studies suggest that the current complement of on-reserve health services does not meet the complex needs of those with disabilities and complex morbidities. Shah, Gunraj, and Hux (2003) documented that residents of reserves in northern Ontario have a much higher rate of hospitalization for ambulatory care sensitive conditions (ACSC) than other residents of Ontario. ACSC are conditions, such as complications related to type 2 diabetes mellitus, that require hospitalization (Manitoba Centre for Health Policy 2003). Shah and colleagues attributed these differences to poorer access to primary health care. In Manitoba, Martens, Sanderson, and Jebamani (2005) documented that the rate of first referral to a specialist for First Nations was only 7 percent higher than that of other Manitobans despite a much heavier burden of disease. The overall rate of specialist consultation was 70 percent that of all other Manitobans. Martens et al. (2002) also documented that the rate of hospitalization for registered First Nations in Manitoba was double that of all other Manitobans (348/1,000 compared with 156/1,000). The study documented that the rate of lower limb amputation in the Manitoba First Nations population was sixteen times that of other Manitobans. At the time, FNIHB did not fund a foot-care program on-reserve. Both studies concluded that structural barriers to accessing primary health care played a major role.

Jurisdictional confusion has historically (Hawthorn 1966) and continually challenged access to health services (Lavoie and Forget 2006; National Advisory Committee on SARS and Public Health 2003; Romanow 2002). The current jurisdictional environment is rooted in the British North America Act, 1867. The act gave legislative authority over Indians and Indian bands to the federal government and authority over health care to the provinces. This was the beginning of a jurisdictional debate that continues to hamper the provision of health services. Lavoie and Forget (2008) have documented that, for the Manitoba health-care system, jurisdictional confusion results in inefficiencies, cost shifting among the federal and provincial governments and First Nations communities, and barriers to accessing health services for an increasing number of Aboriginal people.

Research continues to show that tacit and sometimes overt discriminatory practices and policies continue to marginalize many Aboriginal people in the mainstream health-care system (Browne 2005, 2007; Browne and Fiske 2001; Kaufert and Putsch 1997; Kaufert, Putsch, and Lavallee 1999; Smith, Varcoe, and Edwards 2005). In part, negative health-care experiences stem from encounters with health-care providers who might be relating to Aboriginal patients on the basis of stereotypes or misinformed assumptions.

The above discussion reflects important innovations as well as continued challenges. It is important to ask this question: *overall, are current efforts likely to deliver better health outcomes for Aboriginal peoples?* The evidence is scant at best because (1) self-government and other structural reform activities vary considerably in nature and scope; (2) the populations included in each initiative can be relatively small; (3) most initiatives are relatively recent; and (4) health information systems are not structured to answer this question. Only two references have attempted to address this issue in the Canadian context. The Evaluation of the First Nations and Inuit Health Transfer Policy reported that respondents from eighty-two communities (78 percent) stated that the health of their communities had improved since their local governments had become involved in the management and delivery of health services (Lavoie et al. 2005). These findings echo those reported by Chandler and Lalonde (1998) that communities engaged in self-government activities in all areas, including health services, have a lower prevalence of First Nations youth suicide. It is reasonable to assume that changes that improve service responsiveness, address jurisdictional issues, and promote better integration are likely to yield benefits, including improved access to services and outcomes. Still, it is important to recognize that current efforts will continue to fall short of expectations as long as structural barriers remain.

Policy Responses

Initiatives have emerged across the country to improve access to appropriate and responsive primary health-care services. Most initiatives have focused on First Nations and Inuit. Métis and Aboriginal peoples not recognized under the Indian Act have yet to benefit from these opportunities. Their needs and circumstances remain largely invisible and undocumented.

What policy response might best ensure that all Aboriginal peoples, especially those from rural and remote communities, can access appropriate and responsive primary health-care services? The policy framework that informs Aboriginal peoples' access to health services is limited. At the national level, the Indian Health Policy was adopted in 1979, with one broad objective – "to achieve an increasing level of health in Indian communities, generated and maintained by the Indian communities themselves" (Health Canada 2005). This is the only federal Aboriginal health policy ever adopted. It has remained broad and unchanged for thirty years.

A recent review of Aboriginal health policies in Canada shows that a patchwork of provincial and territorial policies also exists, with important gaps. When looking at territorial and provincial health legislative frameworks, the report noted that no specific provisions exist in Yukon, Northwest Territories, Nunavut, British Columbia, Manitoba, Nova Scotia, and Prince Edward Island. Where provisions exist, they focus on jurisdiction: legislation in Alberta is said to apply to Métis settlements. Legislation in Alberta, Saskatchewan, Ontario, and New Brunswick specifically states that the minister may opt to enter into an agreement with First Nations for the delivery of health services, thereby clearly indicating that the provision of services is outside a province's mandate. Health legislation in Quebec and Newfoundland and Labrador contains provisions related to existing self-government agreements, thereby clarifying roles and responsibilities (Lavoie et al. 2011).

Although federal, provincial, and territorial governments have recognized the value of entrenching provisions in policy, what has emerged is a policy patchwork reflecting different standards, priorities, and partial responses with different Aboriginal groups. To date, only Northwest Territories has publicly released a plan detailing the minimum level of care and the type of services that must be available in all of its communities (Northwest Territories Health and Social Services 2004). The lack of national minimum standards remains a concern.

Closing the gap that exists in the health status of Aboriginal peoples and their national counterparts is a national priority and requires access to appropriate primary health care. Current trends are encouraging but unevenly distributed across Aboriginal peoples, regions, and communities. Although some have benefited from these opportunities and thrived, others have faced exclusion and invisibility. As mentioned, the engagement of civil society and community is key to achieving health gains. A national Aboriginal health policy framework must be created to entrench this principle, guide current and emerging initiatives, and entrench common minimal standards.

Notes

1 A status Indian is a person registered as an Indian under the terms of the Indian Act. Status ensures the right to live on-reserve and access to treaty- and policy-defined benefits. Status is a poor proxy for cultural affiliation.
2 The name of the department responsible for the provision of health services has changed over time. The restructuring of FNIHB in February 2006 has led to confusion over the name of the government department. FNIHB now refers exclusively to the Ottawa office. Regional offices are FNIH. For clarity, we will use FNIH when referring to specific regional offices. FNIHB will be used when speaking in national terms.
3 Although FNIHB required the nurses that it employed to be registered with a provincial or territorial nursing association, FNIHB did not require them to be registered in the province in which they practised. Registered nurses also worked with an expanded scope of practice outside any legislative framework. FNIHB assumed any liability (Lavoie et al. 2005). This practice changed in the past decade. When First Nations sign a transfer agreement, they are required to ensure that their nursing staff meet the registration and scope of practice defined by the nursing association in place in the province or territory in which they practise.

References

Aboriginal Nurses Association of Canada. 2002. *Developing Best Practice Environments: Best Practice Model Development in Aboriginal Communities – Final Report*. Ottawa: Aboriginal Nurses Association of Canada.

Adelson, N. 2005. "The Embodiment of Inequity." *Canadian Journal of Public Health* 96: S45-S61.

Archibald, L. 2006. *Volume III: Promising Healing Practices in Aboriginal Communities*. Ottawa: Aboriginal Healing Foundation.

Bartlett, J.G. 2003. "Involuntary Cultural Change, Stress Phenomenon, and Aboriginal Health Status." *Canadian Journal of Public Health/Revue canadienne de santé publique* 94, 3: 165-66.

Booz, Allen and Hamilton Canada. 1969. *Study of Health Services for Canadian Indians*. Ottawa: Booz, Allen and Hamilton Canada.

Browne, A.J. 2005. "Discourses Influencing Nurses' Perceptions of First Nations Patients." *Canadian Journal of Nursing Research* 37, 4: 62-87.

–. 2007. "Clinical Encounters between Nurses and First Nations Women in a Western Canadian Hospital." *Social Science and Medicine* 64, 10: 2165-76.

Browne, A.J., and J-A. Fiske. 2001. "First Nations Women's Encounters with Mainstream Health Care Services." *Western Journal of Nursing Research* 23, 2: 126-47.

Browne, A.J., J-A. Fiske, and G. Thomas. 2000. *First Nations Women's Encounters with Mainstream Health Care Services and Systems*. Vancouver: British Columbia Centre of Excellence for Women's Health.

Canadian Institute for Health Information (CIHI). 2004. *Improving the Health of Canadians*. Ottawa: CIHI.

–. 2006. *Pan-Canadian Primary Health Care Indicators: Report 1, Volume 1*. Ottawa: CIHI.

Chandler, M.J., and C. Lalonde. 1998. "Cultural Continuity as a Hedge against Suicide in Canada's First Nations." *Transcultural Psychiatry* 35, 2: 191-219.

Church, W., L. Saunders, and R. Pong. 1995. *Organizational Models in Community-Based Health Care: A Review of the Literature Prepared for the Federal/Provincial/Territorial Conference of Deputy Ministers of Health through the Advisory Committee on Health*

Human Resources. Edmonton: Healthcare Quality and Outcomes Research Centre, Department of Public Health Sciences, University of Alberta; Sudbury: Northern Health Human Resources Research Unit, Laurentian University.

Dyck, R.F. 2001. "Mechanisms of Renal Disease in Indigenous Populations: Influences at Work in Canadian Indigenous Peoples." *Nephrology* 6, 1: 3-7.

First Nations and Inuit Regional Health Survey (FNIRHS) National Steering Committee. 1999. *First Nations and Inuit Regional Health Survey.* Ottawa: Health Canada and the Assembly of First Nations.

First Nations Regional Health Survey (FNRHS) National Committee. 2005. *First Nations Regional Longitudinal Health Survey (RHS) 2002/03 Results for Adults, Youths, and Children Living in First Nation Communities.* Ottawa: FNIRHS National Committee.

Hawthorn, H.B. 1966. *A Survey of the Contemporary Indians of Canada: Economic, Political, Educational Needs and Policies Part 1 (The Hawthorn Report).* Ottawa: Indian Affairs Branch.

Health Canada. 2002. *Healthy Canadians: A Federal Report on Comparable Health Indicators 2002.* Ottawa: Health Canada.

–. 2003. *A Statistical Profile on the Health of First Nations in Canada.* Ottawa: Health Canada (FNIH).

–. 2004. *Community Planning Management System (CPMS).* Ottawa: Health Canada (FNIH).

–. 2005. *Annual Report on First Nations and Inuit Control 2002-2003.* Ottawa: Health Canada.

Health Council of Canada. 2005. *The Health Status of Canada's First Nations, Métis, and Inuit Peoples.* Ottawa: Health Council of Canada.

Heeney, H. 1995. *Life before Medicare: Canadian Experiences.* Toronto: Ontario Coalition of Senior Citizens Organizations.

Indian and Northern Affairs Canada (INAC). 2002. *Mandate, Roles, and Responsibilities Indian and Northern Affairs Canada.* Gatineau, QC: INAC.

Kaufert, J.M., and R.W. Putsch. 1997. "Communication through Interpreters in Healthcare: Ethical Dilemmas Arising from Differences in Class, Culture, Language, and Power." *Journal of Clinical Ethics* 8, 1: 71-87.

Kaufert, J.M., R.W. Putsch, and M. Lavallee. 1999. "End-of-Life Decision Making among Aboriginal Canadians: Interpretation, Mediation, and Discord in the Communication of Bad News." *Journal of Palliative Care* 15, 1: 31-38.

Last, J. 1983. *A Dictionary of Epidemiology.* New York: Oxford University Press.

Lavoie, J.G. 2001. "The Decolonization of the Self and the Recolonization of Knowledge: The Politics of Nunavik Health Care." In C.H. Scott, ed., *Aboriginal Autonomy and Development in Northern Quebec and Labrador.* Vancouver: UBC Press.

–. 2006. *Evaluation Report, Norway House Health Services Inc. Health Integration Initiative, FINAL Report, Conducted for Norway House Health Services Inc.* Winnipeg: MFN-Centre for Aboriginal Health Research.

Lavoie, J.G., and E. Forget. 2006. *A Financial Analysis of the Current and Prospective Health Care Expenditures for First Nations in Manitoba.* Winnipeg: Manitoba First Nations Centre for Aboriginal Health Research.

–. 2008. "The Cost of Doing Nothing: Implications for Manitoba Health Care." *Pimatiwisin* 6, 1: 105-19.

Lavoie, J.G., et al. 2005. *The Evaluation of the First Nations and Inuit Health Transfer Policy.* Winnipeg: Manitoba First Nations Centre for Aboriginal Health Research.

Lavoie, J.G., E. Forget, G. Rowe, and M. Dahl. 2008. *Leaving for the City: Report of the Medical Relocation Project, Phase II*. Winnipeg: Manitoba First Nations Centre for Aboriginal Health Research.

Lavoie, J.G., L. Gervais, J. Toner, O. Bergeron, and G. Thomas. 2011. *Aboriginal Health Policies in Canada: The Policy Synthesis Project*. Prince George, BC: National Collaborating Centre for Aboriginal Health.

Manitoba Centre for Health Policy. 2003. *Ambulatory Care Sensitive (ACS) Conditions*. Winnipeg: Manitoba Centre for Health Policy.

Martens, P., et al. 2002. *The Health and Health Care Use of Registered First Nations People Living in Manitoba: A Population-Based Study*. Winnipeg: Manitoba Centre for Health Policy, University of Manitoba.

Martens, P.J., D. Sanderson, and L. Jebamani. 2005. "Health Services Use of Manitoba First Nations People: Is It Related to Underlying Need?" *Canadian Journal of Public Health* 96, Supplement 1: S39-S44.

National Advisory Committee on SARS and Public Health. 2003. *Learning from SARS: Renewal of Public Health in Canada: A Report of the National Advisory Committee on SARS and Public Health October 2003*. Ottawa: Health Canada.

Northwest Territories Health and Social Services. 2004. *Integrated Service Delivery Model for the NWT Health and Social Services System: A Detailed Description*. Yellowknife: Northwest Territories Health and Social Services.

O'Donnell, V., and H. Tait. 2003. *Aboriginal Peoples Survey 2001 – Initial Findings: Well-Being of the Non-Reserve Aboriginal Population*. Ottawa: Statistics Canada.

Public Health Agency of Canada. 2003. *HIV/AIDS among Aboriginal Persons in Canada: A Continuing Concern*. Ottawa: Public Health Agency of Canada.

Reading, J. 1999. *The Tobacco Report: First Nations and Inuit Regional Health Survey*. Ottawa: FNIRHS.

Reading, J.L., A. Kmetic, and V. Gideon. 2007. "First Nations Wholistic Policy and Planning Model." Discussion paper for Commission on Social Determinants of Health, WHO. Ottawa: Assembly of First Nations.

Richmond, C.A., and N.A. Ross. 2008. "The Determinants of First Nation and Inuit Health: A Critical Population Health Approach 1." *Health and Place* 15, 2: 403-11.

Romanow, C.R.J. 2002. *Building on Values: The Future of Health Care in Canada*. Saskatoon: Commission on the Future of Health Care in Canada.

Shah, B.R., N. Gunraj, and J.E. Hux. 2003. "Markers of Access to and Quality of Primary Care for Aboriginal People in Ontario, Canada." *American Journal of Public Health* 93, 5: 798-802.

Smith, D., C. Varcoe, and N. Edwards. 2005. "Turning around the Intergenerational Impact of Residential Schools on Aboriginal People: Implications for Health Policy and Practice." *Canadian Journal of Nursing Research* 37, 4: 38-60.

Smylie, J., and M. Anderson. 2006. "Understanding the Health of Indigenous Peoples in Canada: Key Methodological and Conceptual Challenges." *Canadian Medical Association Journal* 175, 6: 602-5.

Solar, O., and A. Irwin. 2006. "Social Determinants, Political Contexts, and Civil Society Action: A Historical Perspective on the Commission on Social Determinants of Health." *Health Promotion Journal Australia* 17, 3: 180-85.

Statistics Canada. 2004. "Life Expectancy at Birth, by Sex, 1991 and 2001, Canada." Ottawa: Statistics Canada, http://www.statcan.ca/.

–. 2008a. *Aboriginal Identity Population, 2006 Counts, for Canada, Provinces, and Territories – 20% Sample Data*. Ottawa: Statistics Canada.

–. 2008b. *Geographic Units: Rural Areas (RA)*. Ottawa: Statistics Canada.

Tjepkema, M. 2005. "Non-Fatal Injuries among Aboriginal Canadians." *Health Reports* 16, 2: 9-22.

Waldram, J.B., D.A. Herring, and T.K. Young. 2006. *Aboriginal Health in Canada: Historical, Cultural, and Epidemiological Perspectives.* Toronto: University of Toronto Press.

Wesley-Esquimaux, C.C., and M. Smolewski. 2004. *Historic Trauma and Aboriginal Healing.* Ottawa: Aboriginal Healing Foundation.

World Health Organization (WHO). 1978. *Primary Health Care: International Conference on Primary Health Care 1978.* Alma-Ata, Kazakhstan. Geneva: WHO.

—. 2008. "Primary Health Care." Geneva: WHO, http://www.who.int/.

Chapter 22   **Bridging the Gap: Accessing Health Care in Remote Métis Communities**

B. Krieg

Key Points

- Due to federal legislation such as the Indian Act, Métis people in Canada are not afforded the same rights to health care as First Nations people.
- Although First Nations and Métis peoples might share similar experiences in terms of remote location, the unique aspects of Métis communities and culture must be considered when responding to the specific health-care needs of this diverse population.
- The Métis women who participated in our community-based research offered suggestions to address the complex service needs of elderly Métis women in their communities.

The Canadian Institute for Health Information (CIHI) reports that "there are few specific data, including health data, on the Métis population" (2004, 78). In a survey of leading academic health journals, Young (2003) found that, though Métis people account for more than 26 percent of the Aboriginal population in Canada, less than 1 percent of Aboriginal-focused health research was specific to Métis people. As such, health-related issues relevant to Métis people in Canada have not been well documented. Even more limited is the health-related information specific to elderly Métis women in rural and remote locations of

Canada. A review of available literature resulted in little information on the health needs of elderly Métis women in rural and remote areas and the issues surrounding their access to informal health-care services (Romanow 2002).

Health-Care Provisions for Métis People

"Aboriginal peoples" is the collective name used to refer to the original peoples of North America and their descendants. The Constitution Act, 1982 recognizes three distinct groups of Aboriginal peoples in Canada: Indians (commonly referred to as First Nations), Métis, and Inuit. Each group is unique in terms of heritage, language, cultural practice, and spiritual belief (Indian and Northern Affairs Canada [INAC] 2002).

In 2006, the Aboriginal population in Canada was an estimated 1,172,790 people. Of this population, 698,025 people self-identified as First Nations; 389,780 people self-identified as Métis; and 50,480 people self-identified as Inuit. Although the Aboriginal population in Canada spans all parts of the country, the majority of Aboriginal peoples can be found in the prairie provinces, with approximately 30 percent of the Aboriginal population residing in Saskatchewan and Manitoba (Statistics Canada 2008a).

The Indian Act, first passed in 1876 and since amended several times, outlines federal government obligations and regulations relevant to Aboriginal peoples in Canada (INAC 2002). By means of this federal legislation, Métis people in Canada are not privy to the same rights as First Nations people.

Historically, the term "Métis" referred either to the children of French fur traders and Cree women in the Prairies or to English and Scottish traders and Déné women of the North. Through the Indian Act and its imposition of discriminatory legislation regarding marriages between European settlers and Aboriginal peoples in Canada, many First Nations women and their children lost their Indian status and membership, and hence their rights as First Nations people, when they married non-status men (INAC 2002).

After many years of opposition and an intense struggle to eliminate the unfair provisions in the Indian Act, Bill C-31 was introduced to allow Aboriginal women and their children the opportunity to have their lost Indian status reinstated. For those women unable to prove their ancestral ties to their First Nations communities, reinstatement of Indian status for them and their children was denied (Bourassa, McKay-McNabb, and Hampton 2004; Lawrence 2004; Leclair, Nicholson, and Hartley 2003). Consequently, the term "Métis" is now used to describe people of mixed First Nations and European ancestry who identify themselves as Métis, distinct from First Nations, Inuit, or non-Aboriginal people (INAC 2002).

Despite being recognized as a distinct Aboriginal group, Métis people in Canada are at a disadvantage when it comes to the provision of health-care services; they are not afforded the same health benefits as First Nations and Inuit peoples (Bent, Havelock, and Haworth-Brockman 2007). The Non-Insured Health Benefits (NIHB) program, for instance, administered by Health Canada's First Nations and Inuit Health Branch (FNIHB), funds extended benefits to eligible First Nations and Inuit populations for health-care services that are not usually covered by provincial and territorial health-care plans, including prescription drugs, eye and dental care, and counselling (Health Canada 2007).

In Canada, the provinces and territories are responsible for the delivery of health-care services to Métis people. An in-depth discussion of historical dynamics in Chapter 20 of this volume (see also Chapter 21) aids our understanding of how this provincial/territorial responsibility translates into health resources that are not always distributed equally among and within Aboriginal communities (Métis Centre @ NAHO 2004). For instance, in communities with both First Nations and Métis residents, Métis people are at a disadvantage given their limited coverage for health-care services such as medical transportation, support for maternal care, and crisis counselling.

On a federal level, some Aboriginal health initiatives, such as early childhood education and prevention of HIV/AIDS, fetal alcohol syndrome, and diabetes, do include Métis people. For the most part, however, many Métis communities are not afforded the same health-care services as other First Nations and northern communities in Canada. Accordingly, future health policies must be developed to reflect and respect the health issues, needs, and concerns of Métis people in Canada. It is essential that these policy developments be informed by Métis-specific research to ensure that disparities in the delivery of health-care services to Métis people are not overlooked. To date, there has been limited research specific to the health concerns of Métis people in Canada.

Rural and Remote Health

Although we adopt the definition of rural as outlined earlier in this volume, we give further attention to understanding the circumstances of those residing in remote communities (see Chapter 20). MacLeod et al. (2004), for instance, discuss rural and remote health primarily in terms of geographical location, access to health-care services, and quality of care provided. Sutherns, McPhedran, and Haworth-Brockman (2004) further explore rural and remote health in gendered terms, taking into account not only geographical location but also the subsequent impact of isolation on access to and quality of health care. In this case and in previous chapters, rural health is defined in relation to travel time to service centres, and remote health is defined in relation to absolute isolation, limited road access, and restricted communication with outside communities.

As presented throughout the text (see Chapters 9 and 20), remote health is characterized by geographical, social, and professional isolation, whereby health-care professionals maintain an extended practice role, take a strong multidisciplinary approach to health care, and give consideration to the cross-cultural issues that affect practice and everyday life (Wakerman 2004, 212). This understanding of remote health, which appears to encompass the professional concerns of health-care service and nursing communities, emphasizes the isolation that impacts the daily lives of residents and the professional bodies that provide health-care services in these communities.

Rural and Remote Access to Health-Care Services

In 2006, there were an estimated 240,825 Aboriginal people living in rural locations throughout Canada. Of this population, an estimated 14,120 were aged sixty-five years and older, and approximately 7,260 of them were Métis (Statistics Canada 2008b). These statistics are alarming when considered in the context of health concerns relevant to the Métis people living in rural and remote communities and the barriers that they face when trying to access health-care services.

Although this group comprises an estimated 34 percent of the overall Aboriginal population in Canada (Statistics Canada 2008c), Métis people receive limited benefits from Aboriginal health provisions made available through provincial and federal initiatives. The struggle for Métis inclusion in current Aboriginal health policies and programs has been reduced to a "jurisdictional wrangling between the federal and provincial governments" (Métis National Council 2004). Further compounding these issues of inclusion is an ongoing struggle over responsibility for provisions that hinder access due to financial constraints.

Travel poses a barrier to service delivery in terms of both the ability of health-care personnel to get into a community and the feasibility of residents to go outside a community for health purposes. Natural conditions such as limited or unsafe roadways and poor weather conditions (see Chapter 20, this volume), for instance, can have a tremendous effect on the provision of health-care services to rural and remote communities; health-care appointments are often postponed, and visits by health-care professionals to rural and remote communities are repeatedly delayed as a result of interrupted access to and from distant communities (Leipert and Reutter 2005a).

In addition to travel, the physical location of health-care service facilities presents a challenge for rural and remote Aboriginal communities. Since the health-care services offered in distant communities are scarce, community residents are often required to travel out of the community to access specialized services. For elderly Métis people, these trips can become quite taxing given their responsibility to cover their transportation costs for health-care appointments (Métis National Council 2004).

Leipert and Reutter (2005b) mention the cost of homecare services as another deterrent to accessing health-care services. Due to financial hardship and minimum costs applied to services such as housekeeping and home visits, even individuals who are eligible for subsidized health-care services will opt not to use homecare services. This is especially disturbing when the situation for elderly Métis women is considered. Due to women's lower levels of labour force participation and higher levels of unemployment in Métis communities, many elderly Métis women have been left to depend on meagre pension benefits as their sole source of income (Métis National Council 2004). With no leeway for extra spending, many elderly Métis women are forced to go without much-needed home support services.

In looking at the role of geography and gender on the health of women in remote and northern communities, Leipert and Reutter (2005a, 2005b) found that women's vulnerability to health risks was the result of marginalization, characterized by physical and social isolation and limited options for education and health services. Central to this finding are elderly Métis women seeking culturally appropriate health care. In particular, health-care provisions for elderly Métis women must encompass holistic concepts of health and well-being, including social supports and activities, mental and emotional well-being, and education (Métis National Council 2004).

Yet another concern for elderly Métis women in remote communities is social isolation (see Chapter 23, this volume). Isolation has been linked to conditions of boredom, loneliness, and depression, all of which can be associated with poor physical health (McCann, Ryan, and McKenna 2005; Métis National Council 2004). Buchignani and Armstrong-Esther (1999) conducted research on the informal care of Aboriginal seniors. Their findings revealed a need among Aboriginal seniors to engage in social activities such as playing bingo, dancing, attending powwows, and visiting; however, issues related to travel and reduced physical ability often prevented Aboriginal seniors from engaging in the social activities that they desired. Leipert and Reutter (2005b) found that limited opportunities for socialization can also affect health in terms of sharing information, receiving support for diagnoses and treatments, and networking for access to health-care services. It is important to note, however, that the experiences of elderly Métis women residing in rural and remote areas are not unlike those of elderly non-Aboriginal women. Much can be drawn from this study that would be applicable to both populations concerning health-care access in rural and remote communities.

The Métis Community of Buffalo Narrows

Buffalo Narrows is a small, remote community in northern Saskatchewan. Although it is home to both Aboriginal and non-Aboriginal people, the majority of residents are Métis (Keewatin Yatthé Regional Health Authority 2006). In 2006, Buffalo Narrows had an estimated population of 1,080 people. Approximately 955 people in this population self-identified as Aboriginal (Statistics Canada 2008d).

Buffalo Narrows has a very young population. In 2006, 52 percent of the population were under the age of 30 years; 28 percent were between 30 and 50 years of age; 13 percent were between the ages of 50 and 65 years; and only 6 percent were over the age of 65 years. Women comprised 76 percent of this elderly population (Statistics Canada 2008d). In 2001, approximately 18 percent of the Canadian population over the age of 15 years were providing informal care for elderly persons; in Buffalo Narrows, this figure was an estimated 28.5 percent. Overall, 60 percent of these people providing informal care to elderly persons were women (Statistics Canada 2008e).

Health-care services available to elderly Métis women in Buffalo Narrows include both community-based programs and health-care services offered outside the community. The majority of community-based programs, run out of the local homecare office, include supportive living programs such as Meals on Wheels and homecare to enable independent living for elderly residents. Nursing staff are also available to address health concerns such as diabetes. As well, the local Friendship Centre facilitates community activities and gatherings and organizes local transportation for elderly women (Keewatin Yatthé Regional Health Authority 2006). All of these community-based programs offer respite services to family members who provide informal care to elderly persons. Buffalo Narrows does not have a personal care home for its elderly residents.

Health-care services in Buffalo Narrows appear to be extensive; however, many services are accessible only through referral from a visiting physician who makes scheduled trips to the community. Residents needing specialized health care such as optical or dental care must travel to appointments outside the community. Depending on the location of practitioners, travel time to appointments can range from two to six hours.

The Buffalo Narrows Métis Women's Health Research Project

In the spring of 2004, a group of Métis women from Buffalo Narrows got together to discuss plans for a research project focusing on the provision of health-care services to elderly Métis women in the community. These women formed the Métis Women's Research Committee to oversee the Buffalo Narrows Métis Women's Health Research Project. During their initial discussions, the research team identified key issues relevant to the project.

- Fiscal restraint, health-care restructuring, and limited investment in homecare infrastructure might save the health system money but at the expense of both clients and caregivers.
- Family members are expected to provide homecare support as an extension of their domestic work and family responsibilities.

- The stress of caring for an elderly family member affects everyone in the family, but women and men recognize and respond to stress differently.
- The community lacks good-quality, long-term care with which to replace existing informal care services.

The Métis Women's Research Committee carried out their research in partnership with the Prairie Women's Health Centre of Excellence. As demonstrated in earlier chapters (e.g., Chapter 9), this research was designed to empower research participants to work toward a vision of accessible, good-quality health care with which to meet the needs of elderly Métis women receiving care and their informal care providers. Participatory action research and qualitative research methods were used to gather information from community women on the need for, and access to, homecare and long-term health-care services for elderly Métis women in the community.

In response to the proposed project, women from the community expressed a desire for the research to be carried out in a manner that reflected Métis cultural values. Specifically, the women wanted to have the interviews conducted by a local Métis woman and to participate in the research using their own languages. Hence, a Métis woman from the community was hired as a community researcher, and an Aboriginal research coordinator was contracted to conduct the research, using Cree, Dené, Michif, and English dialects.

A semi-structured interview guide was developed in consultation with the Métis Women's Research Committee and included questions regarding the type and quality of health and social services available, the type and quality of services that were lacking, barriers to accessing services, and recommendations to improve the quality and accessibility of services. Twelve women were interviewed, including six elderly Métis women who were users of formal and informal health-care services, three younger Métis women who provided informal care to family members, and three younger Métis women who provided formal health-care services in the community.

Interviews were audiotaped to ensure accuracy of the information collected and analyzed using qualitative analysis software, Atlas ti. From this thematic analysis of the data collected, the research identified several shortcomings in the health-care services available for elderly Métis women in Buffalo Narrows. Although these findings are not representative of the experiences of all elderly Métis women, they do present some of the challenges that these women can encounter when trying to access health-care services in remote communities such as Buffalo Narrows.

Personal Concerns of Elderly Métis Women in Buffalo Narrows

Through their discussions with the research participants, the research team learned that geographical location and economic position were relevant to the concerns of elderly Métis women in the community. The isolation of living in a remote location limited their opportunities to fulfill their desires for social interaction. As one care recipient put it, "gatherings at other ladies' houses to just have coffee and visit each other; because it gets quite lonesome being home alone and nobody to talk with. Nobody visits anymore; they just phone and see how you are."

The elderly women experienced a lack of availability and affordability of services in Buffalo Narrows, and family members appeared to play vital roles in filling the service gaps in the community. Even so, some concern was expressed over elderly women having to depend on family members for transportation and assistance with household tasks.

You're forgotten people when you turn sixty-five ... [It's] pretty sad, because to me the elders are forgotten people. When you turn sixty-five, you get a good kick in the butt, and you stay there. (care recipient)

And their travel, if you don't have family taking you, and like, most of the time, you still have to help out a little bit with gas, even if family takes you. (formal caregiver)

I need to take her myself because I get no help from anyone in the community. They know she is getting older, and it gets harder for me to take her out in public because she tends to act up once in a while, but they don't make any attempt to come to my home and see how she is doing. (informal caregiver)

Although elderly women would sometimes challenge their lack of independence by "acting out," they did acknowledge the difficult position that they would be in if they did not have family members to rely on for assistance. The women were especially reliant on family members for assistance with transportation to social activities, to appointments within the community, and to urban centres for specialized health-care attention. As one informal caregiver noted, "yeah, it is just her family that takes her; if she had no kids, no one would take her. She would just have to stay home." In fact, transportation was a recurrent theme throughout the discussions with the research participants. It became obvious that transportation services offered by non-family members were not only expensive but also frustrating and inconvenient.

> *We get transportation just to your [hotel] rooms. Where that guy stops, that's where you're supposed to stay, I guess. From there on, you need to take a taxi to your appointments everywhere; take a taxi back to the hotel. [He] doesn't take you anywhere, and that's wrong ... When they take you on a medical trip, you should be taken to your appointments in the mornings and picked up again. (care recipient)*

In spite of their concerns, elderly women expressed gratitude that they were able to rely on family members for support. In addition to providing them with a means to engage in social interaction, family members helped to ease elderly women's financial burdens of having to cover out-of-pocket expenses to attend health-care appointments. Still, even in the absence of medical expenses, the women's monthly pension benefits were barely enough to cover their costs of living.

> *And they think you are getting such a big cheque at the end of the month, because you're not; if that's what it comes down to, most of these people don't even have enough to last 'til the fifteenth of the month. Even the ones that don't smoke, that don't drink, they still have to eat. (care recipient)*

Improving Health-Care Services for Elderly Métis Women in Buffalo Narrows

The aim of the research was to identify, in gender-specific terms, the strengths and limitations of the current health-care situation in Buffalo Narrows and to determine how these health-care services affect elderly Métis women and their families in the community. The research participants offered many good suggestions to meet better the health-care needs of elderly Métis women in the community. The suggestions put forth address service concerns at both individual and community levels.

Individual Service Needs

It was apparent from the conversations with the research participants that elderly Métis women in the community would have safer independent living if they had additional supports to allow them to carry out their daily tasks more autonomously, without having to rely so heavily on family members for support. Assistance with transportation, for instance, was identified as an area where additional support should be provided to elderly Métis women.

The women liked the idea of having reliable and affordable transportation to, from, and between appointments. As well, they were keen on the idea of implementing a travel subsidy program to assist with the out-of-pocket expenses often incurred with distant health-care appointments.

> *[It] would be nice if the elderly had some kind of coverage for their drugs and for travel. For example, when we need to go to, let's say, Saskatoon for a doctor's appointment, we need to pay for gas and hotel rooms, meals, and it gets costly. It would be nice if we could have a taxi take us and we had coverage like the social assistance clients do. (care recipient)*

Medical escorts were also identified as a much-needed service, especially for elderly women who did not have readily available support from family members. In this case, medical escorts could accompany the women to their appointments and provide them with physical assistance when needed as well as assistance with language translation to overcome communication barriers.

> *It would be good for the seniors if they did have [a translator] because a lot of them don't ask for, well, they can't; they don't know how to ask for it. They don't even know what the name of it is, until the interpreter gets the information from them and tells the doctor, "this is what she needs; she has this kind of pain; this is where it hurts." And then they know what medication to administer. (formal caregiver)*

In terms of personal support at home, the research participants identified a need for elderly women in the community to have consistent and readily available home support. These support services were recommended to include assistance with household chores such as grass cutting and snow removal as well as companionship for often isolated elderly women. One care recipient noted that, "yeah, the ones who don't go out very much, at least once a week. There should be some-body going into these homes to visit, you know, or make it a whole week; but choose different people."

Community Service Needs

It was evident from the discussions with the research participants that elderly women in the community commonly experience bouts of lone-liness as a result of being at home alone. Regularly scheduled social activities were identified as a possible means to address elderly women's mental and physical concerns.

> *They should even meet once a week somewhere and have these crafts or storytelling, anything to get together. (care recipient)*

> *Even if the library could come here to bring them books from the library. Like, they should have access to Cree books. I'd like my mother to know about social studies, how the world's changing, 'cause she has no idea. If they ordered Cree books ... she could read that because she reads Cree Bibles. So why can't the library have those kinds of books? (informal caregiver)*

The research participants also acknowledged the absence of readily available health-care services in the community. Consequently, resi-dents often had no choice but to travel long distances to medical ap-pointments or to pick up prescription medications. In response, the participants recommended the operation of a health-care services van to assist in meeting urgent health needs. As well, it was suggested that the van be used to take elderly Métis women shopping for groceries and other essential household items.

> *Well, it would be nice to have our pharmacy back. Since we lost the pharmacy, we need to go to Île-à-la-Crosse for our medication if there is no doctor coming to Buffalo, and it gets costly for gas to go back and forth. (informal caregiver)*

> *If she wanted to live independently by herself, it would be nice if our stores offered free delivery for the seniors. You know, like, they would phone them and say, "do you need groceries today?" Like, if they did it once or twice a week, and then they would deliver it, and she would pay. (informal caregiver)*

In addition to implementing subsequent programs, the research participants identified the need for increased funding to hire more personnel to expand existing programs. It was also suggested that subsidized programming be introduced to assist elderly Métis women in meeting their much-needed community supports, such as meal programs and homecare services.

> *Home health-care services, I think, should be free for the elders; they are being charged now, I guess, what is it, $2.50 per hour? (informal caregiver)*

> *They are short of workers. I find it hard to do the work, so homecare comes in and does the rest of the work that I can't do. (care recipient)*

> *Homecare would be good if they had someone where they stayed overnight. Say, what if I got sick, and there was no other family members ... someone here to take care of her while I'm gone? (informal caregiver)*

> *There is lots left to be seen if they do implement more programs for the elderly, but I guess only time will tell, and they do need more staff. (formal caregiver)*

Discussion

Despite recognition that a holistic framework is an appropriate means to respond to the health concerns of Métis women (Métis National Council 2004), the results of this research suggest that there is some danger in incorporating both Métis and Aboriginal communities into the same framework. Due to distinct historical and cultural factors, funding for health care is different for Métis people. Although First Nations and Métis peoples might share similar experiences in terms of location, the unique aspects of Métis communities and culture must be considered when responding to the specific health-care needs of this diverse population.

Furthermore, the Métis National Council (2004) emphasizes the importance of Métis women being involved in determining issues in and responses to health services for Métis women. Despite the small sample size informing these results, this project presents research inclusive of a Métis perspective, from approach through to dissemination. The responses of the elderly Métis women are unique in that they recognize traditional Métis values of collective and personal well-being.

The Métis women whose voices are profiled in this chapter call for more formal, affordable, and comprehensive health-care services for elderly women living in Buffalo Narrows. Currently, gaps in formal and informal service provision prevent elderly residents from having many of their health-related needs met. The Métis women who participated in the research offered suggestions to address the complex service needs of elderly women in their community. With this information, the research team was in a good position to inform policy and propose recommendations to improve health-care services for elderly Métis women in remote communities such as Buffalo Narrows.

Recommendations

The women interviewed thought that homecare programming should be better funded to support elderly Métis residents in a more comprehensive and affordable way. They recommended, for instance, that costs for services such as meal delivery and home maintenance should be eliminated for elderly Métis residents. They also suggested that homecare providers should become more involved in developing and implementing services to meet the unique needs of each community. In addition, the women called for extended home health-care services, such as overnight care.

Overall, the women talked about the need for more home visits and broader community support for the elderly residents of Buffalo Narrows as a way to address their feelings of loneliness and isolation. One major concern of elderly residents related to the lack of available social resources, regardless of existing social supports. They suggested a variety of activities that could help in this regard, including visits from schoolchildren, craft-making gatherings, exercise programs (e.g., walking and swimming programs), and grocery delivery. Other suggestions included having a gathering place where elders could socialize and having access to Cree-language library books to help them keep up with the changing world. Finally, the women thought that the community should have a free medical van service to assist elderly women in emergency situations or to get them to and from health-care appointments, to pick up prescriptions and groceries, and to meet other transportation needs.

The participants thought that with these additional supports elderly Métis women would be better able to live independently and be less reliant on their families to help them with transportation, household chores, and social activities. Personal assistants are needed for those who do not have family members to escort them to appointments outside the community. Women thought that this person could also act as a mediator between clients and health personnel by addressing language barriers and ensuring clear and accurate communication. They further suggested that elderly clients would benefit from help with activities such as banking, making a will, cutting grass, and shovelling snow. Elderly women also need access to affordable medical equipment that would allow them to live safely and independently.

Acknowledgments

The Prairie Women's Health Centre of Excellence wishes to acknowledge Diane Martz, Kay Wilson, and the women of Buffalo Narrows who dedicated their time and energy to this project.

References

Bent, K., J. Havelock, and M. Haworth-Brockman. 2007. *Entitlements and Health Care Services for First Nations and Métis Women in Manitoba and Saskatchewan*. Winnipeg: Prairie Women's Health Centre of Excellence.

Bourassa, C., K. McKay-McNabb, and M. Hampton. 2004. "Racism, Sexism, and Colonialism: The Impact on the Health of Aboriginal Women in Canada." *Canadian Women's Studies* 24, 1: 23-39.

Buchignani, N., and C. Armstrong-Esther. 1999. "Informal Care and Older Native Canadians." *Aging and Society* 19: 3-32.

Canadian Institute for Health Information (CIHI). 2004. *Improving the Health of Canadians*. Ottawa: CIHI, http://www.cihi.ca/.

Health Canada. 2007. *Population Health Approach*. Ottawa: Health Canada, http://www.hc-sc.gc.ca/.

Indian and Northern Affairs Canada (INAC). 2002. *First Words: An Evolving Terminology Relating to Aboriginal Peoples in Canada*. Ottawa: INAC.

Keewatin Yatthé Regional Health Authority. 2006. *Buffalo Narrows Service Directory*. Buffalo Narrows: Keewatin Yatthé Regional Health Authority, http://www.kyrha.ca/.

Lawrence, B. 2004. *"Real" Indians and Others: Mixed Blood Urban Native Peoples and Indigenous Nationhood*. Vancouver: UBC Press.

Leclair, C., L. Nicholson, and E. Hartley. 2003. "From the Stories that Women Tell: The Métis Women's Circle." In *Strong Women Stories: Native Vision and Community Struggle,* edited by K. Anderson and B. Lawrence, 55-69. Toronto: Sumach Press.

Leipert, B., and L. Reutter. 2005a. "Developing Resilience: How Women Maintain Their Health in Northern Geographically Isolated Settings." *Qualitative Health Research* 15, 1: 49-65.

–. 2005b. "Women's Health in Northern British Columbia: The Role of Geography and Gender." *Canadian Journal of Rural Medicine* 10, 4: 241-53.

MacLeod, M., et al. 2004. "The Nature of Nursing Practice in Rural and Remote Canada." *Canadian Nurse* 100, 6: 27-31.

McCann, S., A. Ryan, and H. McKenna. 2005. "The Challenges Associated with Providing Community Care for People with Complex Needs in Rural Areas: A Qualitative Investigation." *Health and Social Care in the Community* 13, 5: 462-69.

Métis Centre @ NAHO. 2004. *National Aboriginal Health Organization.* Ottawa: Métis Centre @ NAHO, http://www.naho.ca/.

Métis National Council. 2004. Canada-Aboriginal Peoples Roundtable: Métis National Council Health Policy Session, Ottawa, 3 and 4 October.

Romanow, R. 2002. *Building on Values: The Future of Health Care in Canada.* Saskatoon: Royal Commission on the Future of Health Care in Canada.

Statistics Canada. 2008a. "Aboriginal Identity Population, 2006 Counts, Percentage Distribution, Percentage Change for Both Sexes, for Canada, Provinces, and Territories – 20% Sample Data." In *2006 Census: Data Products; Highlight Tables; Aboriginal Peoples.* Ottawa: Statistics Canada, http://www12.statcan.ca/.

–. 2008b. "Aboriginal Identity, Area of Residence, Age Groups, and Sex for the Population of Canada, Provinces, and Territories, 2006 Census – 20% Sample Data." In *2006 Census: Data Products; Highlight Tables; Aboriginal Peoples.* Ottawa: Statistics Canada, http://www12.statcan.gc.ca/.

–. 2008c. *Aboriginal Peoples in Canada in 2006: Inuit, Métis, and First Nations, 2006 Census Aboriginal Peoples, 2006 Census.* Catalogue No. 97-558-XIE. Ottawa: Statistics Canada, http://www12.statcan.gc.ca/.

–. 2008d. *Community Profiles: 2006 Census.* Ottawa: Statistics Canada, http://www12.statcan.ca/.

–. 2008e. *Community Profiles: 2001 Census.* Ottawa: Statistics Canada, http://www.census2001.ca/.

Sutherns, R., M. McPhedran, and M. Haworth-Brockman. 2004. *Rural, Remote, and Northern Women's Health: Policy and Research Directions Final Summary Report.* Winnipeg: Centre of Excellence for Women's Health.

Wakerman, J. 2004. "Defining Remote Health." *Australian Journal of Rural Health* 12: 210-14.

Young, T.K. 2003. "Review of Research on Aboriginal Populations in Canada: Relevance to Their Health Needs." *British Medical Journal* 327: 419-22.

Part 7: Aging in Rural Contexts

Chapter 23 Diversity among Older Adults in Rural Canada: Health in Context

N. Keating and J. Eales

Key Points

- Rural communities are diverse in size, density, and distance from service centres. Some communities have excellent resources to support older residents, whereas some have impoverished service and social environments.
- Older rural adults differ in their physical health, social connection, and community engagement.
- The interaction of type of older adult and community context is what helps to define the person-environment fit that is the hallmark of healthy aging.
- Community-active and stoic seniors have the resources to age well. Community-active seniors are in good health, well connected to others, and net contributors to their communities. Stoic seniors ask little of their communities, are not joiners, and might refuse services because of their strong sense of independence.
- Marginalized and frail seniors have higher support needs that are difficult to meet in rural communities. Marginalized seniors have precarious health and financial status and poor social connections. Frail seniors have significant health concerns but differ in their approaches to meeting their health challenges.

Increasing importance is attached to the geographies of rural areas (Cloke, Milbourne, and Thomas 1997) because rural places are seen as having powerful influences on those who live in them. Stark contrasts exist in beliefs about the nature of these influences. Rural settings are viewed both as hinterlands bereft of basic amenities and opportunities and as idyllic pastoral settings (Wiebe 2001).

The situation of older rural adults mirrors these tensions. Rural communities are often thought of as disadvantaged, with few services to support older residents (Joseph and Cloutier-Fisher 2005). Although seniors living in urban settings might take for granted essential services such as grocery stores, post offices, health clinics, and pharmacies, these services might not be available or accessible to seniors living in rural communities (Hodge 2008). Availability of essential services has declined, levels of homecare and mental health services are low (Skinner and Rosenberg 2006), and small towns have 22 percent of the population but only 10 percent of physicians (Society of Rural Physicians of Canada 2008). Similarly, the number of RNs working in rural Canada has decreased while the number of people living in rural and small-town Canada has increased (Canadian Institute for Health Information [CIHI] 2002).

Older adults are particularly vulnerable to service loss because of their lower incomes, reduced geographical mobility, and health needs. Although older rural adults tend to age in place, there is long-term out-migration of young people from rural communities (Stockdale 2004; Wenger and Keating 2008).

Despite these changes, rural communities are also seen as excellent places in which to grow old (Keating 2008). Rural communities are viewed as closely knit and supportive with good community connections and stable networks of friends and neighbours who provide older adults with familiarity and continuity (Bull 1998). Family ties are significant and meaningful to older rural adults (Keating, Swindle, and Foster 2005), who typically have social networks that include these family ties as well as friends and neighbours who provide a good basis for support if needed (Dobbs et al. 2004). Close ties are evidence of this contrasting stereotype of rural Canada as an idyllic place where older adults are buffered from lack of services by the caring support of family, friends, and neighbours.

Part of the contemporary discourse on older rural Canadians is a concern about their health. Older adults are over-represented in rural places, and their proportion of the population is growing faster than in urban areas. More than 20 percent of older Canadians now live in rural communities (Schellenberg and Turcotte 2007). A combination of rapid population aging and growing numbers of older adults in rural Canada (see Chapter 24, this volume) makes it imperative to understand better what might be important in optimizing their health.

Contemporary definitions of health are often multi-faceted, grounded in a belief in the importance of physical status, maintaining active social contacts, and meaningful involvement in community activities (Bryant, Corbett, and Kutner 2001; Damron-Rodriguez et al. 2005). Based upon this definition, good health might be seen as a state of positive physical status, strong personal connections, and high levels of community engagement. Yet such a "positive state" view of health seems rather exclusive, including only those who have the good fortune to have avoided major chronic health problems, who are sufficiently gregarious to seek and maintain social connections and involvement, and who live in a setting where all of these end states are possible. We prefer a more inclusive view of health that takes into account the variety of personal resources and settings of older adults that might determine the relative importance of each of these three elements of health (Chapman 2005).

This chapter provides information on the ways in which rural communities in Canada influence the health of older adults who live in them. We begin by drawing on current literature on diversity in rural contexts in Canada and among older adults in terms of their physical health, social connections, and community engagement. We describe data on which the chapter is based and use these data to illustrate four profiles of older adults in Canada: (1) community-active, (2) stoic, (3) marginalized, and (4) frail seniors. These profiles have distinctive patterns of elements of health that define how seniors live in their rural communities. We conclude with a discussion of health in context: the interaction of type of older adult and community context that defines the hallmark of good health for each group.

Diversity in Rural Contexts

How rural is viewed has an influence on how one thinks about the health of older adults. We draw on the definition of "Rural and Small Town" (see Chapter 1, this volume), emphasizing diversity among rural communities. Such communities in Canada vary considerably in their characteristics. Among the 2,759 rural communities in Canada, hamlets predominate. The average population size is 1,736, with 52 percent of communities having fewer than 1,000 residents.[1]

The majority of rural communities (60 percent) are close enough to urban centres for some residents to commute to work. Although most older adults are not in the labour force, those who live in such communities can be advantaged by having access to services that might not be available in the 40 percent of rural communities that are outside commuting range of a larger centre. Service accessibility is an important issue to all rural residents but especially to those for whom travel might be restricted because of physical health, climate, or income. Chapters 18 and 25 of this book offer powerful narratives of the challenges of providing services to older adults in culturally and geographically remote areas of the country.

Similarly, access by rural residents to neighbours and friends is influenced by population density. On average, rural communities in Canada have ninety-nine people per square kilometre. However, almost one-fifth of rural communities have a population density of one person (or fewer) per square kilometre, and the top 20 percent have 174 or more people per square kilometre. Chapter 22 speaks to the sense of social isolation of Métis women in remote communities who are at high risk of loneliness and depression.

The physicality of rural settings creates challenges in developing sound social and health policy and delivering services to small, dispersed communities. There is great concern about older adults who have poor access to health and social services (Joseph and Cloutier-Fisher 2005; Skinner and Rosenberg 2006) and who might need to leave their homes to move to distant communities if they need residential care.

Diversity among Older Adults in Rural Canada

Similar to rural places, older rural adults are diverse. This diversity is often invisible given the themes of self-reliance, strong family ties, and good community connections (Dorfman et al. 2004) associated with them. Strong values related to caring for other community members, privacy, and frugality contribute to use of services as a last resort (Shenk et al. 2002). These characteristics suggest a "families first/services last" approach to meeting health and other basic needs.

Yet there is ample evidence that older adults in rural places vary considerably. A generation ago Scheidt (1984) found four main groups of older rural adults who differed considerably in physical and mental health, connections to people, and community engagement. There has been relatively little subsequent research on diversity among older rural adults. We draw on current findings from research on different elements of the health of older adults to illustrate possible areas of diversity among current cohorts of older rural adults.

Physical Health

One body of research that informs our understanding of the health of older rural Canadians is evidence of physical challenges in later life related to high levels of chronic health problems and disability. Most older adults (81.9 percent) living in their own homes have some activity limitation due to a chronic health condition, and 22.2 percent are often restricted in their daily activities as a result of health problems (Schellenberg and Turcotte 2007). Older rural adults have poorer health status than do those living in urban areas (Smith, Humphreys, and Wilson 2008). Physical health status has been the basis for current concern about older rural adults' access to acute and chronic health services.

Older rural adults with high levels of chronic health problems likely have functional status limitations that result in compromised ability to perform daily tasks such as housekeeping or personal care. Yet most live in the community, relying on assistance from their families and friends to help them remain at home (Keating et al. 1999; van Groenou and van Tilburg 2003). As their health and personal resources deteriorate, home and neighbourhood environments of these older adults become less able to compensate for their losses (Gustavson and Lee 2004), requiring those with high levels of disability to seek residential care. Nursing home residence is associated with decreased levels of social participation and engagement (Washburn, Sands, and Walton 2003), especially problematic if seniors must leave their communities to find residential care options.

Social Connections

In addition to physical status, high-quality personal relationships are seen as essential elements of health (Lucey 2007). Reduced health services in rural areas and difficulties in providing services to dispersed populations have meant that older adults in rural areas are especially reliant on family members and friends. Some older rural adults have rich social networks in late life, whereas others have few people to call on (Wenger and Keating 2008). Strong social connections are often forged through activities in social and community groups (Manthorpe, Malin, and Stubbs 2004). Those who are active and engaged are often the providers of various forms of support to their family members, friends, and neighbours (Stobert and Cranswick 2004).

In sharp contrast to the literature on social connections of older adults is a growing body of knowledge on isolation of older adults who have weak links to others in their communities. Isolation can result from a combination of financial constraints, fragility of social connections, and acute health problems (Scharf and Bartlam 2008). Typically, these seniors have few close ties, are protective of their privacy, and interact only with a small number of people (Wenger and Burholt 2004). They are especially dependent on vigilant family members to help them remain in the community, though some are lifelong isolates (van Groenou and van Tilburg 2003). Isolation is of particular concern given Canada's vast physical context and the challenges of access to services and people in rural Canada (Skinner and Rosenberg 2006).

Community Engagement

In the past decade, there has been a great deal of interest in the engagement and contributions of older adults in areas such as community activities and provision of unpaid family labour (Fast et al. 2006). Rural residents are more likely to spend their time on unpaid volunteer work than their urban counterparts (Turcotte 2005). There is a current though contentious belief that active engagement is the key to aging well (Martinson and Minkler 2006). Many devote considerable time and skill to community organizations or management of community events.

At its best, volunteerism is a mechanism through which people establish connections to others (Wilson 2000). Indeed, older volunteers "play critical roles in maintaining strong communities and effective family functioning" (Warburton and McLaughlin 2005, 726). Active older adults might be the most likely to volunteer. By connecting with others such as frail seniors through volunteering, they can also enhance the links among other older adults in the community.

In conclusion, the different bodies of literature briefly reviewed here might correspond to seniors in quite different circumstances: those who are in poor health, those who are active and engaged, or those who are isolated from others. Explicit comparisons across these areas are rare. Hence, it is difficult to determine whether they represent distinct groups of older adults. Furthermore, it might be that rural community settings make it more or less difficult for people with these various characteristics and approaches to rural life to experience a "good fit" in terms of their health.

Methods

This chapter is based on data from a national program of research on older adults in rural Canada in which we investigated how rural Canada is supportive of its older residents. The Rural Seniors program[2] had three phases: an analysis of the 2001 census to determine level of supportiveness of rural communities of older adults, a national telephone survey of older adults, and a case study of three rural communities. Data for this chapter were drawn from a community case study in 2004-5 of three Canadian rural communities: Oyen, Alberta; Bobcaygeon, Ontario; and Parrsboro, Nova Scotia. Each case community approximated the size of the average rural Canadian community (see Table 23.1). Because we were interested in older adults, we chose communities that had higher than (provincial) average proportions of older adults. Reflecting diversity among rural communities, case communities differed in terms of region, distance from urban centres, migration patterns, labour force participation, and income. Oyen is a farming community in southeastern Alberta, 190 kilometres from Medicine Hat, a larger service centre; Bobcaygeon is an affluent retirement community along the Trent Severn Waterway, fifty-nine kilometres northwest of Peterborough; and Parrsboro, a seasonal tourist community along the northern shore of the Bay of Fundy in Nova Scotia, has the lowest average income of the three communities and is fifty-five kilometres from the nearest service centre of Amherst.

Case study approaches assume that a complex phenomenon is best understood by being immersed in the setting over time and by exploring the phenomenon using diverse methods and multiple perspectives (Yin 2003). Data collection extended over one year and included stakeholder interviews, community consultations, archival analyses, and photographs. Guiding questions focused on older adults' ability to have their needs met, their connections to people, and their participation in community activities. Interviewers recorded field notes after each interview. Guiding focus group questions used in the community consultations validated initial findings of four groups of older adults (described

Table 23.1   Characteristics of case study rural communities, 2001

Characteristic	Oyen, AB	Bobcaygeon, ON	Parrsboro, NS
Population and population history			
Population (2001)	1,020	2,854	1,529
Population change (1961 to 2001)[1]	23.5	57.6	-19.9
Distance (km)			
Nearest small city (population of 10,000 to 99,999)	190	32	55
Nearest large city (population of 100,000 or more)	308	156	186
Age			
Population 65 and older (%)	22.6	41.0	23.2
Median age of population (years)	39.0	59.7	44.0
Labour force			
Unemployment rate (%)[2]	1.8	6.8	17.2
Income			
Median household income	$44,926	$40,544	$25,886
[Provincial median household income]	[$52,524]	[$53,626]	[$39,908]
Incidence of low income in the population in private households (%)	9.7	14.4[3]	31.4

1 Census of Canada, 1961 and 2001.
2 Unemployment rate refers to the percentage of those who are not working but actively looking for work divided by the labour force (the population 15 years of age and over who are working or looking for work) in the week (Sunday to Saturday) prior to census day (15 May 2001).
3 Because Bobcaygeon and all other municipalities in Victoria County were amalgamated in January 2001 to form the City of Kawartha Lakes, some data are not reported separately for Bobcaygeon in the 2001 census. In this table, Bobcaygeon data from the 1996 census are reported for incidence of low income in the population in private households.
Source: Statistics Canada (2001).

in the next section) and deepened understanding of diversity among older adults in these communities. Data gathered were analyzed through a continuous, iterative, and comparative process (Patton 2002; Silverman 2000). Coding and analysis began as soon as sufficient transcripts were available and continued parallel to interviewing. Careful reading of transcriptions and field notes led to the first phase of coding organized into broad categories of older adults' ability to meet their needs, interactions with family members and friends, participation in community activities, and personal resources.

Following Bryman (2001), within each code, data were analyzed with the intention of building general patterns through a process of breaking down, examining, comparing, conceptualizing, and categorizing data. New codes were developed that were grounded in the data and particularly relevant to questions of diversity among rural older adults and their experiences of "fit." Within-case analyses were conducted to map the diversity among rural older adults in the same community. For each case, a densely descriptive picture was developed (Patton 2002; Yin 2003), with data coded for themes including personal resources such as physical health, connections to others, and community engagement. Comparisons among interviews were conducted to identify a set of characteristics that defined a particular group of older adults by virtue of their personal resources, interactions with people, and level of and approach to engagement in community activities. Subsequent cross-case analysis was used to compare the different groups of older adults, looking for commonalities among the groups across the three case communities. Validation of the initial findings of four groups of older adults that emerged from the data was an important feature of the community consultations.

Profiles of Older Adults in Rural Canada

Among the older adults in the case communities, there were four groups who differed in terms of physical health, social connections, and community engagement: community active, stoic, marginalized, and frail. The groups had distinctive patterns of elements of health that, as a whole, defined their styles of living in their communities.

Community-Active Seniors

Defining features of community-active seniors are their engagement in their communities in a wide range of formal and informal activities and their large social networks. They enjoy being active and fully engaged in their communities, and they have resources that allow them to do so, such as health, energy, skills, and money. Volunteering is one important method of engagement. Providing support to people in need, contributing to community culture, or helping friends, they get a great sense of satisfaction from their community engagement.

> *Keeping busy and being involved whether it's the church or seniors or friends or what[ever] ... If I can get out for a walk or visit somebody, I usually do. I think that's why I'm so busy all the time.*

[They are] the movers and the shakers. They get the stuff done in this community.

If you want to live in a certain type of community, you have to make a contribution to making it that kind of community ... And to get involved is the way to do that.

Community-active seniors are well connected, maintaining broad social networks of family members and many friends, both with those nearby and with those at a distance. They describe their communities as places "where all my friends are" and where they have "real good friends." Community-active seniors' extensive involvement in supporting friends, volunteering, and participating in community activities and organizations contributes to the diversification of their social networks and to their strong sense of connectedness.

We go up to [city, a two-hour drive away] to visit our daughter, and I have a brother there and old friends, but we stay a couple of days, and we hurry back to [rural community].

I have a friend that has never driven a car, and I'm her wheels.

There's a group of us that meet up on a Friday night and go out for supper. We have a different group there that meets up on a Tuesday or Wednesday. And now the Tim Hortons has opened. You get somebody ringing up, saying, "let's go to Tim Hortons for coffee," which I think is a nice thing. We usually have friends who call us, and I think it's nice.

Stoic Seniors

Defining characteristics of stoic seniors are their strong work ethic, their purposeful and often limited community engagement, and their practical and reserved social connections. When they are not working in their homes, yards, or shops, stoic seniors engage in solitary pursuits with tangible outcomes. They are not joiners. They have limited involvement in community organizations and events, though they might be engaged in their local churches. They are careful in their selection of community projects. Only those seen as worthy of their time will get them engaged. Staying home is an acceptable alternative.

She's very practical ... She'd rather work than sit on the couch and talk to someone. She doesn't join the clubs; she just has other priorities.

I do not go and golf, and I do not curl. I do not belong to the Legion. I do not belong to the seniors' centre's association, and I don't want to.

Tomorrow there's a supper, with ham and beans and potato scallop and pies and cakes galore, of course. So I'll be going to work at that. I'll either be cutting pies or doing something like that ... It keeps us busy making money for the church.

Stoic seniors' social connections are focused on family members and close friends who are nearby. They are familiar with people but not intimate in their social relationships. They become connected to others through their work, their everyday routines in a small rural community, or their chance social encounters with other community members.

Oh, if I needed them [family members], they're right there. [Interviewer: Are they?] Yup, but I try not to bother them.

A lot of them you just take as you see them. Some of them are people that you'd stand and chat with, and some of them aren't. I mean, everybody doesn't want to talk all the time.

[It's] too hard to make friends.

Marginalized Seniors

Defining characteristics of marginalized seniors are their limited social connections to people in the community other than family members, their limited incomes, and their lack of personal agency. Some have health concerns that add to the precarious nature of their lives.

Nothin' else going for me, I got no kids, never was married. That's probably why nobody ever comes around and visits.

[We have to be] very economical to live on a pension. That's basically what we do. It's not that we have a lot of money; it's just that we have to pinch pennies.

> *The only time we go out is if we're invited to your birthday party or something ... Our kids pick us up for dinner or supper or whatever.*

Marginalized seniors' social connections are narrowly focused and passive. "Being near your family" was most important. Some lived at a distance from their family members, and others had moved to be closer to theirs. Marginalized seniors have few friends, and they rely heavily on family members to initiate social interactions. Often they are socially isolated, invisible in their communities until a crisis arises.

> *When you have your family, it's everything as far as I'm concerned – having family around and having them care about you. They know the hard things you're going through ... When you're not feeling good, they [children] tend to, or mine do, take over sort of to help me out, not moneywise maybe – they're no better off than I am – but they're just there for you. You need that.*

> *I don't know who the neighbours are here ... I don't talk. I just wave at them.*

Economic vulnerability permeates marginalized seniors' everyday lives, constraining their choices and levels of community engagement. They frequently report modest incomes and try to adjust their lifestyles and expectations to available financial resources. They might worry about making ends meet.

> *We've always been on a tight budget ... We find we don't do too much of it [shopping] here ... because we find the stores are too expensive here, far as groceries [go] ... It's cheaper to drive to [the city].*

> *There are lots of recreation opportunities for seniors here if you can afford to go.*

Frail Seniors

The defining characteristic of frail seniors is the presence of significant health concerns. All needed support because of their health challenges. They differed in their approaches to meeting these challenges. Some "made do," some relied on family members or friends, and some paid for assistance.

I would never call a taxi in this town, I'd have to be desperate, absolutely desperate, I'd take my walker and try to make it with my walker before I'd call a taxi.

Peter[3] periodically comes over and sees if there's something we would like done, changing lightbulbs, things like that. He often does that. He's a good friend of the family.

I'm able to hire some of the work done if I need it ... They could do the things that I just am not able to do ... I got the maid [to] come in and clean the windows and move out some furniture that I thought I couldn't move out now.

Frail seniors differed as well in terms of the strength of their social connections and their interactions with family, friends, and neighbours or willingness to call on them for support.

When you get to be a senior, you're more or less by yourself, you know.

Once in a while some of the grandchildren [visit] but not very often ... They all have got a life of their own. I understand that.

Once in a while I might speak to one of the neighbours on the phone. I have other friends that I do keep in touch with by telephone in town and outside of town. I have family, like nieces and nephews and a sister-in-law in Ontario. I talk to them on the phone.

We [frail senior and sister] usually get into town one day a week, if the weather is good. In the summer, it's no problem. We go to church on Sundays, and we go to the restaurant for lunch after church, and we also get out one day a week to do the grocery shopping. Buy stamps, go to post, go to mail, go to the bank, I mean, you know, get the little things done we have to get done.

Despite their significant physical health problems, frail seniors differ considerably in their interest in community engagement. Some put great effort into maintaining their engagement, adapting their activities as required. Others find that frailty precludes their ability to go out with friends and participate in community activities.

I like playing cards. Now I can't see unless they get the big cards.

[My sister] and I [are] planning a dance for our church group. So that'll be nice. I like music, I love music, I've always been involved with it, you know. Singing and dancing, can't dance anymore, but I can do it in my mind!

Probably at one point, they were probably fairly active, in the community, but you know things happen, you get arthritis ... you get this and the other thing. And you just can't get out anymore.

I miss it [church] ... I'd like to go.

The defining characteristics of health – physical health, social connections, and community engagement – distinguish four groups of rural older adults: community-active, stoic, marginalized, and frail seniors. These profiles provide a more nuanced understanding of the diversity among them. Some rural older adults have good resources across elements of health, whereas others struggle. Rural communities too are diverse. The question of whether rural communities are healthy places for older adults to live is best addressed by critically examining the fit between the defining features of the groups of older adults and the resources available to them in rural communities.

Health in Context

The interaction of type of older adult and community context is what helps to define the person-environment fit that is the hallmark of good health. Each has been described in the previous section. In this final section, we consider person-environment fit for each group. Table 23.2 summarizes the issues of fit for groups of seniors by health domain. "Best fit" requires consideration of physical health, social connections, and community engagement in relation to community resources.

Community-active older adults have high levels of personal agency. They have skills to seek out and use services that they need either within or outside their communities. For them, having local access to health and other services is useful but not necessary. They have broad social connections with people inside their communities and elsewhere and thrive on these interactions.

Table 23.2   Facilitating the "good health" of rural older adults

Group of seniors	Health domain		
	Physical	Social connections	Community engagement
Community-active seniors	Can and will access services at a distance	Maintain broad social connections with others near and far and have the resources to do so	Want opportunities to be socially active, volunteer, and keep busy without feeling stretched or conscripted by a lack of community resources
Stoic seniors	Rely on goods and services available locally	Need proximate family members or close friends	Have little need for community recreation and leisure programs
Marginalized seniors	Need access to basic necessities that are affordable Need subsidized health-care and emergency services	Rely on proximate family members for agency	Need community programs that are affordable and offer companionship and an invitation to participate
Frail seniors	Need local health services and supportive housing options	Need long-standing family members and friends nearby to provide support and link to broker services	Level of community engagement varies with pathway to frailty and current physical health

The main issue for them is to have satisfying levels of engagement in their communities without undue personal costs. In retirement communities such as Bobcaygeon, with a large pool of volunteers, these older adults have choice and flexibility in their participation, confident that there will continue to be a robust voluntary sector. In contrast, communities with fewer resources, such as Parrsboro, have a sense of "compulsory volunteerism" in which older adults do more than they would like or can easily manage. Those who live in places where the population is stable or declining worry that they will not be able to sustain their contributions as they grow older and that there might not be younger people who will take over. Here the greatest need might be for community-level interventions that would reduce pressure on the voluntary sector.

Stoic seniors seem ideally adapted to living in rural communities with limited resources. They "make do" with available goods and services, expect little from their few social connections, and are very judicious in their community engagement. At question is how to support these elements of their health given that they are fiercely independent and self-reliant. Proximate social connections that otherwise are not actively sought can be very useful. Family members and close friends can provide support if and when needed. In communities in which the local economy is thriving, stoic seniors' children might have employment opportunities and remain nearby. However, if the local economy is lagging, stoic seniors might have few proximate social connections, and formal services might be of little use in bridging the gap. Homecare workers commented that stoic seniors often refuse services, saying that they do not need assistance or are managing fine, even when they might not be.

Although opportunities for community engagement are of little concern to stoic seniors, it is important that they be close to adequate basic health services. In remote communities, stoic seniors might be unwilling to drive long distances to seek specialist care or obtain prescriptions. Living in rural communities such as Parrsboro and Bobcaygeon that are within commuting distance of larger urban centres can increase the likelihood that stoic seniors will obtain the health services that they require.

In many ways, older adults who are marginalized have the poorest fit with their rural communities because of their limited resources and personal agency. They seem to reflect the profile of older adults who are socially isolated: fragile health, poor financial resources, and limited or no social connections. They might be reluctant to access health services because of worry about costs. Some have always been on a tight budget and fare better in communities, such as Parrsboro, where local services are affordable. Others have seen their retirement incomes eroded because of increasing costs of housing and local services. Prices of basic goods such as food and clothing might be beyond reach in newly affluent retirement communities such as Bobcaygeon.

Marginalized seniors can benefit from living in rural communities with stable populations where long-term neighbours will watch for problems. Having family members nearby can also reduce the risk of social isolation. Access to kin is reduced in communities with high unemployment or that, like Oyen, are remote from larger centres that have employment for adult children.

Frail seniors with high levels of chronic health problems are most in need of access to acute and continuing care services within their communities and to proximate family members and friends who will help them to maintain their independence, provide support, and broker services. Frail seniors are well suited to communities, such as Oyen, that have physicians, a hospital, and a range of residential housing options for older adults. Yet aging in place can be difficult to achieve in rural communities that have experienced hospital closures or that struggle to retain health-care professionals. Under these conditions, the availability of family and friends becomes even more important in providing frail seniors with the assistance that they need to remain in their communities. The next chapter describes the challenges facing both family and formal caregivers to frail seniors with dementia.

The diversity that we see among frail older adults in social engagement and health domains provides evidence that frail older adults may previously have been either community active, stoic, or marginalized. Thus, despite commonalities that stem from high levels of chronic health conditions, frail older adults might have more in common with those other groups in their preferences for social connections and community engagement.

Viewing health in context provides a more detailed view of how some features of rural communities are better suited to a particular group of rural seniors than other aspects. Although access to health professionals and services is essential, for some distance is not a great barrier. In times of limited health services and declining pools of professionals in rural areas, regional health boards might look to the mix of older adults in their communities to plan targeted interventions. Proximate nursing services can best serve those who are marginalized and unable to gain access to larger centres. Holistic views of health that include both physical and social elements require interventions that acknowledge the relevance of both. Employment programs to enhance job opportunities for adult children, community development initiatives to enhance voluntary capacity, or infrastructure to improve highway access – all can be important in maintaining good health. One size does not fit all. Understanding diversity among people and contexts takes us further toward ensuring quality of life for an aging rural Canada.

Notes

1 All data on rural communities in this section are from the 2001 census analysis. See Keefe et al. (2004).
2 The Caring Contexts of Rural Seniors research program was funded by Veterans Affairs Canada (September 2002-March 2006) and led by Norah Keating, University of Alberta; Janice Keefe, Mount St. Vincent University; and Bonnie Dobbs, University of Alberta.
3 Real names have been replaced with pseudonyms to maintain confidentiality.

References

Bryant, L.L., K.K. Corbett, and J.S. Kutner. 2001. "In Their Own Words: A Model of Healthy Aging." *Social Science and Medicine* 53, 7: 927-41.

Bryman, A. 2001. *Social Research Methods.* New York: Oxford University Press.

Bull, C.N. 1998. "Aging in Rural Communities." *National Forum* 78, 2: 38-41.

Canadian Institute for Health Information (CIHI). 2002. "Supply and Distribution of Nurses in Rural and Small Town Canada, 2000." Ottawa: CIHI, http://secure.cihi.ca/.

Chapman, S.A. 2005. "Theorizing about Aging Well: Constructing a Narrative." *Canadian Journal on Aging* 24, 1: 3-18.

Cloke, P., P. Milbourne, and C. Thomas. 1997. "Living Lives in Different Ways? Deprivation, Marginalization, and Changing Lifestyles in Rural England." *Transactions of the Institute of British Geographers* 22, 2: 210-30.

Damron-Rodriguez, J.A., J.C. Frank, V.L. Enriquez-Haass, and D.B. Reuben. 2005. "Definitions of Health among Diverse Groups of Elders: Implications for Health Promotion." *Generations* 29, 2: 11-16.

Dobbs, B., J. Swindle, N. Keating, J. Eales, and J. Keefe. 2004. *Caring Contexts of Rural Seniors: National Telephone Survey of Rural Older Adults.* Final report to Veterans Affairs Canada. Edmonton: Dobbs et al.

Dorfman, L.T., S.A. Murty, R.J. Evans, J.G. Ingram, and J.R. Power. 2004. "History and Identity in the Narratives of Rural Elders." *Journal of Aging Studies* 18: 187-203.

Fast, J., M. Charchuk, N. Keating, D. Dosman, and L. Moran. 2006. *Participation, Roles, and Contributions of Seniors.* Final report to Human Resources and Social Development Canada, Knowledge and Research Directorate. Edmonton: Fast et al.

Gustavson, R., and C.D. Lee. 2004. "Alone and Content: Frail Seniors Living in Their Own Home Compared to Those Who Live with Others." *Journal of Women and Aging* 16, 3-4: 3-18.

Hodge, G. 2008. *The Geography of Aging.* Montreal: McGill-Queen's University Press.

Joseph, A.E., and D. Cloutier-Fisher. 2005. "Ageing in Rural Communities: Vulnerable People in Vulnerable Places." In *Ageing and Place: Perspectives, Policy, Practice,* edited by G.A. Andrews and D.R. Phillips, 133-46. Oxon, UK: Routledge.

Keating, N., ed. 2008. *Rural Ageing: A Good Place to Grow Old?* Bristol: Policy Press.

Keating, N., J. Fast, J. Frederick, K. Cranswick, and C. Perrier. 1999. *Eldercare in Canada: Context, Content, and Consequences.* Statistics Canada Catalogue No. 89-570-XPE. Ottawa: Statistics Canada.

Keating, N., J. Swindle, and D. Foster. 2005. "The Role of Social Capital in Aging Well." In *Social Capital in Action: Thematic Policy Studies,* 24-51. Ottawa: Social Development Canada.

Keefe, J., P. Fancey, N. Keating, J. Frederick, J. Eales, and B. Dobbs. 2004. *Caring Contexts of Rural Seniors: Census Analysis.* Final report to Veterans Affairs Canada. Edmonton: Keefe et al.

Lucey, P. 2007. "Social Determinants of Health." *Nursing Economics* 25, 2: 103-9.

Manthorpe, J., N. Malin, and H. Stubbs. 2004. "Older People's Views on Rural Life: A Study of Three Villages." *International Journal of Older People Nursing* 13, 6: 97-104.

Martinson, M., and M. Minkler. 2006. "Civic Engagement and Older Adults: A Critical Perspective." *Gerontologist* 46, 3: 318-24.

Patton, M.Q. 2002. *Qualitative Research and Evaluation Methods.* 3rd ed. Thousand Oaks, CA: Sage.

Scharf, T., and B. Bartlam. 2008. "Ageing and Social Exclusion in Rural Communities." In *Rural Ageing: A Good Place to Grow Old?,* edited by N. Keating, 97-108. Bristol: Policy Press.

Scheidt, R.J. 1984. "A Taxonomy of Well-Being for Small-Town Elderly: A Case for Rural Diversity." *Gerontologist* 24, 1: 84-90.

Schellenberg, G., and M. Turcotte. 2007. *A Portrait of Seniors in Canada.* Ottawa: Statistics Canada.

Shenk, D., B. Davis, J.R. Peacock, and L. Moore. 2002. "Narratives and Self-Identity in Later Life: Two Rural American Older Women." *Journal of Aging Studies* 16: 401-13.

Silverman, D. 2000. "Analyzing Talk and Text." In *Handbook of Qualitative Research,* edited by N.K. Denzin and Y.S. Lincoln, 821-34. Thousand Oaks, CA: Sage.

Skinner, M.W., and M.W. Rosenberg. 2006. "Managing Competition in the Countryside: Non-Profit and For-Profit Perceptions of Long-Term Care in Rural Ontario." *Social Science and Medicine* 63, 11: 2864-76.

Smith, K.B., J.S. Humphreys, and M.G.A. Wilson. 2008. "Addressing the Health Disadvantage of Rural Populations: How Does Epidemiological Evidence Inform Rural Health Policies and Research?" *Australian Journal of Rural Health* 16, 2: 56-66.

Society of Rural Physicians of Canada. 2008. *Society of Rural Physicians of Canada.* Shawville, QC: Society of Rural Physicians of Canada, http://www.srpc.ca/.

Statistics Canada. 2001. *Community Profiles.* Ottawa: Statistics Canada, http://www12. statcan.ca/.

Stobert, S., and K. Cranswick. 2004. "Looking after Seniors: Who Does What for Whom?" *Canadian Social Trends* 74: 2-6.

Stockdale, A. 2004. "Rural Out-Migration: Community Consequences and Individual Migrant Experiences." *Sociologia Ruralis* 44, 2: 167-94.

Turcotte, M. 2005. "Social Engagement and Civic Participation: Are Rural and Small Town Populations Really at an Advantage?" *Rural and Small Town Canada Analysis Bulletin* 6, 4: 1-23.

van Groenou, M., and T. van Tilburg. 2003. "Network Size and Support in Old Age: Differentials by Socio-Economic Status in Childhood and Adulthood." *Aging and Society* 23, 5: 625-45.

Warburton, J., and D. McLaughlin. 2005. "'Lots of Little Kindnesses': Valuing the Role of Older Australians as Informal Volunteers in the Community." *Ageing and Society* 25: 715-30.

Washburn, A.M., L.P. Sands, and P.J. Walton. 2003. "Assessment of Social Cognition in Frail Older Adults and Its Association with Social Functioning in the Nursing Home." *Gerontologist* 43, 2: 203-12.

Wenger, G.C., and V. Burholt. 2004. "Changes in Levels of Social Isolation and Loneliness among Older People in a Rural Area: A Twenty-Year Longitudinal Study." *Canadian Journal on Aging* 23, 2: 115-27.

Wenger, G.C., and N. Keating. 2008. "The Evolution of Networks of Rural Older Adults." In *Rural Ageing: A Good Place to Grow Old?,* edited by N. Keating, 33-42. Bristol: Policy Press.

Wiebe, N. 2001. "Rewriting the Rural West." In *Writing Off the Rural West,* edited by
    R. Epp and D. Whitson, 325-30. Edmonton: University of Alberta Press.
Wilson, J. 2000. "Volunteering." *Annual Review of Sociology* 26: 215-40.
Yin, R.K. 2003. *Applications of Case Study Research.* 2nd ed. Thousand Oaks, CA: Sage.

Chapter 24   **Looming Dementia Care Crisis:
Are Canadian Rural and Remote
Settings Ready?**

D.A. Forbes and P. Hawranik

Key Points

- The looming dementia crisis will place greater challenges on rural
  and remote family caregivers. In addition, contrary to beliefs of
  health-care providers that rural residents are embedded in strong
  networks of family and friends, family caregivers reported that they
  feel isolated from family and friends.
- Recruitment, retention, and available and appropriate dementia training and continuing educational opportunities for health-care providers are increasing challenges, especially for First Nations communities
  and the resource hinterland.
- The models of delivery of rural and remote services must address
  the uniqueness of the community by taking into account the social,
  economic, and cultural history and traditions that influence the need
  for, availability of, and quality of supports and care for persons with
  dementia.
- Various forms of technology are needed and can play a key role in
  reducing the impacts of distance and dispersion in rural and remote
  communities and in meeting the needs of persons with dementia.
- Flexible, respectful, and culturally sensitive care is needed by persons with dementia and their family caregivers to enable them to
  remain in their homes and communities for as long as possible.

Many rural and remote Canadian communities are experiencing a faster-growing proportion of seniors than in urban areas because of the out-migration of youth, the lack of in-migration, and the attractiveness of some rural communities for retirees (see the previous chapter). In addition, the 9.9 million baby boomers (those born between 1947 and 1966) are beginning to turn sixty, and they are entering the age of greater risk of being afflicted with dementia (Foot and Stoffman 2004). Eight percent of Canadians sixty-five years of age and older and 34.5 percent over the age of eighty-five years have or will have dementia (Canadian Study of Health and Aging [CSHA] Working Group 2000). Approximately 60,000 new cases of dementia are diagnosed each year. This chapter presents the challenges faced by Canadian rural and remote family and friend caregivers and their formal care providers in meeting the needs of older adults with dementia, and it offers models of health service delivery and dementia care best practices that address these challenges.

The definition of rural used in this chapter is that of "Rural and Small Town" (du Plessis et al. 2002) provided in Chapter 1. Dementia is defined as acquired impairment in short- and long-term memory, associated with impairment in abstract thinking, judgment, and other disturbances of higher cortical function or personality changes (American Psychological Association [APA] 1995; McKhann et al. 1984). This definition of dementia is the most widely used in practice (Robillard 2007) and will be used here. As in Chapter 17, this chapter focuses on the provision of dementia care as it transpires primarily within the home (place) in rural and remote settings (space).

Challenges Facing Rural and Remote Family and Friend Caregivers of Persons with Dementia

Over the past two decades, the proportion of older adults who have been receiving care in institutions has been declining. In 2001, less than 10 percent of senior women and 5 percent of senior men resided in health-care institutions (Cranswick and Thomas 2005). Thus, greater numbers of persons with dementia are living in their communities, with up to 90 percent of their in-home care provided by family and friends (Keating et al. 1999). Advanced dementia results in progressive impairment of cognition, function, and behaviour (Herrmann, Gauthier, and Lysy 2007). Persons with dementia eventually become dependent on others for every aspect of their care. Those caring for a family member with dementia are more likely to experience social isolation, chronic health problems, and depression than those caring for cognitively intact elderly persons (CSHA Working Group 1994; O'Rourke, Cappeliez, and Guindon 2003). Specifically, these caregivers are more likely than non-caregivers to experience fair to poor health, with high levels of stress hormones, reduced immune function, slow wound healing, and newly diagnosed hypertension and coronary heart disease (Alzheimer's Association 2008). Additionally, 41 percent of Canadian caregivers report that they use personal savings to survive while caregiving (Pollara Research 2007).

Forbes et al. (2008a) analyzed a subset of the 2003 Canadian Community Health Survey (Statistics Canada 2004) to explore use of and satisfaction with health-care services by Canadians diagnosed with dementia. Men with severe dementia were found to be living in their homes longer and receiving fewer homecare services than women with dementia, implying that caregivers of men (often their wives) are willing to provide care longer with fewer services than those caring for women with dementia. Thus, those caring for men with dementia are particularly vulnerable to negative health outcomes. Furthermore, less than a third of Canadians with dementia received publicly funded homecare services. This finding is a concern given that all participants were diagnosed with dementia, 42 percent were over the age of eighty, the majority reported needing help with activities of daily living, and nearly half had difficulty dealing with an unknown person and with initiating and maintaining conversation. Availability and quality of services are two reasons cited for the low use of publicly funded homecare. Almost half reported the availability of health services in the community as "poor" or "fair," and a quarter rated the quality of services as also "poor" or "fair."

Rural and remote caregivers have additional challenges in caring for their family members with dementia: difficulty accessing available services, and lack of health-care services and providers. Recent studies (Forbes et al. 2008b; Jansen et al. 2009) examined the role of rural and urban homecare in Ontario, Manitoba, and Saskatchewan using an interpretive descriptive design. Focus groups ($n = 12$) and personal interviews ($n = 3$) with formal care providers and rural and urban family caregivers of persons with dementia were conducted. The data specific to rural family and friend caregivers and formal care providers are discussed in this section. Access to available limited health-care services was reported to be complicated by weather, distance, and lack of transportation. Inability to access appropriate health care can result in delayed diagnosis and difficulty in receiving available services and treatments for persons with dementia and respite services for their family caregivers. Caregivers reported a lack of health-care services such as intermediary resources (e.g., publicly funded housing that would meet the needs of those with moderate levels of dementia and those with modest incomes, Meals on Wheels, and respite programs), specialty services (e.g., geriatricians), and long-term-care beds. Anticipatory guidance related to the disease process, available support resources, and knowing how to deal with difficult behaviours were also identified as lacking yet needed (Forbes et al. 2008b). The lack of these services often leads to premature admissions to more expensive acute care facilities or long-term-care settings (Canadian Home Care Association [CHCA] 2006; McCracken et al. 2005; Skinner et al. 2008) that often are not available in one's home community. Entering health-care facilities at a distance from the home community contributes to loneliness and depression in persons with dementia and reduced caregiver interactions due to the time and costs incurred with visiting (McCracken et al. 2005).

This three-province study (Forbes et al. 2008b; Hawranik et al. 2008) also revealed that, contrary to beliefs that rural residents are embedded in strong networks of family and friends, rural caregivers reported that they do not have the energy to socialize and feel isolated from family and friends.

> It's frustrating for the family because everyone pulls away. It's because people don't know what to say. (Hawranik et al. 2008)

> Sometimes even as a caregiver, because you've put in all of this energy, and you're exhausted, and you don't even want to go out. It would be nice if somebody dropped by. (Hawranik et al. 2008)

On the other hand, homecare providers claimed that rural family and friend networks are supporting persons with dementia, and therefore homecare services are not needed:

> Like in some of the smaller rural areas people didn't ask us for formal services so much because the informal caregiving network kicked in. (Hawranik et al. 2008)

A person who is slowly dementing actually lasts longer independently in a rural community than they do in an urban community. If it's a local, little rural community store, you can rely on the fact they'll take care of you even when you can't articulate your needs anymore. (Hawranik et al. 2008)

Statistics Canada (2005) reported similar findings: differences between rural and urban residents are smaller than expected in terms of social engagement and isolation from family, friends, and helping others. Indeed, rural caregivers and older adults with dementia might be in a more vulnerable situation than those in an urban setting. Rural residents with dementia are less likely to have an adult child to help them compared with their urban counterparts (Anderson 2006). Thus, rural persons with dementia rely more heavily on their spouses and friends, who are likely elderly. Their need for formal support and care appears as great as that of their counterparts living in urban settings.

Because of short-term and possibly long-term memory problems of persons with dementia, having a consistent homecare provider was described by family caregivers as an essential component of developing trusting and partnering relationships. Although this was less likely to be an issue in small rural and remote communities since caregivers and their family members with dementia often knew their formal care providers, inconsistency of care providers was often cited as the reason for not accepting or discontinuing homecare services (Forbes et al. 2008b; Hawranik et al. 2008). It was viewed as more of a hindrance than a help. Inconsistent care providers resulted in negative outcomes for the person with dementia (e.g., increased anxiety and agitation and refusal to participate in bathing) and the caregiver (e.g., interference with employment; Forbes et al. 2008b; Hawranik and Strain 2007).

There's gotta be a way that we can have more consistency in the care so that somebody like me might access it. I didn't access it because I didn't want different people coming all the time for Mom, which doesn't help her, that would probably make things worse. (Hawranik et al. 2008)

In small rural and remote communities, people have relationships that often extend back several generations and can be both a facilitator of and a barrier to the development of relationships between formal providers and caregivers (Chappell, Schroeder, and Gibbens 2008;

Sims-Gould and Martin-Matthews 2008). Thus, to enhance the quality of care provided and received, the "fit" among the care provider, care recipient, and family caregiver should be taken into consideration when assigning health-care providers to clients.

Other aspects of care that were important to rural caregivers but often lacking were receiving a comprehensive assessment of their family members that included the caregivers' perspectives, appropriate treatment, and individualized, respectful, and sensitive care from health-care providers knowledgeable in dementia care (Forbes et al. 2008b; Hawranik and Strain 2007; Morgan et al. 2002). Chapter 17 of this book reported that family caregivers caring for a dying relative in a rural setting had similar dissatisfying experiences with many of their physicians. An ethnographic study (Neufeld, Kushner, and Rempel 2007) revealed that caregivers also identified needing a "coach" to facilitate the whole caregiving experience by informing them of resources and supports, helping them to navigate the health-care system, and being their advocate. The lack of these services often leads to premature admissions to more expensive acute care facilities or long-term-care settings (CHCA 2006; Skinner et al. 2008) that often are not available in one's own rural community.

Reasons for the under-utilization of rural health-care services include the belief that service use carries with it an image among community members of accepting welfare (Anderson 2006); the stigma of dementia; a lack of privacy (Chapter 23, this volume); beliefs and attitudes (e.g., acknowledging that a family member has dementia and is unable to manage); a lack of awareness; and inflexibility in and inadequacy of service delivery (care often needed twenty-four hours a day) (Forbes et al. 2008b; Hawranik and Strain 2007; Markle-Reid and Browne 2001; Morgan et al. 2002). Chapter 17 also found that volunteer services related to palliative care in rural settings were under-utilized. Rural caregivers' stoicism (see the previous chapter), self-reliance, feelings of obligation and commitment, and psychological distress also contribute to the under-utilization of health-care services (Forbes et al. 2008b). As one rural caregiver noted, "rural people who have never had the privileged life have always done for themselves and are actually quite reluctant to accept outside help because you always take care of your own" (Hawranik et al. 2008). The previous chapter referred to this as a "families first/services last" approach to meeting health and other basic needs.

Challenges Facing Rural and Remote Health-Care Providers

The proportion of health-care services and providers has been declining in rural areas (Halseth and Ryser 2006; Chapter 25 of this volume). The Canadian Rural Revitalization Foundation's New Rural Economy project (Halseth and Ryser 2006) tracked service availability in nineteen Canadian rural and small towns from 1998 to 2005. Sites included forestry, mining, fishing, farming, manufacturing, and tourism towns. The availability of most health-care professional services in all of the communities reduced over time. The proportion of sites with reduced available nurses (52.6 percent in 1998 to 36.8 percent in 2005) and social workers (42.1 percent in 1998 to 26.3 percent in 2005) over time was particularly dramatic. Areas with available nursing homes also decreased from 26.3 percent in 1998 to 21.1 percent in 2005; however, nearly 80 percent of the sites had access to a nursing home within thirty minutes. A reverse trend was observed with homecare visits; the proportion rose from 47.4 percent in 1998 to 68.4 percent in 2005.

Chapter 25 of this book reports additional challenges with providing services for older adults living in the resource hinterland that has become a retirement community (e.g., Elliot Lake, Ontario). The research reveals that members of these communities experience increasing health and social needs but have fewer family members to provide support and care, volunteer burnout, nurses leaving when their spouses find work elsewhere, and limited sharing of resources and knowledge as residents compete for the same funding and at times have conflicting priorities (e.g., new retirees versus long-time residents).

The Aboriginal Nurses Association of Canada (2000) reported that 60 percent of northern nurses considered their workplaces understaffed. In response, temporary nursing staff are assigned to northern communities. However, frequent nursing turnover affects continuity of care, which results in compromised follow-up, client disengagement, illness exacerbation, and increased burden on family and community members (Minore et al. 2005). Specifically, for persons with dementia and their family caregivers, the shortage of supportive and specialized health-care services often means having to be placed on a wait list for diagnostic services and supportive community care and having no available day centre, respite, and palliative services (Jansen et al. 2009). These shortages can lead to negative consequences for both the persons with dementia and their family caregivers (Forbes et al. 2008b) and result in premature admissions to hospitals or long-term-care facilities for longer periods of time, thus placing a strain on these services (CHCA 2006) and increasing the costs of health care for this population (Hux et al. 1998; Ostbye and Crosse 1994).

Additional challenges include making available appropriate training and continuing educational opportunities related to dementia care assessments, treatments, and resources for rural and remote formal care providers. In the Forbes et al. (2008b) study, 65 percent of all formal care participants reported that they were not completely confident that their training had adequately prepared them to care for persons with dementia (Jansen et al. 2009). A recent study that examined dementia care in northern Saskatchewan Aboriginal communities revealed that only a small number of the nurses reported that they were providing care to, or knew of, older adults with dementia (Andrews 2008). Dementia care was not a component of their work; more urgent issues that "walked through the door" of the nursing station took priority. Although this finding can be related to the smaller number of persons with dementia in northern communities, other issues that could have contributed to this response were limited, senior-specific services and resources (including dementia care); hiring practices of northern nurses based on acute care knowledge and skill; and nurses' limited ability to communicate in the native languages of older adults and their cultural differences. These challenges support the need for Aboriginal health-care workers and para-professionals who speak the language, have a sense of belonging and commitment to the community, and can assess older adults in their homes and in their social interactions within the community.

Rural and Remote Health Service Delivery Models

Since the early 1970s, urban-based health service delivery models on efficiency and market parameters have been increasingly extended into rural service areas (Williams 1996). However, the application of such urban- and market-based models is often unsuited to the needs and realities of rural settings (Halseth and Ryser 2006; Leipert et al. 2007; Williams 1996). The consequences have been closure of health-care facilities or discontinuation of services that can have significant effects on community social and economic sustainability (Halseth and Ryser 2006). The models of rural health service delivery need to be different from those in urban settings, recognizing that there will always be a limited number and range of resources (MacLeod 1999).

Successful rural and remote service delivery models are based on the following assumptions regarding interdisciplinary teams: they are grounded in a "health" model rather than a "medical" model; they are rooted in the principle of social justice; and they are committed to solutions based on the needs of the community and its residents (Jensen and Royeen 2002). Health human resource planning should be based on needs for care rather than traditional methods of capacity-based approaches (i.e., based on current or targeted provider-population ratios; Tomblin Murphy, Birch, and MacKenzie 2007). Minore and Boone (2002) correctly argue for health-care teams in the North that include both professionals and para-professionals. Combining the knowledge, skills, and judgment of health professionals (most of whom are non-Aboriginal) with Aboriginal para-professionals' cultural and community awareness will ensure the delivery of culturally appropriate health services in these communities. Addressing the needs of persons with dementia would be facilitated by these mixed teams since nurses in the North have little contact with each other and limited opportunities to address their needs (Andrews 2008). Including community Aboriginal para-professionals who know the residents, speak the language, and understand the culture of the elders could result in earlier identification of the behavioural problems associated with dementia and initiation of assessment and treatment options. However, these mixed teams are not without their challenges (e.g., lack of clarity about their own and others' roles, lack of appreciation of their respective "equal but different knowledge," and lack of confidence in one another's competence (Minore and Boone 2002). Addressing these interdisciplinary issues within health science education programs will enhance the functioning of these teams in rural and remote settings.

Another essential assumption in delivering health-care services is that rural and remote communities are diverse. Social, economic, and cultural history and traditions all influence the need for and availability of supports and care for persons with dementia. For example, although the health status of Aboriginal seniors at any given age tends to be lower than that of other seniors (McCracken et al. 2005), there is some suggestion that Aboriginal persons are less likely to be afflicted with dementia than their Caucasian counterparts (Forbes, Morgan, and Janzen 2006; Hendrie et al. 1993). Chapter 18 of this volume reported that dementia appears to be virtually non-existent among the Inuit. However, other factors, such as the cultural perception of dementia (e.g., no Cree word for dementia) and the limited diagnostic assessments in the Aboriginal population (Andrews 2008), can contribute to the finding of lower incidence of dementia among Aboriginal people.

A self-managed care model in which caregivers are provided with funding to purchase and manage services needed by their family members with dementia was recommended by caregivers and health-care providers (Forbes et al. 2008b; Jansen et al. 2009). This model can be especially useful in rural and remote areas, where the family caregiver would best know the residents of the community and be able to hire the most appropriate person to assist in meeting the needs of the person with dementia. The homecare case manager, who might not reside in the community, would likely not have this knowledge (Leipert et al. 2007).

Best Practice Rural and Remote Dementia Care

Unique rural features of successful best practice approaches include the notion that economic development infrastructure precedes service delivery; new and innovative programs developed to serve clear, unmet needs; staffing, planning, and program delivery coordinated and integrated at the local level with support (not direct involvement) from upper levels of government; services based on principles of equity, choice, and quality that might require inducements and financial incentives not necessary in urban areas; and community and regional models of service delivery built from the bottom up (Anderson 2006; Bushy 2002). Residents, nurses, and other health-care providers are acutely aware of the needs of community members and therefore should be involved in advocating for and formulating health policies and planning for service delivery (Raphael 2000).

Information technology (IT) is a key tool for reducing the impacts of distance and dispersion in rural and remote communities (CHCA 2008b) and in meeting the needs of persons with dementia and their caregivers. Telemonitoring devices allow health-care providers in a central office to view clients in their homes in order to monitor vital signs, medication use (Anderson 2006), disruptive behaviours, and responsive approaches. IT such as two-way video-conferencing can be used to assess, monitor, consult, and support rural persons with dementia, their family caregivers, and health-care providers (CHCA 2008b;

Morgan et al. 2005). Telephone support groups among isolated persons caring for family members (Stewart et al. 2006) are another example of supportive use of IT.

Such technology can also assist in addressing the number one challenge in rural and remote settings: insufficient supportive and specialized health-care providers. Training of health-care professionals, paraprofessionals, and family and friend caregivers, providing services, decreasing isolation, and building health-care teams can all be accomplished through technology (CHCA 2008b). However, Kulig et al. (2002) caution that the use of technology can increase the liability of practitioners and the risk of security and confidentiality breaches.

Additional strategies to address insufficiently supportive and specialized health-care providers include leveraging partnerships to optimize local resources; building required capacity among local residents through training programs; and utilizing case management as a strategy for systems integration to maximize community resources, access resources outside the community, and share resources across communities and regions (CHCA 2006, 2008a). When recruiting for skilled health-care providers, maximizing the "fit" between the professional (the extrinsic motivation of a career or job opportunity) and the personal (an intrinsic comfort) aspects of living in a rural or remote area (MacLeod 1999), and examining the "fit" between the professional's personality, needs, and expectations and those of the rural community (Bushy 2002), can enhance retention rates. Community members rather than only a recruitment agency should be involved in the recruitment process.

The challenges of delivery of continuing education in rural and remote areas can only partially be met through IT. Nurse practitioners in rural and remote areas identified multiple delivery modes such as networking as also being important (Tilleczek, Pong, and Suzanne 2005). Encouraging learners to integrate proactively their practice networks into a support system for learning, identifying and establishing mentors in the practice setting (Gibb, Anderson, and Forsyth 2004), and connecting with other health-care professions with expertise in the content area were all strategies for building learning networks (Tilleczek, Pong, and Suzanne 2005). Additional approaches to providing education and consultation include a mobile memory clinic van that could visit rural communities on a rotating basis to offer assessment, treatment, monitoring, and consultation services to persons with dementia and their caregivers (Hawranik et al. 2006).

458

The Internet can also be an important resource for rural and remote health-care providers and family caregivers of persons with dementia who specifically reported a lack of information on the disease process, support resources, and how to deal with difficult behaviours (Forbes et al. 2008b). For example, the Saskatchewan Alzheimer Society offers information on its website on the availability of support groups in rural areas for caregivers and persons with early memory loss (http://www.alzheimer.sk.ca); the Alzheimer Society of Toronto offers the First Link program, which connects persons with dementia and their caregivers to a community of learning, services, and supports early in their Alzheimer journey (http://www.alzheimertoronto.org); the *Dementia Guide* helps caregivers to create, track, and communicate symptom profiles (http://www.DementiaGuide.com); and the Saskatchewan Alzheimer Society (http://www.alzheimer.sk.ca) and the Kenneth G. Murray Alzheimer Research and Education Program (http://www.marep.uwaterloo.ca) offer virtual resource libraries. However, individuals in rural and remote areas often do not have access to the Internet. Training and educational programs can assist users to take full advantage of available technology (CHCA 2006).

Other best practice approaches that support persons with dementia and their caregivers to remain in their homes and communities for as long as possible are flexible services (e.g., adequate number of hours and types of respite provided within the home and at other sites) and consistent, respectful, and culturally sensitive supportive care (e.g., personal care, housework, meal assistance; Forbes et al. 2008b). Building retirement homes within rural communities that have graduated levels of support services, ranging from independent living to full nursing care, will also allow persons with dementia to remain in their home communities (McCracken et al. 2005). With the looming dementia crisis, the time is now to implement these models and approaches in rural and remote settings.

References

Aboriginal Nurses Association of Canada. 2000. *Survey of Nurses in Isolated First Nations Communities: Recruitment and Retention Issues*. Ottawa: Aboriginal Nurses Association of Canada.
Alzheimer's Association. 2008. "2008 Alzheimer's Disease Facts and Figures." *Alzheimer's and Dementia* 4, 2: 110-33.
American Psychological Association (APA). 1995. *Diagnostic and Statistical Manual of Mental Disorders*. 4th ed. (DSM-IV). Washington, DC: APA.

Anderson, A. 2006. *Delivering Rural Health and Social Services: An Environmental Scan.* Toronto: Alzheimer Society of Ontario, http://alzheimerontario.org/.

Andrews, M.E. 2008. "Dementia Care in Remote Northern Communities: Perceptions of Registered Nurses." PhD diss., University of Saskatchewan.

Bushy, A. 2002. "International Perspectives on Rural Nursing: Australia, Canada, USA." *Australian Journal of Rural Health* 10: 104-11.

Canadian Home Care Association (CHCA). 2006. *The Delivery of Home Care Services in Rural and Remote Communities of Canada: Identifying Gaps and Examining Innovative Practice.* Ottawa: CHCA.

–. 2008a. *Integration of Care: Exploring the Potential of the Alignment of Home Care with Other Health Care Sectors: Final Report.* Ottawa: CHCA.

–. 2008b. *Integration through Information Communication Technology for Home Care in Canada: Final Report.* Ottawa: CHCA.

Canadian Study of Health and Aging (CSHA) Working Group. 1994. "Patterns of Caring for People with Dementia in Canada." *Canadian Journal on Aging* 13, 4: 470-87.

–. 2000. "The Incidence of Dementia in Canada." *Neurology* 55: 66-73.

Chappell, N.L., B. Schroeder, and M. Gibbens. 2008. "Respite for Rural and Remote Caregivers." In *Rural Ageing: A Good Place to Grow Old?,* edited by N. Keating, 1-10. Bristol: Policy Press.

Cranswick, K., and D. Thomas. 2005. "Elder Care and the Complexities of Social Networks." In *Canadian Social Trends,* Statistics Canada Catalogue No. 11-008, 10-16. Ottawa: Statistics Canada.

du Plessis, V., R. Beshiri, R. Bollman, and H. Clemenson. 2002. *Definitions of "Rural."* Statistics Canada Catalogue No. 21-601-MIE. Ottawa: Statistics Canada, http://www.statcan.ca/.

Foot, D.K., and D. Stoffman. 2004. *Boom, Bust, and Echo: Profiting from the Demographic Shift in the 21st Century.* Toronto: Footwork Consulting.

Forbes, D., L. Jansen, M. Markle-Reid, P. Hawranik, D. Morgan, S. Henderson, B. Leipert, S. Peacock, and D. Kingston. 2008a. "Canadians with Dementia: Gender Differences in Use and Availability of Home- and Community-Based Health Services." *Canadian Journal of Nursing Research* 40, 1: 38-59.

Forbes, D., M. Markle-Reid, P. Hawranik, S. Peacock, D. Kingston, D. Morgan, S. Henderson, B. Leipert, and L. Jansen. 2008b. "Availability and Acceptability of Canadian Home- and Community-Based Services: Perspectives of Family Caregivers of Persons with Dementia." *Home Health Care Services Quarterly* 27, 2: 75-99.

Forbes, D.A., D. Morgan, and B. Janzen. 2006. "Rural and Urban Canadians with Dementia: Use of Health Care Services." *Canadian Journal on Aging* 25, 3: 321-30.

Gibb, H., J. Anderson, and K. Forsyth. 2004. "Developing Support for Remote Nursing Education through Workplace Culture that Values Learning." *Australian Journal of Rural Health* 12: 201-5.

Halseth, G., and L. Ryser. 2006. "Trends in Service Delivery: Examples from Rural and Small Town Canada, 1998-2005." *Journal of Rural and Community Development* 1: 69-90.

Hawranik, P., D. Forbes, D. Morgan, B. Leipert, M. Markle-Reid, S. Henderson, D. Kingston, S. Peacock, L. Jansen, and S. Normand. 2008. "The Perspectives of Rural Formal and Informal Caregivers on Community Dementia Services." Paper presented at the Thirty-Seventh Annual Scientific and Educational Meeting of the Canadian Association on Gerontology, London, ON, 23-26 October.

Hawranik, P., C. Lengyel, R. Grymonpre, and P. St. John. 2006. "Barriers to the Delivery of In-Home Services to Older Adults in Rural Manitoba." Paper presented at the Thirty-Fifth Annual Scientific and Educational Meeting of the Canadian Association on Gerontology, Quebec City, October.

Hawranik, P.G., and L.A. Strain. 2007. "Giving Voice to Informal Caregivers of Older Adults." *Canadian Journal of Nursing Research* 39, 1: 156-72.

Hendrie, H.C., K.S. Hall, N. Pillay, D. Rodgers, C. Prince, J. Norton, et al. 1993. "Alzheimer's Disease Is Rare in Cree." *International Psychogeriatrics* 5: 5-14.

Herrmann, N., S. Gauthier, and P.G. Lysy. 2007. "Clinical Practice Guidelines for Severe Alzheimer's Disease." *Alzheimer's and Dementia* 3: 385-97.

Hux, M.J., B.J. O'Brien, M. Iskedjian, R. Goerce, M. Gagnon, and S. Gauthier. 1998. "Relation between Severity of Alzheimer's Disease and Costs of Caring." *Canadian Medical Association Journal* 159: 457-65.

Jansen, L., D. Forbes, M. Markle-Reid, P. Hawranik, D. Kingston, S. Peacock, D. Morgan, S. Henderson, and B. Leipert. 2009. "Formal Service Providers' Perceptions of In-Home Care: Informing Dementia Service Quality." *Home Health Care Services Quarterly* 28, 1: 1-23.

Jensen, G.M., and C.B. Royeen. 2002. "Improved Rural Access to Care: Dimensions of Best Practice." *Journal of Interprofessional Care* 16, 2: 117-28.

Keating, N., J. Fast, J. Frederick, K. Cranswick, and C. Perrier. 1999. *Eldercare in Canada: Context, Content, and Consequences.* Ottawa: Statistics Canada.

Kulig, J.C., E. Thomlinson, F. Curran, M. MacLeod, N. Stewart, and R. Pitblado. 2002. *Recognizing and Addressing the Challenges: The Impact of Policy on Rural and Remote Nursing Practice. Documentary Analysis Interim Report: Policy Analysis for the Nature of Nursing in Rural and Remote Nursing Practice in Canada.* Lethbridge: University of Lethbridge.

Leipert, B., M. Kloseck, C. McWilliams, D. Forbes, A. Kothari, and A. Oudshoorn. 2007. "Fitting a Round Peg into a Square Hole: Exploring Issues, Challenges, and Strategies for Solutions in Rural Home Care Settings." *Online Journal of Rural Nursing and Health Care* 7, 2: 5-20, http://www.rno.org/.

MacLeod, M. 1999. "'We're It': Issues and Realities in Rural Nursing Practice." In *Health in Rural Settings: Contexts for Action,* edited by W. Ramp et al., 165-78. Lethbridge: University of Lethbridge.

Markle-Reid, M., and G. Browne. 2001. "Explaining the Use and Non-Use of Community-Based Long-Term Care Services by Caregivers of Persons with Dementia." *Journal of Evaluation in Clinical Practice* 7, 3: 271-87.

McCracken, M., K. Tsetso, B. Jean, K. Young, D. Huxter, G. Halseth, and M. Green. 2005. *Seniors in Rural and Remote Canada: Position Paper.* Ottawa: Canadian Rural Partnership Advisory Committee on Rural Issues, http://www.rural.gc.ca/.

McKhann, G., D. Drachman, M. Folstein, R. Katzman, D. Price, and E.M. Stadlan. 1984. "Clinical Diagnosis of Alzheimer's Disease: Report of the NINCDS-ADRDA Work Group under the Auspices of Department of Health and Human Services Task Force on Alzheimer's Disease." *Neurology* 34: 939-44.

Minore, B., and M. Boone. 2002. "Realizing Potential: Improving Interdisciplinary Professional/Paraprofessional Health Care Teams in Canada's Northern Aboriginal Communities through Education." *Journal of Interprofessional Care* 16, 2: 139-47.

Minore, B., M. Boone, M. Katt, P. Kinch, S. Birch, and C. Mushquash. 2005. "The Effects of Nursing Turnover on Continuity of Care in Isolated First Nation Communities." *Canadian Journal of Nursing Research* 37, 1: 86-100.

Morgan, D., K. Semchuk, N. Stewart, and C. D'Arcy. 2002. "Rural Families Caring for a Relative with Dementia: Barriers to Use of Formal Services." *Social Science and Medicine* 55, 7: 51-64.

Morgan, D.G., N. Stewart, M. Crossley, C. D'Arcy, J. Biem, A. Kirk, and D. Forbes. 2005. "Dementia Care in Rural and Remote Areas: The First Year of a CIHR New Emerging Team." *Canadian Journal of Nursing Research* 37, 1: 177-82.

Neufeld, A., K.E. Kushner, and G. Rempel. 2007. "Men Negotiating the Maze of Care for a Relative with Dementia." Paper presented at the thirty-sixth Annual Scientific and Educational Conference of the Canadian Association on Gerontology, Calgary, 1-3 November.

O'Rourke, N., P. Cappeliez, and S. Guindon. 2003. "Depressive Symptoms and Physical Health of Caregivers of Persons with Cognitive Impairment: Analysis of Reciprocal Effects over Time." *Journal of Aging and Health* 15, 4: 688-712.

Ostbye, T., and E. Crosse. 1994. "Net Economic Costs of Dementia in Canada." *Canadian Medical Association Journal* 151: 1457-64.

Pollara Research. 2007. *Health Care in Canada Survey: A National Survey of Health Care Providers, Managers, and the Public.* Ottawa: Canadian Healthcare Association, http://www.cha.ca/.

Raphael, D. 2000. "Health Equalities in Canada: Current Discourses and Implications for Public Health Action." *Critical Public Health* 10: 193-216.

Robillard, A. 2007. "Clinical Diagnosis of Dementia." *Alzheimer's and Dementia* 3: 292-98.

Sims-Gould, J., and A. Martin-Matthews. 2008. "Distance, Privacy, and Independence: Rural Home Care." In *Rural Ageing: A Good Place to Grow Old?,* edited by N. Keating, 43-51. Bristol: Policy Press.

Skinner, M.W., R.W. Rosenberg, S. Lovell, J.R. Dunn, J.C. Everitt, N. Hanlon, and T.A. Rathwell. 2008. "Services for Seniors in Small-Town Canada: The Paradox of Community." *Canadian Journal of Nursing Research* 40, 1: 80-101.

Statistics Canada. 2004. *CCHS Cycle 2.1 (2002-2003): Public Use Microdata File Documentation.* Ottawa: Statistics Canada.

Stewart, M., A. Barnfather, A. Neufeld, S. Warren, N. Letourneau, and L. Liu. 2006. "Accessible Support for Family Caregivers of Seniors with Chronic Conditions: From Isolation to Inclusion." *Canadian Journal on Aging* 25, 2: 179-92.

Tilleczek, K., R. Pong, and C. Suzanne. 2005. "Innovations and Issues in the Delivery of Continuing Education to Nurse Practitioners in Rural and Northern Communities." *Canadian Journal of Nursing Research* 37, 1: 146-62.

Tomblin Murphy, G., S. Birch, and A. MacKenzie. 2007. *Needs-Based Health Human Resources Planning: The Challenge of Linking Needs to Provider Requirements.* Ottawa: Canadian Nurses Association and Canadian Medical Association.

Williams, A. 1996. "The Development of Ontario's Home Care Program: A Critical Geographical Analysis." *Social Science and Medicine* 42, 6: 937-48.

Chapter 25   **Health- and Social-Care Issues in Aging Resource Communities**

M. Skinner, N. Hanlon, and G. Halseth

Key Points

- "Resource frontier aging" is a new phenomenon with immediate implications for rural service provision, community support, and older people's abilities to age in place.
- Current service provision challenges in rural communities include the changing service environment, accessibility of services, limited financial resources, recruitment and retention of staff and volunteers, and maintenance of networks and partnerships to mobilize community support.
- Public policy and program decisions must take into account the irrevocable link between service deprivation and resource economy restructuring.
- Relying on the social nature of community will not be enough to sustain older people in aging rural resource communities in the long term.

Meeting the health- and social-care needs of older people is a challenge for rural and remote communities across Canada (Skinner et al. 2008). Along with the long-standing problems of servicing smaller and dispersed populations, with low-order facilities and family caregiver shortages, rural communities face disproportionately the growing demands of the aging population in an era of economic transition and welfare system reform (Hanlon and Halseth 2005). This situation is described poignantly in the literature as a double jeopardy of caring for increasingly vulnerable rural people in increasingly vulnerable rural places (Joseph and Cloutier-Fisher 2005), and it resonates with concern for the capacity of rural and remote communities to cope (see Chapters 11, 17, 22, and 24, this volume). How this burdensome scenario plays out among different types of rural places, however, is only beginning to become clear (e.g., Halseth and Williams 1999).

Extending the concern for aging in rural contexts (Section 7), this chapter contributes to the links among rural and remote aging, service provision, and community support by examining health and social care in Canada's resource hinterland, a unique context in which the socio-economic dynamics of single-industry dependence and transition present a significant departure from general experiences of aging rural communities (Hanlon and Halseth 2005). Drawing on the empirical cases of two communities in northern parts of British Columbia and Ontario, we consider implications for the provision of services, over both shorter and longer terms, in Canada's aging resource communities. Our purpose is to describe the major issues and challenges facing these communities as they respond to health- and social-care needs under conditions of resource frontier aging. That is, we want to understand how older people are faring in communities not originally equipped to provide services for seniors. This is not only a crucial rural service question but also an important policy question about how to meet health- and social-care needs in communities that have never before dealt with population aging.

Service Provision Issues in Rural and Remote Communities

Dotted among Canada's rural and northern landscapes are small towns and communities where people's lives and livelihoods, for better or worse, are linked to resource development (Lucas 1971). Although consistent with the "Rural and Small Town" definition outlined in Chapter 1, the resource hinterland, as these spaces and places are generally known, represents a unique setting in which the combined impacts of boom-and-bust economies, rural service deprivation, and population decline make the provision of health and social care problematic (Bryant and Joseph 2001). Service provisioning in resource-based communities occurs within a context of employment instability and geographical isolation as well as gaps in the social support networks normally associated with rural people and places (Hanlon et al. 2007).

Of particular concern in this chapter are the distinct types of rural and remote communities known as "instant towns" that have populated Canada's resource frontier since the early 1950s (Bollman 1992). Unlike resource boom towns of the late nineteenth century and early twentieth century that typically developed in an ad hoc manner around a new mill or mine, post-World War II resource towns across Canada's provincial norths were purposefully created under guidance from provincial governments. Drawing on comprehensive planning principles, the provinces were interested in managing the costs of both the towns and the supporting public infrastructure (Halseth and Sullivan 2002). The goal was to have fully functioning towns and local governments in place on the day that the mill or mine opened. These post-World War II resource towns are collectively called "instant towns" in reference to British Columbia's Instant Towns Act. The defining features of instant towns are that they were planned purposefully not only to house the labour forces of new resource industries in sectors such as mining but also to create attractive and diverse resource-based communities and that they often comprise small settlements isolated from major urban centres (Halseth and Sullivan 2004). Because of their very economic nature, these types of rural communities face instability and inevitable transition (Halseth 1999), and many are caught in the downward spiral of economic restructuring because of industry closures and population decline due to out-migration of unemployed, working-age families (Randall and Ironside 1996). Alongside these changes are the longer-term impacts of the aging population, which are most pronounced in rural and remote communities (Bryant and Joseph 2001) but take on a unique pattern in the resource hinterland where the historical growth through in-migration of young families has been replaced by population decline and aging in place of older residents (Halseth and Sullivan 2002; Mawhiney and Pitblado 1999). Unlike the previous experiences of aging in other parts of rural Canada (e.g., see the contributions to Keating 2008 as well as Chapter 23), however, many instant towns are struggling to meet the growing demands for care specifically because they were not originally designed to provide services for older people (Pong, Salmoni, and Heard 1999). The relatively new phenomenon of "resource frontier aging" (Hanlon and Halseth 2005, 7) thus raises critical questions about the capacities and abilities of resource-based communities to respond to health- and social-care needs.

As demonstrated in various parts of this book, most rural and remote communities across Canada have problems providing services, whether they are public services such as health care and education, private consumer services, or volunteer-based community services (Hanlon and Halseth 2005). Similar to their urban and metropolitan counterparts, rural and remote service providers face increasing demands for care, funding constraints, and an ever-changing system of government mandates and divested responsibilities (Skinner and Rosenberg 2006). What makes the rural and remote situation distinct are the physical, technical, and economic barriers to servicing a small, isolated clientele, the critical lack of qualified health-care and allied professionals, and the often over-estimated capacity for volunteers to meet the needs of the community (Skinner 2008). Further distinguishing the instant town context are the changes associated with resource-based community development (Halseth and Ryser 2006a), whereby rural providers are caught between meeting the immediate demands of older people aging in place, the longer-term decline in local capacity both public and private, and the more recent out-migration of younger families, reducing the already strained pool of potential volunteer caregivers (Joseph and Cloutier-Fisher 2005). For many rural people and places, especially those in the resource hinterland, the challenge thus has become how to sustain both their services and their communities.

From a rural health perspective, the problem of providing services for older people in the resource hinterland is as much about the social dimensions of community as it is about the formal availability of services (Hanlon et al. 2007). Indeed, recent studies, including the palliative and end-of-life care research described in Chapters 12, 17, and 18, have highlighted that a mix of formal and informal supports and services is key to building service-rich communities as well as the importance of understanding rural aging in relation to the social determinants of health (e.g., Skinner et al. 2008). Although the latter has become a guiding framework for the study of health and social care in Canada and elsewhere (see the contributions to Raphael 2004), social determinants research remains urban in focus, and the potential contributions toward understanding aging and health in rural Canada, let alone the resource hinterland, have been all but ignored. With these gaps and issues in mind, we now consider the local dynamics of service provision for older people living in Canada's resource frontier.

Researching the Service Challenges of Resource Frontier Aging

To understand the issues, challenges, and responses associated with providing health and social care for older people in the resource hinterland, we consider the empirical case of service provision in two of Canada's aging instant towns: Elliot Lake (population 11,500), a former uranium-mining town in northeastern Ontario, and Tumbler Ridge (population 2,500), a former coal-mining town in northeastern British Columbia. The communities are excellent examples of the long-standing tradition of resource-based instant towns in Canada and their significant decline over the past two decades (Halseth and Sullivan 2002; Mawhiney and Pitblado 1999). Although established three decades apart, they have a similar history of industry- and government-funded planned development, growth through in-migration of young families, and subsequent economic and demographic transition in the years following closure of their mining industries in the 1990s and 2000s, respectively. Indeed, there is an irrevocable link between community and resource development in these two locales (Halseth and Sullivan 2004; Robinson and Wilkinson 1995), highlighted by the fact that mines in both towns were at one time owned and operated by the same company (Denison Mines Corporation). The post-mining transition of Elliot Lake and Tumbler Ridge away from single-industry dependence, however, is well under way. It is within the more recent context of change that we seek to understand the challenges facing the communities as they respond to the health- and social-care needs of their older residents.

The research reported here is part of ongoing work on the social determinants of rural health in rural and northern parts of British Columbia and Ontario. Specifically, we draw on findings from Elliot Lake and Tumbler Ridge in the form of case studies of services for seniors undertaken in the early and mid-2000s. The case studies were completed separately but followed a similar mixed-methods research approach that complemented secondary data on demographic change and service availability in the communities with primary data collected through semi-structured interviews, focus groups, and surveys with a range of key informants, including community leaders, service providers, volunteers, and older residents. Table 25.1 summarizes the research methodologies, further details of which are published elsewhere (Halseth and Ryser 2006b; Reschny et al. 2007; Ryser, Halseth, and

Hanlon 2008; Waldbrook, Herron, and Skinner 2007, 2008). In essence, the case studies are successive, with the experiences from the initial research in British Columbia informing the design of the research in Ontario for comparative purposes (Waldbrook, Herron, and Skinner 2008). In the sections that follow, the results of thematic analyses of interview, focus group, and survey data from Elliot Lake and Tumbler Ridge are integrated with secondary data, and local examples and verbatim quotations are used to highlight specific perspectives and circumstances. Indeed, the similar socio-economic trajectories in northern parts of these provinces, combined with the prevailing neoliberal policy environments within which the provincial health- and social-care systems are evolving, make BC-Ontario comparisons of considerable analytical interest (Chouinard and Crooks 2008). To understand the challenges facing instant towns and their consequent responses as they come to terms with the double jeopardy of rural aging and service deprivation, we start with the backdrop of industrial restructuring and socio-economic change in northern British Columbia and northern Ontario.

Community Trajectories of Aging and Renewal

Elliot Lake is located 160 kilometres west of Sudbury (population 155,000) in northern Ontario's Algoma District (Statistics Canada 2007a). It has evolved from its origins as a boom-and-bust mining town to its present form as an affordable retirement community. The town site was established in 1955 in conjunction with twelve uranium mines designed to supply North America's growing nuclear industry. Similar to other instant towns, it was a planned community from the start, with infrastructure and housing built for 25,000 people who were estimated to live and work there eventually (Bucksar 1965). Such growth proved elusive as Elliot Lake's population experienced dramatic changes because of the fluctuating uranium market, at times growing to almost 20,000 with the higher levels of production in the 1980s, then declining almost by half with the final closure of mines in the mid-1990s (Mawhiney and Pitblado 1999). Instead of becoming a typical ghost town with the exodus of its unemployed working-age population, the community transformed itself into a retirement destination; however, the population has been slowly declining ever since (e.g., a decline of 3.4 percent from 2001 to 2006). The combined trends of

Table 25.1   Summary of research methodologies

	Elliot Lake, ON	Tumbler Ridge, BC
Site profile	Population 11,500 (est. 1955)	Population 2,500 (est. 1986)
Study design	Case study of services for seniors	Case studies of services for seniors
Research team	Trent University	University of Northern British Columbia
Timeline	2007	2007-8
Primary data	Semi-structured key-informant interviews	Focus groups and household key-informant interviews
Secondary data	Statistics Canada, local government, service organizations, and community group documents	Statistics Canada, local government, service organizations, and community group documents
Participants	29 community leaders, service providers, and volunteers	52 older residents (10 focus groups) 524 household representatives
Research themes	Local context; formal and informal services; community resources; issues and challenges	Local context; formal and informal services; community resources; issues and challenges
Analytical approach	Thematic analysis based on social determinants of rural health	Thematic analysis based on social determinants of rural health

out-migration of youth and in-migration of older people have led to rapid population aging, with the median age now almost fifty-five years and the proportion of seniors in the community reaching almost one-third, leading some commentators to label Elliot Lake a harbinger of Canada's aging rural population (Whyte 2007). In response to a changing economic and demographic reality, the community rallied around its retirement industry and actively developed services for older people, including expansion of the local hospital, establishment of new long-term-care beds, and creation of recreational activities aimed at the senior population. Despite these initiatives, the significant challenge of supporting the new demographic reality with limited resources remains.

Tumbler Ridge was founded in 1986 under the provincial government's Instant Town legislation (Halseth and Sullivan 2002), in association with British Columbia's last resource development "megaproject." Tumbler Ridge is located on the eastern foothills of the Rocky Mountains in northeastern British Columbia, approximately 400 kilometres from Prince George (population 72,000) (Statistics Canada 2007b).

Figure 25.1   Increasing proportion of population over sixty-five years old, 1996-2006

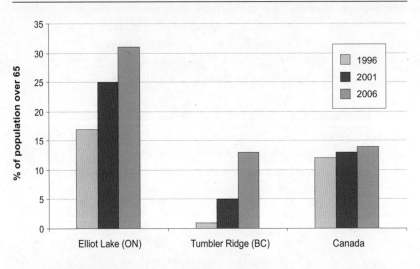

Source: Statistics Canada (1997a, 1997b, 2002a, 2002b, 2007a, 2007b).

Planning for Tumbler Ridge and the area's coal mine developments began in 1975. The local economy was originally developed around two open-pit coal mines, Quintette and Bullmoose, whose markets were Japanese steel mills. The provincial government managed the planning and development of the community, and extensive efforts were put into the design, layout, and servicing of the town site as a stable mining town to attract and retain a skilled labour force. Global commodity prices and corporate restructuring have affected Tumbler Ridge almost since its opening, culminating in the closure of both mines within a few years of each other in the early 2000s. Originally designed to accommodate up to 10,000 residents, Tumbler Ridge's population peaked in the early 1990s at just over 4,500 people but declined to 1,851 residents in 2001 (Statistics Canada 2002b). Much like Elliot Lake, however, former residents and newcomers were in the process of moving into the community as part of a successful housing sales campaign targeted at retirees, and the 2006 census reported just under 2,500 residents (Statistics Canada 2007b). Consequently, the composition of the Tumbler Ridge population has changed further (see Figure 25.1), with an aging population of seniors, in-migration of workers for two recently opened small coal mines, and continued out-migration of younger residents. Similar to the situation in Elliot Lake, the combination of population decline and aging has generated important implications for planning and community development, including the provision of recreational, educational, health, and seniors' services.

Limited Capacities to Support Older People Aging in Place

It is against the backdrop of economic renewal imperatives and population aging demands that the local capacities to support older people in Elliot Lake and Tumbler Ridge have evolved. As shown in Table 25.2, both communities have a range of government agencies, private businesses, and community organizations across the various types of health- and social-care sectors. As demonstrated in Chapters 17 and 24, among others, the presence of support services is crucial in sustaining elderly residents in their homes and communities. Although some of the services were established during the growth periods of the towns, others were created more recently in response to the particular needs of the aging communities.

In Elliot Lake, for instance, some service providers and organizations have been providing services in the community since it was established more than forty years ago (e.g., St. Joseph's General Hospital), whereas the services offered by other providers and organizations such as the Elliot Lake Palliative Care Program are relatively new. Almost one-quarter of the agencies, organizations, and groups have been delivering services for more than fifteen years, and one-fifth have been providing services in the community for at least five years. These historical patterns coincide with some of the major growth periods in the development of the community as a mining town in the 1950s and 1960s, whereas the more recent growth in services relates to when Elliot Lake was promoted as a retirement community in the mid-1990s, such as services for seniors and those with mental health needs.

Much newer and smaller in population, Tumbler Ridge has a more limited range of services, programs, and personnel to support an aging population. Most health services are located in the Tumbler Ridge Health Centre, including family physician practices, public health nurses, homecare, speech therapy, and physiotherapy. Although services were originally planned for a much younger population, in recent years there has been an effort to develop services and supports for older residents, such as the 49 Forever Club, a hospice, a palliative care society,

Table 25.2   Inventory of health- and social-care services for older people

Service type	Sector	Elliot Lake, ON	Tumbler Ridge, BC
Advocacy	municipality, non-profit organization	✓	✓
Community health centre	private business, public sector	✓	✓
Community support	community, non-profit organization, municipality	✓	✓
Counselling	public sector	✓	✓
Education, literacy	community, non-profit organization	✓	✓
Ethno-cultural groups	community	✓	
Health care	private business, public sector	✓	✓
Health promotion	non-profit organization		✓
Homecare	non-profit organization	✓	
Hospice, palliative care	non-profit organization, public sector	✓	✓
Hospital	public sector	✓	
Housing	non-profit organization	✓	
Long-term care	non-profit organization, private business	✓	
Medical equipment	non-profit organization, private business	✓	✓
Mental health	public sector	✓	✓
Nutrition	non-profit organization, private business	✓	✓
Pharmacy	private business	✓	✓
Personal health	non-profit organization, private business	✓	✓
Public health	public sector	✓	✓
Recreation	community, municipality	✓	✓
Retirement services	non-profit organization	✓	
Social clubs	community	✓	✓
Social support	non-profit organization	✓	✓
Therapies	private business	✓	✓
Women, family health	community, non-profit organization, public sector	✓	✓

grievance counselling, and advocacy by and support from the Tumbler Ridge Cares organization. Several gaps and challenges remain, however, particularly in regard to the availability of specialized health care. The community is not seen to have sufficient population to support an acute care hospital or long-term-care facility. Other gaps include the availability of housing suited to the needs of older residents and various support services to allow aging residents to remain in their homes, and in the community, for as long as possible.

Challenges for Service Providers

Various factors affect the ability to deliver services in rural and remote Canada, including changing government policies, access to financial and human resources, and relationships within the community itself (see Chapters 11 and 22). Based on our integrated thematic analysis of the perspectives from Elliot Lake and Tumbler Ridge, there are five major challenges facing the provision of services in the resource hinterland: (1) the changing service environment; (2) accessibility of services; (3) limited financial resources; (4) recruitment and retention of staff; and (5) networks and partnerships to mobilize community support. For the purposes of this chapter, we provide only a general overview of what these challenges mean for service provision in the 2000s. Accounts of similar rural and remote service provision challenges are provided in Chapters 7 (training), 10 (technology), and 26 (gender), for instance.

Changing Service Environment

Our two study communities experienced major changes in their service environments over the past decade related to local economic upheavals and their resulting demographic impacts. Mine closures in both locations led to depopulation and accelerated aging in place. An influx of retirees in search of cheap housing, on the other hand, has offset population losses somewhat and helped to attract new programs, service providers, and organizations in both locales. Yet population aging added stresses to already overstretched health and social services, and concerns about future impacts on services were foremost in the minds of many informants. As a provider in Elliot Lake stated, "we see a client population with more needs, but fewer family members are there to provide the service they need, especially in Elliot Lake, where people move to retire. They are healthy when they first get there, but they have no family members to take care of them when their health declines." In response to this changing environment, a number of informants spoke of the need for broad changes in the mindsets of community service providers in the health- and social-care sectors and in wider spheres such as retail, public works, and land use planning.

Access to Services

Various factors were cited as challenges to accessing health- and social-care services for those living in Elliot Lake and Tumbler Ridge, where long-distance travel is often necessary to access most specialist services. Ongoing issues of staff retention mean that seniors in resource communities cope with periodic gaps in primary-level health services. For example, during our study of Tumbler Ridge, residents were without a local dentist, chiropractor, and physiotherapist. In addition, recreational and cultural programs and other non-medical services were cited as reasons for travel, signalling the pervasive challenge of isolation and distance in remote areas. In response to service inaccessibility, regional health organizations have made specific efforts to be available to their rural and remote clients; however, outreach initiatives such as satellite offices are constrained by the lack of human and financial resources in the health- and social-care sector.

Financial Resources

Financial resources have a significant impact on the ability to deliver services. Because of government reforms in recent years, the amount of public funding and resources available to health- and social-care providers in provinces such as British Columbia and Ontario have been negatively affected. Within this context, alternative sources of funding have been necessary, although options are often limited, with community organizations competing for the same funding opportunities. As an informant explained, "there are not really enough resources to meet the demand of local groups and organizations. Many groups in the area are competing for the same amount of funding. For example, the ATV club wants money put into trails, while others want money put into the pool." Overwhelmingly, however, informants in both communities thought that the biggest funding gaps were in the areas of long-term and continuing care. Indeed, in an era of rationalization and centralized control of health- and social-care funding, the informants were very concerned about their longer-term ability to provide services for their aging populations.

Staff Recruitment and Retention

The ability to find and retain qualified paid and volunteer staff in rural and remote towns often poses considerable challenges to service delivery. In both of our study sites, chronic shortages of physicians, registered nurses, and allied health-care professionals have resulted from difficulties in both recruitment and retention of staff. This problem is due to the combination of the northern and remote locations of the communities and their aging and retired populations. In addition, informants raised concerns about volunteer burnout and a recruiting crunch as the available pool of volunteers ages along with the rest of the population. As an informant from Elliot Lake commented, "the nature of our services can cause volunteer burnout, and the age[s] of our volunteers have an impact on the services available." An underlying issue for health and social service providers is the degree to which health human resources are affected by resource economy restructuring in the local and regional economies. Recent studies of nursing recruitment and retention highlight the importance of family status and remote practice (Betkus Henderson and MacLeod 2004). That is, most nurses in rural and remote settings are married females who were "recruited" because their spouses or partners moved to the area to work in the resource sector. In times of resource industry restructuring and downsizing, many nurses leave if their spouses find work elsewhere. The intersection of these labour force and household dynamics poses important challenges for places such as Elliot Lake and Tumbler Ridge, which view a stable health and social services workforce as an important tool both to diversify their economic bases and to attract new residents.

Networks and Partnerships

Networks and partnerships are often fundamental in providing services in rural and remote communities, where resources and funding are limited. Some informants saw shared resources and knowledge as a challenge because of competing and at times conflicting priorities of community partners. For example, informants in Elliot Lake highlighted the challenge of meeting the conflicting demands of "new retirees" in search of active retirement living versus "long-time residents" with established connections to the community. In both study sites, however, there is ample evidence that local groups can mobilize in the face of episodic crises, such as mine closures, major market down-turns, or announced cuts to social programs. As one informant succinctly put it, "in the North, if you don't collectively do things, things don't get done." Whether existing networks, and the knowledge acquired from these major events, can develop and adapt to the more gradual and long-term impacts of population aging is yet to be determined. The lessons from both study sites are clear; partnerships have proven essential to community development efforts in these two challenging environments.

Discussion: Lessons from the Aging Resource Frontier

The research described above showcases the service provision challenges related to population aging in the unique context of Canada's resource hinterland. Since our focus was on elucidating service provision challenges, however, the findings reflect only one side of the story, and we acknowledge that a full appreciation of resource frontier aging would require further analysis of the perspectives of the various service users (including non-seniors); informal caregivers such as friends and family members (including adult children who live outside the community where their parents retired to); and women, who play a central role as service providers, caregivers, and elderly residents in rural, remote, and resource-based communities. These limitations notwithstanding, the descriptive findings from northern British Columbia and northern Ontario provide lessons on important service questions for rural and remote Canada and on important policy questions about how to meet health- and social-care needs in places not originally equipped for aging residents.

First, the case studies revealed a convergence of issues, challenges, and local outcomes in the resource hinterland despite the historical and geographical differences between the evolution of services in places as far apart as Elliot Lake and Tumbler Ridge. In both cases, the community response to rapid economic decline was centred on revitalization through the retirement industry and the development of senior-friendly amenities, and in both cases the demands for services exceed existing service capacities. In Elliot Lake, for instance, the voluntary sector led the conversion to a senior-oriented housing market (Elliot Lake Retirement Living, a non-profit organization), while volunteer-based services are struggling to keep up with the growing demands for care in the community. We cannot assume that other resource-based communities

will have the opportunity or capacity to follow these examples of renewal; the ensuing challenges of meeting the needs of elderly residents
as they age in place are clear and should not be underestimated by governments at all levels.

Second, the case studies also revealed a convergence of service provision issues and challenges in the resource hinterland and other parts
of rural and remote Canada, where, as outlined in Chapter 1, aging is
already a pervasive and long-standing trend. Similar to the informants
in previous chapters, those from Elliot Lake and Tumbler Ridge highlighted issues such as lack of government funding, staff recruitment and
retention, and distance and isolation as key barriers to service provision,
all part of the historical continuity of rural service challenges across the
country (Bryant and Joseph 2001; Halseth and Ryser 2006a). Besides
being unprepared for the aging population, what sets the resource hinterland cases apart from other types of rural and remote communities,
however, is the link between service capacity and resource economy
restructuring. As noted in Tumbler Ridge, the major downsizing in the
mining sector led to the exodus of health providers who moved with
their families after their spouses were laid off and left the community to
seek work elsewhere. The interdependence of labour force and household dynamics is therefore a crucial factor for places such as Elliot Lake
and Tumbler Ridge that are seeking to diversify their economic bases,
especially given the importance of health and social care in attracting
new (older) residents.

Third, the case studies revealed the critical importance of "community" for ensuring sustainable services and for maintaining the independence of seniors as they age in place. The significance of social networks
for healthy aging is well recognized, especially in the context of rural
and remote Canada, where other services and supports are lacking
(Skinner 2008; see also Chapter 23, this volume). Yet it is paradoxical
that, as resource-based communities transition into retirement destina-
tions for seniors, the major sources of social support (families) are dwin-
dling or located in faraway urban centres. In places such as Elliot Lake
and Tumbler Ridge, the solution seems to lie in creating opportunities
to foster networks of support in the larger community, such as through
the establishment of seniors' associations and centres. It remains to be
seen, however, whether the social nature of community will be enough
to support the aging population in resource-turned-retirement communities, especially given the demands associated with the demographic
transition from the newly retired to the frail elderly. For instance, how

will these communities cope with the end-of-life and dementia-related challenges outlined in Chapters 17, 18, and 24?

And fourth, along with highlighting the crucial link between sustainable services and communities, the case studies revealed several other sources of concern about future health- and social-care issues in the aging resource frontier. They include the increasing demands placed on provincial and municipal infrastructure (hospitals, highways, etc.), the potential escalation of conflicting interests among newly retired and long-time residents, and the inevitable challenges of caring for growing numbers of frail elderly within an already limited service environment. In both Elliot Lake and Tumbler Ridge, steps have been taken to anticipate and resolve these issues, such as the palliative care and hospice care initiatives, but each community will need considerable support to meet the demands of the double jeopardy of rural aging in the years to come.

Concluding Comments

It is in the unique context of Canada's resource hinterland where the phenomenon of resource frontier aging emerges and where older people are aging in rural and remote places not originally designed to support them. Although the socio-economic dynamics of the transition away from single-industry instant towns and toward retirement-oriented communities diverge from the general experiences of aging in rural communities outlined elsewhere in this book, there are several lines of convergence with regard to service provision, including the long-standing barriers associated with rural and remote services and the important role that community plays in creating supportive environments for aging in place. The very nature of resource dependency, however, makes communities such as those in northern British Columbia and northern Ontario that we examined especially vulnerable. Indeed, we see the irrevocable link among economic restructuring, local service capacity, and aging as the most important policy issue with regard to sustaining health and social care in resource hinterland communities. It is here that future research on resource frontier aging should prove useful, including in-depth comparative analyses of the sustainability of other instant towns and retirement communities as it relates to local response strategies to support seniors. In terms of addressing the broader rural and remote health research agenda (Kulig 2005), we finish by reinforcing the need to increase understanding of how the burdensome scenario of caring for increasingly vulnerable rural people in increasingly vulnerable rural places plays out across rural and remote Canada and elsewhere.

Acknowledgments

The research reported here was funded by the Social Sciences and Humanities Research Council of Canada (Standard Research Grant No. 410-2007-0597) (Skinner) and the New Emerging Team for Health in Rural and Northern BC, funded by the Canadian Institutes of Health Research (Halseth and Hanlon). Local support for the studies in Tumbler Ridge also came from the Peace River Regional District and the Tumbler Ridge Mayor's Task Force on Seniors' Needs. We are grateful for the participation of the anonymous informants from Elliot Lake and Tumbler Ridge. The views expressed are entirely our own.

References

Betkus Henderson, M., and M. MacLeod. 2004. "Retaining Public Health Nurses in Rural British Columbia: The Influence of Job and Community Satisfaction." *Canadian Journal of Public Health* 95: 54-58.

Bollman, R.D., ed. 1992. *Rural and Small Town Canada*. Toronto: Thompson.

Bryant, C., and A.E. Joseph. 2001. "Canada's Rural Population: Trends in Space and Implications in Place." *Canadian Geographer* 45: 132-37.

Bucksar, R.G. 1965. "Elliot Lake." *Habitat* 8: 175-81. [Reprinted in *Little Communities and Big Industries: Studies in the Social Impact of Canadian Resource Extraction,* edited by R.T. Bowles, 175-81. Toronto: Butterworth Publishing, 1982.]

Chouinard, V., and V.A. Crooks. 2008. "Negotiating Neoliberal Environments in British Columbia and Ontario, Canada: Restructuring of State-Voluntary Sector Relations and Disability Organizations' Struggles to Survive." *Environment and Planning C: Government and Policy* 26: 173-90.

Halseth, G. 1999. "'We Came for the Work': Situating Employment Migration in B.C.'s Small, Resource-Based, Communities." *Canadian Geographer* 43: 363-81.

Halseth, G., and L. Ryser. 2006a. "Trends in Service Delivery: Examples from Rural and Small Town Canada, 1998-2005." *Journal of Rural and Community Development* 1: 69-90.

–. 2006b. *Service Provision in Rural and Small Town Places: A Report for Tumbler Ridge, British Columbia*. Montreal: Initiative on the New Economy, Canadian Rural Revitalization Foundation, Concordia University, http://www.unbc.ca/cdi/.

Halseth, G., and L. Sullivan. 2002. *Building Community in an Instant Town: A Social Geography of Mackenzie and Tumbler Ridge, British Columbia*. Prince George: UNBC Press.

–. 2004. "From Kitimat to Tumbler Ridge: A Crucial Lesson Not Learned in Resource-Town Planning." *Western Geography* 13-14: 132-60.

Halseth, G., and A. Williams. 1999. "Guthrie House: A Rural Community Organizes for Wellness." *Health and Place* 5: 27-44.

Hanlon, N., and G. Halseth. 2005. "The Greying of Resource Communities in Northern British Columbia: Implications for Health Care Delivery in Already-Underserviced Communities." *Canadian Geographer* 49: 1-24.

Hanlon, N., G. Halseth, R. Clasby, and V. Pow. 2007. "The Place Embeddedness of Social Care: Restructuring Work and Welfare in Mackenzie, BC." *Health and Place* 13: 466-81.

Joseph, A.E., and D. Cloutier-Fisher. 2005. "Aging in Rural Communities: Vulnerable People in Vulnerable Places." In *Aging and Place: Perspectives, Policy, and Practice,* edited by G.J. Andrews and D.R. Phillips, 133-55. New York: Routledge.

Keating, N., ed. 2008. *Rural Ageing: A Good Place to Grow Old?* Bristol: Policy Press.

Kulig, J.C. 2005. "Rural Health Research: Are We beyond the Crossroads?" *Canadian Journal of Nursing Research* 37: 7-13.

Lucas, R.A. 1971. *Minetown, Milltown, Railtown: Life in Canadian Communities of Single Industry.* Toronto: University of Toronto Press.

Mawhiney, A-M., and J. Pitblado, eds. 1999. *Boom Town Blues: Elliot Lake Collapse and Revival in a Single-Industry Community.* Toronto: Dundurn Press.

Pong, R.W., A. Salmoni, and S. Heard. 1999. "Aging in a Hurry: Changing Population Profile in Elliot Lake." In *Boom Town Blues: Elliot Lake Collapse and Revival in a Single-Industry Town,* edited by A-M. Mawhiney and J. Pitblado, 204-18. Toronto: Dundurn Press.

Randall, J.E., and R.G. Ironside. 1996. "Communities on the Edge: An Economic Geography of Resource-Dependent Communities in Canada." *Canadian Geographer* 40: 17-35.

Raphael, D., ed. 2004. *Social Determinants of Health: Canadian Perspectives.* Toronto: Canadian Scholars' Press.

Reschny, J., C. Hoffman, D. Manson, G. Halseth, and N. Hanlon. 2007. *Peace River Regional District Seniors' Needs Project: Methodology Report.* Prince George: Community Development Institute, University of Northern British Columbia.

Robinson, D., and D. Wilkinson. 1995. "Sense of Community in a Remote Mining Town: Validating a Neighborhood Cohesion Scale." *American Journal of Community Psychology* 23: 137-48.

Ryser, L., G. Halseth, and N. Hanlon. 2008. *Tumbler Ridge Mayor's Task Force on Seniors' Needs: Final Report on Focus Groups.* Prince George: Community Development Institute, University of Northern British Columbia, http://www.unbc.ca/cdi/.

Skinner, M.W. 2008. "Voluntarism and Long-Term Care in the Countryside: The Paradox of a Threadbare Sector." *Canadian Geographer* 52: 188-203.

Skinner, M.W., and M.W. Rosenberg. 2006. "Managing Competition in the Countryside: Non-Profit and For-Profit Perceptions of Long-Term Care in Rural Ontario." *Social Science and Medicine* 63: 2864-76.

Skinner, M.W., M.W. Rosenberg, S.A. Lovell, J.R. Dunn, J.C. Everitt, N. Hanlon, and T.A. Rathwell. 2008. "Services for Seniors in Small Town Canada: The Paradox of Community." *Canadian Journal of Nursing Research* 40: 80-101.

Statistics Canada. 1997a. Elliot Lake, ON. *1996 Community Profiles.* 1996 Census. Ottawa: Statistics Canada, http://www.statcan.ca/.

–. 1997b. Tumbler Ridge, BC. *1996 Community Profiles.* 1996 Census. Ottawa: Statistics Canada, http://www.statcan.ca/.

–. 2002a. Elliot Lake, ON. *2001 Community Profiles.* 2001 Census. Ottawa: Statistics Canada, http://www.statcan.ca/.

–. 2002b. Tumbler Ridge, BC. *2001 Community Profiles.* 2001 Census. Ottawa: Statistics Canada, http://www.statcan.ca/.

–. 2007a. Elliot Lake, ON. *2006 Community Profiles.* 2006 Census. Ottawa: Statistics Canada, http://www.statcan.ca/.

–. 2007b. Tumbler Ridge, BC. *2006 Community Profiles.* 2006 Census. Ottawa: Statistics Canada, http://www.statcan.ca/.

Waldbrook, N., R. Herron, and M. Skinner. 2007. *Services for Seniors in Ontario's Ageing Rural Communities: Pilot Study of Elliot Lake, Preliminary Results.* Peterborough: Department of Geography, Trent University. Available from markskinner@ trentu.ca.

–. 2008. "Pilot Study of Services for Seniors in Ontario's Ageing Rural Communities." In *Proceedings from the CIHR New Emerging Team for Health in Rural and Northern BC (NETHRN-BC) 12 December Conference,* edited by R. Raygada Watanabe, G. Halseth, and N. Hanlon, 19-29. Prince George: University of Northern British Columbia.

Whyte, P. 2007. "Elliot Lake: A Glimpse into the Future of Our Aging Nation." *Globe and Mail,* 30 July, L4.

Chapter 26   **Rural Women's Health Promotion Needs and Resources: A Photovoice Perspective**

B. Leipert, T. Landry, C. McWilliam,
M.L. Kelley, D. Forbes, P. Wakewich,
and J. George

Key Points

- The rural context, age, personal history, abilities and interests, community resources, economics, and other factors interact to affect rural older women's health promotion needs and resources.
- The experiences, history, and memories of living in rural and small towns are very important to rural older women. Changing rural demographics, limited infrastructure, and other rural changes shape rural older women's health and their experiences of living rurally.
- Photovoice can act as both a research method and an empowerment intervention with diverse groups of rural women. Photovoice facilitates interest in research, recruitment, data collection and dissemination, consciousness raising, social support, speaking up, and speaking out.
- Photographic depictions of rural life can become a means of both registering and shaping rural reality. (Casey 2009, 157)

Older women are one of the fastest growing segments of the female population (Ministry of Industry 2006) and comprise a substantial number of seniors in rural Canada (Statistics Canada 1999). Yet knowledge about older rural women's social and health promotion needs and resources is very limited. Enhanced knowledge of social and health promotion needs and resources for older rural residents has been identified as an urgent national need (Ministerial Advisory Council on Rural

Health 2002). In this chapter, we present findings from a study that used the photovoice method to explore aging and social and health promotion needs and resources of older rural women in Ontario. For this study, older is defined as sixty-five years of age or older, and the definition of rural is adopted from that presented in Chapter 1.

Health and Rural Contexts

"Community and regional models for serving rural older people should be built from the bottom up" (Anderson 2006, 7). Thus, to be effective, health-care delivery requires significant input from rural residents, including seniors. Yet little is known about the health-related needs of rural older people, particularly older rural women. What is known about their health needs and the contexts of their lives reveals that this population is growing (Ministry of Industry 2006), often marginalized (Chapter 23, this volume), and in need of enhanced health care that involves them as partners in their care (Chapter 17, this volume; Leipert 2006a). In Ontario, rural elderly who are isolated, living at home, with relatives, or in need of homecare present particular challenges for under-resourced rural public health and home health care (Anderson 2006).

In some rural communities in Canada, seniors comprise up to 40 percent of the population (Statistics Canada 2001). In southwest Ontario, there is a slightly greater proportion of residents aged sixty-five and older than in the province as a whole (Sarkella 2005). The number of older women in Canada far exceeds the number of older men, primarily as a result of women's longer life spans (Pringle 2008). Older residents often prefer to age in place in rural settings (Hodge 2008), and urban seniors might seek retirement in more tranquil and manageable rural environments (Keating 2008). Thus, rural communities consist and will continue to consist of large populations of older women. These older rural women, who often live alone, are likely to experience isolation, depression, and stress (Thorndyke 2006) as they attempt to manage challenging geographical, socio-cultural, and climatic rural contexts and care for themselves and others (see Chapters 17 and 22).

The health of older rural women is affected by geographical, health-care delivery, and socio-cultural environments (Anderson 2006; Coward, et al. 2006; Hodge 2008; Keating 2008). Distance, weather, and transportation limitations exacerbate mobility issues that can already be problematic for frail older residents and limit their ability to be active and socially connected (Anderson 2006; Chapter 23, this volume). As a result, rural seniors can have more difficulty maintaining appropriate weight, physical ability, and independence (Parrett 2006); they can also experience greater isolation and mental health issues such as depression and anxiety (Thorndyke 2006). Other concerns include inappropriate care (Leipert 2006b; Leipert and George 2008) or limited care to address issues of prevention, health promotion, rehabilitation, and treatment important to rural women (Forbes and Janzen 2004; Sutherns, McPhedran, and Haworth-Brockman 2004). As a result, rural women might not be able to access care, or they might postpone or forgo it (Leipert 2006b). They might experience a greater number of, and more severe, health issues; live with health-care issues longer; and have less ability to recover from health issues following treatment (Leipert 2006b) compared with their urban counterparts.

Socio-culturally, although there is diversity in rural women's experiences, in many rural settings the roles of women are often more constrained (Leipert and George 2008; Thorndyke 2006). Rural women are often expected to engage in caregiving and other gendered roles with little recognition, remuneration, or support (Forbes and Janzen 2004; Leipert and Smith 2008). Rural older women often live in poverty and are one of the most economically deprived populations in Canada (Ministry of Industry 2006). In addition, the rural legacy and expectation of being resilient, independent, and hardy (Chapter 19, this volume; Leipert 2006b; Wirtz, Lee, and Running 1998) can cloud rural women's ability to detect and address mental and physical health issues.

These are serious health issues for rural settings, now and for the future. By 2025, Canada will be one of the top ten countries with the highest proportion of seniors (World Health Agency 2002). By 2021, one in four seniors will live in a rural setting (Health Canada 2002); since women live longer than men, there are more older women than men living in rural settings, and this will become more pronounced in the future (Hodge 2008).

Social Exclusion, Social Support, the Rural Context, and Aging

Rural older residents in southwest Ontario can experience four key aspects of social exclusion (Sarkella 2005; Scharf and Bartlam 2008). In terms of *exclusion from material resources,* women and the elderly in southwest Ontario are at risk of living in low-income and poverty situations, which limit their ability to access resources (Sarkella 2005). In terms of *exclusion from social relations,* southwest Ontario has a higher proportion of seniors living alone than does the province as a whole, with one in three seniors living alone (Sarkella 2005). Furthermore, Ontario has the highest number of farms in Canada (Karpan and Karpan 2002), and the majority of them are in southwest Ontario. Because male farmers tend to die before female partners, more women than men are left alone to age in rural communities (Hodge 2008; Keating 2008). *Exclusion from services* is experienced because about 30 percent of rural older people in Canada live in settings with no physician and pharmacy (Dobbs et al. 2004), and the provision of rural homecare and public health nursing services is difficult and often non-existent (Leipert et al. 2007; McCracken et al. 2005). Lack of transportation, limited ability to drive, isolation due to distance, and challenging weather all compound the difficulties in reaching local and distant services. *Exclusion from community* for older rural women can occur due to de-population and out-migration of younger rural residents who can support the development of community and rural women's involvement in it (see Chapter 23). In addition, undervalued or invisible contributions of older women as well as their limited voice and power in rural communities serve to exclude them from the community (Leipert and Smith 2008).

Nonetheless, the social support that rural people provide often serves to offset social exclusion and greatly assists in dealing with rural aging issues (see Chapters 17, 22, and 23). Rural social support can help older women to access resources, relationships, services, and community events (Clark and Leipert 2007). Indeed, in spite of the challenges of living rurally, rural women often prefer it to urban living (Leipert and George 2008; Sutherns, McPhedran, and Haworth-Brockman 2004), and they might not see rurality as a threat to their health (Thurston and Meadows 2003).

Research Questions

This study sought to address two research questions. What do older rural women experience as needs and resources related to the promotion of their health? What are the socio-cultural, economic, geographical, and community environments in which rural older women's health promotion is located?

Study Design

This study builds on a regional photovoice pilot study conducted in two communities in southwest Ontario (Leipert and Smith 2008) by extending the scope of the research to include more southwestern and northern Ontario communities. The chapter presents findings from the portion of the study conducted in southwest Ontario.

The Photovoice Method

Photovoice is a unique research method developed initially for research with rural women (Wang, Burris, and Ping 1996). In photovoice, cameras are provided to participants, and they "create and discuss photographs as a means of catalyzing personal and community change" (Wang et al. 1998, 75). Participants thus have greater control over the research and can photograph, reflect on, depict, and dialogue about strengths and problems in their rural communities (Wang 1999), thereby providing powerful visual representations of community issues that can be used to influence practitioners and policy makers as well as local residents themselves. Photovoice also provides research opportunities to participants with low literacy and limited English abilities, which can exist for older rural women with limited formal education and for immigrant rural women.

In addition to cameras, the photovoice method includes the use of log books and focus groups. Log books provide opportunities for sharing details about experiences and perspectives of a sensitive nature that participants might not wish to reveal in focus group situations. Log books are particularly useful in rural research where participants are known to each other since they facilitate the provision of information in a confidential manner. Focus groups provide opportunities for collective sharing of, reflection on, and comparison of experiences, perspectives, issues, solutions, and empowerment (Leipert and Smith 2008; Morgan and Krueger 1998). Thus, photovoice, in its use of photographs, log books, and focus groups, provides diverse opportunities for in-depth and extensive data provision and reflection.

Theoretical Perspective

This study is guided by a feminist theoretical perspective that informs understanding of rural older women's social and health promotion needs and resources in terms of power, control, and inclusion as they relate to personal and collective health and the individual, socio-cultural, economic, and contextual factors that influence healthy aging (Leipert and Smith 2008; Ward-Griffin and Ploeg 1997). Principles that underlie feminist research include valuing women's experiences from their perspectives, representing diverse women's experiences, pro-moting reflexivity by investigators and participants during data collec-tion and analysis and sharing reflections through dialogue, and fostering change at individual and societal levels (Olesen 2000).

Data Collection and Analysis

The study was conducted in four southwest Ontario counties: Chatham-Kent, Elgin, Lambton, and Norfolk. Farmland covers 75 percent of the area, a higher proportion than in any other region of Ontario as well as most regions of the country (Turner and Gutmanis 2005). The farms of southwest Ontario produce major shares of many of Canada's agricul-tural products, including cereal crops, dairy products, vegetables, and fruit (Caldwell et al. 2006).

Recruitment

Following approval from the University of Western Ontario Research Ethics Board, older rural women were recruited using purposeful snowball sampling (Patton 2002) whereby information about the study was provided to groups, such as the Federated Women's Institutes of Ontario and seniors' groups, and to women living in rural commun-ities. Two research assistants from rural communities, including a First Nations reserve and a Mennonite community, facilitated recruitment. Women were included in the study if they were sixty-five years of age or older (though on-reserve women were included if they were fifty-five years of age or older as there were few women sixty-five years of age or older); had expressed interest in participating; and were willing and able to use a camera, following demonstration.

Data Collection

After receiving written consent, data were collected from five groups of older rural women in their communities. Each group consisted of four to eight women who participated in two focus group sessions. In the first one-hour audio-recorded orientation session, participants introduced themselves, the researchers explained the purpose and nature of the research, and participants were provided with disposable cameras and demonstrations and instructions on their use. The inclusion of personal introductions, an extension of the method learned as a result of experiences gleaned from a pilot study (Leipert and Smith 2008), ensured that important personal and contextual information was provided.

Participants were asked to take pictures in their neighbourhoods, towns, or farms that depicted health promotion needs and resources pertinent to older rural women. Participants were also asked to provide a letter of information and to obtain written consent from individuals whose pictures they wished to take. A log book was provided to each participant to record information about pictures that she had taken or wanted to take and for any other perspectives and experiences regarding rural health promotion needs and resources. Due to their concerns about English-language literacy, the Mennonite women asked that the log books be omitted in data collection from them. A woman from the local Mennonite community support centre provided interpretation services, although the participants required little translation from English to Low German and vice versa. The week after the orientation session, each participant was telephoned to determine and encourage progress. Two weeks after the orientation session, the cameras and log books were retrieved, and print photographs (one copy for the participant and one copy for the researchers) and digital versions on CD were obtained.

Participants were then invited to a second focus group session, approximately two hours in length and audio-recorded. At this session, each participant was asked to select from her photographs two pictures, one that best represented a health promotion need and one that best represented a health promotion resource. These pictures formed the basis of the subsequent group discussion.

The groups were moderated by B. Leipert using a semi-structured interview guide to elicit perceptions of the pictures, their meaning, and their significance. Examples of questions asked included "why did you select the photo you did?," "what message about health promotion needs or resources do you want your picture to convey?," and "what title would you give your picture?" The last question helped to elicit the meaning and significance that participants attributed to their pictures. At the end of the second focus group, participants completed a brief written questionnaire to provide socio-demographic information.

Data Analysis

Three processes were used to analyze the qualitative data (see Table 26.1). The *first* process (Wang and Burris 1997) was captured in the audio-recordings of the group interviews that were transcribed verbatim; the transcriptions were checked for accuracy by reviewing them with corresponding log books and tapes. In the *second* process, NVIVO (QSR International 2006), a qualitative data computer program, assisted with labelling and retrieving codes and themes. Concurrent with the above analyses, a *third* four-stage analysis process (Oliffe et al. 2008) was used to enhance interpretation of the photos. Descriptive statistics were used to summarize information provided in the written questionnaires.

Rigour and trustworthiness of the study were attended to in several ways: focus group interviews were recorded and transcribed verbatim; transcribed data were edited to present recorded data accurately; participants' pictures, perspectives, and language formed the bases of the analysis; transcribed information was analyzed by a minimum of two investigators to facilitate interpretive consistency; and an audit trail was created by keeping raw data and analytical memos for a minimum of seven years.

Findings

The study sample consisted of thirty-one women who ranged from fifty-five to eighty-nine years of age. Five women claimed First Nations heritage, and four women were Mennonite; the remaining participants did not claim an ethnic background. The majority of women were widowed ($n = 18$), lived on farms ($n = 4$) or in small towns of 250-7,500 people ($n = 18$), and had annual incomes of less than $40,000 ($n = 19$). Fifteen women had less than grade 9 education, nine had graduated from high school, and ten had completed some postsecondary education.

Participants took a total of 593 pictures, 18 of which were excluded from the study due to lack of clarity of meaning or picture depiction, and 14 of which could not be included for public presentation due to

Table 26.1 Data analysis

Method	Process
1. *Wang and Burris (1997)*	
Identifying key data	Participants select photos for discussion.
Contextualizing data	Participants explain meanings of photos, which promotes discussion.
Codifying data	Participants identify issues, concepts, themes, and theories arising from discussion.
2. *Leipert and Smith (2008)*	
Identifying codes	Line-by-line analysis of transcripts is undertaken by a minimum of two researchers; analysis of picture titles also assists in determining meaning and codes.
Identifying emerging themes	Codes are compared across transcripts.
Understanding complexities, commonalities, and differences	Themes are compared across transcripts, cultures, and geographical locations represented in the study.
3. *Oliffe et al. (2008)*	
Stage 1: Preview	Photos and perspectives are initially viewed in context to understand participants' interpretations.
Stage 2: Review	Photos are viewed again to broaden and enhance understanding of participants' perspectives and to account for contradictions or explanations.
Stage 3: Cross-photo comparison	All of the participants' photos are viewed together and sorted into categories and themes based on participants' comments, log book entries, and picture titles.
Stage 4: Theorizing	More abstract understanding is developed by linking themes and categories to theory.

lack of consent, although they were included in the analysis. Thus, 575 pictures were analyzed. The majority of the pictures reflected health promotion resources rather than health promotion needs or problems.

Health Promotion Resources

By far the largest number of pictures was of garden and other natural environments. This might reflect the time of year of the study (July and August). The titles of pictures and words of participants also reflected the importance of home gardens, lawns, local parks, lakes, birds, flowers, trees, and plant nurseries. Some of the titles included "Peace/ Happiness," "My Sanctuary," and "A Fine Crop of Seagulls." Gardens provided opportunities for physical activity and contributed to mental health, appreciation of nature and beauty, and pride of place and effort. Participants commented, "gardening beautifies your home, gives you exercise, and is relaxing," and "my little garden creates a feeling of peace and enjoyment which of course makes me happy and healthy." For Mennonite women, home represented their primary domain, the place where they spent the most time and felt the most comfortable, and the place where they socialized.

Churches emerged as important for faith, mental and spiritual health, socializing, and beauty as depicted in pictures of stained-glass windows and captivating architecture. For Mennonite women, pictures of the prominent locations of Bibles in their homes together with the titles of these pictures, "The Roadmap to Heaven" and "We Shall Be Joyful Even in Sorrow," indicated the importance of these items to their spiritual and mental health.

Women stayed active by walking and caring for their pets, which also provided company for those who lived alone or were isolated. Indeed, pets were "My Buddy," "My Pick-Me-Upper," and "The Loves of My Life." A Mennonite participant whose husband had recently been admitted to a long-term-care facility commented, "my bird gives me much happiness ... When I come home, I am welcomed by him ... If I had two birds, they would be mates, but [I have] only one bird, [so he is like my] mate." Participants' pictures illustrated other activities, such as biking, golfing, lawn bowling, swimming in summer, and exercise classes in winter. In addition, pictures of motorized scooters revealed their importance in facilitating mobility in town (but not farm) environments.

Other pastimes and hobbies included basket weaving, macramé, flower arranging, watching TV, playing cards, cooking and baking, quilting, knitting, doing puzzles, reading, collecting, biking and motorbiking, flying airplanes (in younger years), square dancing, travelling, researching and enjoying cultural heritage, and enjoying others enjoying themselves (e.g., a husband and son who collect vintage cars). A Mennonite participant described the depth and breadth of meaning of her hobby of quilting: "I [have made] several hundred quilts ... They help me care for my family, help them remember me; quilting is something to do, and it is fun." Titles for these pictures included "Sports for Seniors" and "Family Tradition." These activities and pastimes fostered social relationships, physical health, self-esteem, and a sense of personal and collective history. As a result, these activities were very important to participants, who often spoke with emotion when discussing them.

Community resources and infrastructures that participants valued included safe walking trails, parks, restaurants, homemaking assistance, local mail service, schools, shops, hairdressing services, banking facilities, community centres, and swimming pools. One participant commented, "the [outdoor] swimming pool is only open two months a year, would be nice to have it year round." These resources were valued for their accessibility and thus their ability to foster independence and social inclusion, contribute to the sustainability of the rural community, and support seniors' health needs.

Some resources were particularly appreciated. Pictures of telephones, radios, televisions, computers, and cars revealed the importance of these resources as "My Best Companion" for "Freedom" and to help participants address issues such as "Lack of Access to Health Care Resources, Need to Travel," and "Fear of Isolation." As one participant noted,

> *Having transportation here is a ... vital necessity ... I have seen many women in the community lose their ability to drive or to purchase or maintain a vehicle. This has created a hardship for many women. Living in the country, we need a vehicle to shop, go to appointments, attend recreational activities, visit friends, and on and on.*

Other participants commented, "in the future, if I couldn't drive ... I would have to leave my home and find something closer to where everything is," and "without wheels we're stuck." As a result, transportation access to resources was critical for physical and mental health.

Participants commented on the importance of past employment on the farm and as nurses, nursing aides, and teachers. One participant described the importance of nursing aide training: "It changed my life ... I worked for twenty-nine years ... It gives me more incentive for living now [when I'm retired]." A retired nursing assistant noted, "I used to work nights all the time ... I loved to come home and jump on the tractor and go out to the fields and think for myself, this is freedom, I can watch the birds ... the trees ... how relaxing to get away from stressful work." This participant so valued her farm life that she continued to farm at the age of eighty-nine years. Titles such as "The Love of John Deeres" and "Accomplishment" reveal the importance of employment to study participants (see Figure 26.1)

Ready access to pharmacies and hospitals, alternative therapies such as reflexology and massage, community health centres, and long-term-care facilities were all deemed essential in helping older women obtain

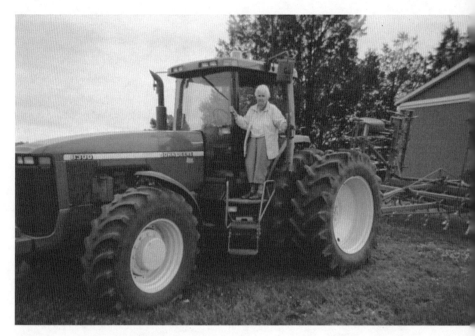

Figure 26.1   The love of John Deeres

the health care that they needed, when they needed it, without needing transportation or having to worry about roads and weather. Picture titles included "Reassurance of Rural Home Care by a Rural Nurse," "Importance of Rural Health Care Providers," and "Loss of Rural Pharmacy: Importance of Delivery." These pictures also catalyzed comments about the importance of quality care and access: "We are an aging society. Medical help and assistance are a necessity. Otherwise, the cemeteries will overcome [us]." Thus, exclusion from local services would have significant effects on the health and peace of mind of rural residents.

Findings unique to this group of rural women related to personal and geographical landmarks. Pictures of abandoned farm buildings and war memorials reminded participants of valued experiences and people. War memorials were often used as central locations for community events and thus facilitated a sense of belonging and inclusion in community as well as collective history and identity. First Nations participants' pictures included those of a house where a participant had lived, entitled "Memories," reminiscent of both good and bad times, and images of the unique local geographical stone formations, called kettles, were also prominent. These pictures represented a connection with culture, the past, and place.

Health Promotion Needs

Pictures and comments often reflected health promotion needs as well as resources. A picture of a former Indian day school represented "Childhood Sadness," as this participant noted:

> You hear a lot about the residential schools, and the Indian day schools were not much better, except we got to go home at night ... I certainly know there's been a lot of physical abuse because I've seen it ... [Our teacher would say] "do you want to be a stupid Indian all your life?" ... All my years working ... I never forgot that. I was always trying to prove to myself that I wasn't a stupid Indian.

Pictures of an army base on reserve property reminded First Nations participants of the appropriation of their land and of disrespect and unresolved cultural and land ownership issues. One participant noted, "I used to live there, and the army took over ... booted us out ... life was changed. [That] hurt the people ... The house they gave my dad – he was promised a new home for his family – it was condemned, an old house with broken windows. They lost a lot." An older First Nations participant was especially eloquent about historical issues and their effects on her and the community in her poem "Broken Promise" (see Box 26.1).

These comments reveal the nature and effects of social exclusion that First Nations people have experienced. This exclusion was largely based on culture, poverty, and power differentials, with the First Nations people being less valued and experiencing extreme poverty and limited power. The effects of these past experiences on First Nations women who are now aging continue to be significant, as these comments reveal.

Health-care issues and effects on community were particularly concerning to First Nations participants whose pictures and comments revealed a "Community Disaster" because of substance abuse and the almost community-wide need for methadone and frequent ambulance services: "Here They [Ambulances] Come Again." Participants remarked on known houses on reserves where drugs were sold and noted the effects of drug use: "There's a lot of partying and noise ... It is very difficult to sleep ... Plus they steal ... and violent things [occur

BOX 26.1   Broken Promise

Little did we know
As we lived in peace
Upon the land we loved
Little did we know
The heartaches and sorrow
Of the future to come
Little did we know
The broken dreams
Our children would share
Little did we know
Our new beginnings
Would be of divisions
Little did we know
The land we loved
Would be taken from beneath our feet

– A First Nations Participant

that] didn't really occur [before]." Pictures of billboards at the entrance to a reserve community warned of problem gambling and advised not to drink and drive; flags at half mast, a frequent occurrence on reserves, depicted deaths often due to substance abuse, accidents, or acts of violence. These pictures and comments reveal the social exclusion that First Nations people often feel among themselves and between themselves and non-First Nations people.

Participants also discussed several limitations regarding rural long-term care. A participant commented extensively and emotionally on the difficulties that she and her husband experienced with his care in a "Nursing Home [Chosen] out of Convenience." They chose this home because it was close to where they lived and thus facilitated daily visits, although care was minimal. A move to a facility that was "Better Than the Other One" resulted in improved physical care, but it had fewer staff, less sensitive care, and was more distant and thus difficult to visit. This experience revealed significant distance and travel issues that contributed to social exclusion (from her husband) and difficulties in remaining connected to a loved one.

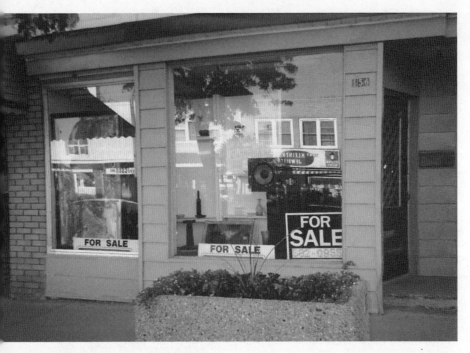

Figure 26.2   Sign of the times

Rural infrastructure problems for participants included sidewalks in poor repair and unsafe park paths, which were "Beautiful but Dangerous" and "Accident[s] Waiting to Happen." Several participants took pictures of and remarked on the lack of indoor pools in the winter. One participant was especially distressed over the "Lack of Resources to Care for Cemeter[ies]," especially in winter, which to her represented "Unforgiven Priorities" and lack of care and respect for grieving families and friends. Pictures of "For Sale" signs of businesses and boarded-up buildings revealed the loss of infrastructure, and thus decreased access to goods and services, that is occurring in many rural towns (see Figure 26.2).

Churches also represented changing rural demographics and consequent effects on health, as revealed by the many photos of churches and extensive, heartfelt comments about their closures: "The church is ... the centre of everything ... The children, they were christened [there] ... the weddings, the funerals ... It belongs to you ... the memory," and "I don't know ... what I'll do when they [churches] close ... It's a tragedy."

Participants also remarked on the "Worries of a Rural Woman" and the "Anxiety of Farming": "You know if you've got a husband ninety-four years old and he is on a tractor ... I am worried all the time ... It's quite stressing," and "with farming ... you worry about them all the time ... I guess that's just something we do, farm women do." Several women took pictures of and commented on their concerns about "New Technology and Spraying," which contributed to contaminated environments of "Tainted Serenity": "I think sprays are a big danger to our health ... because the spray drift is gonna go for several miles, so it's gonna get ... organic food ... I don't think it would be organic because of spray."

Participants took pictures and noted effects of political issues, such as "Heroes Laid to Rest," a photo of a newspaper headline reporting ongoing war. War was stressful and "very, very upsetting that our boys are getting killed [overseas]," especially as participants' children and grandchildren were actively serving overseas and participants were concerned about their welfare. First Nations women commented on their pictures of the Ipperwash Inquiry report and on the "Promise of Return [of Property] by Our Government." These issues reveal the impacts of historical and ongoing political issues on participants' emotional health and of participants' concerns regarding their families and communities.

Study Limitations

The photovoice method has many strengths, bringing a new depth to the investigation of human experience and empowering rural women to promote their health through a process of consciousness raising and speaking out. However, some limitations merit consideration. As noted above, some participants were reluctant to use the log books because they were uncomfortable expressing themselves in a written format. Others experienced some difficulties using the cameras for distance photos due to visual problems, and others wanted more time and more film to take all of the pictures they wished.

Some participants thought that obtaining consent from others for photographs was an obstacle or created suspicion. A participant explained, "it's just that some didn't want their pictures taken ... They think ... they're going to get sucked into something." A few participants thought that explaining the study to people was too much, so they refrained from taking pictures of people. Written and signed consent issues arose for participants who took a picture of a picture of a person who lived far away, requiring them to obtain consent via email or telephone.

Discussion and Implications

The photovoice method, by including participants' photographs together with more traditional focus group and log book data, provided an enriched way to obtain information and to give voice to rural older women's experiences. The visual element of photographs helped to initiate and focus the dialogue; there was power in the visual, allowing participants to critique their experience in a unique way that enhanced thinking and discussion. Indeed, camera work involves entering into aspects of representation, expression, and social power (Casey 2009).

Participants in this study revealed significant resources to promote their health, including gardens, churches, pets, active lifestyles, access to health care, and personal and community history. Participants also noted health promotion needs in the form of churches closing, lack of quality long-term-care facilities, health-care issues, cultural issues, rural infrastructure changes, farming issues, and political problems. Many of these needs have been noted for other groups (Canadian Institute for Health Information [CIHI] 2006; Romanow 2002), but this study is important in that it highlights the particular health promotion needs and resources of rural older women, a population much neglected in the literature.

This study concurs with others (Chapter 25, this volume; Keating 2008; McPherson and Wister 2008) in that growing older in rural settings poses problems as well as satisfactions and opportunities. For older rural women, issues related to loneliness due to the loss of a spouse and limitations in transportation and access to supports are particularly noteworthy. In addition, limited long-term care in rural settings problematizes women's ability to maintain connections with spouses and friends since they might need to travel to visit them. The "social convoy" phenomenon noted by Wenger and Keating (2008) was noted in this study as well in that many of the women had lived in the same community for several decades; thus, they knew some of each other's needs and strengths and could provide relevant social and other supports to each other. However, in more transient rural communities or where older residents might be newcomers, such as retirees, they might not be aware of or willing to support other older residents or wish to ask for assistance for themselves. Thus, the nature of the rural experience, such as length of time and familiarity among residents, has implications for the nature of the health promotion needs and resources of older rural women.

Regarding social exclusion, participants experienced economic and social circumstances that affected their ability to access material resources and services and to be included in some social and community activities. For example, modest incomes restricted the ability of some participants to own and operate a vehicle and to travel, and living alone as a widow contributed to an increased need for social and other types of support, which were limited in small towns and farm settings, especially in winter. Nonetheless, the women in this study tended to emphasize their health promotion resources rather than their needs or restrictions. For the most part, they were happy or at least relatively satisfied to remain living in their rural communities. Several explanations can be offered for this satisfaction, but it was obvious that most participants enjoyed assets (e.g., communities that are relatively close geographically) that rural women elsewhere might not have. These assets enriched the quantity and diversity of available resources (e.g., social supports), which enhanced quality of life and perhaps facilitated decisions to remain in a rural community that had limitations. In addition, it might be that the whole is greater than the sum of its parts; in other words, taken holistically, connection to the rural community and social supports there might outweigh inconveniences and lack of resources. Clearly, more research is needed to understand the relationship between social exclusion and the social and health promotion needs and resources of rural older women. In addition, enhanced understanding of the resilience of rural older women in coping with social exclusion and other limitations and making the best of strengths inherent in rural settings could assist these women in participating more fully in economic, social, and health resources in their communities (Leipert 2006b). Better understanding of rural older women's resilience could also assist health-care providers and others in providing more effective health promotion resources and services in rural settings for older women.

In this study, the photovoice method acted as an incentive to recruitment, especially of vulnerable and marginalized populations who rarely participate in research. We believe that the intrigue of using a camera and being able to keep the pictures was attractive to the Mennonite and First Nations women – indeed, to all of the participants – and encouraged and sustained their participation in the study. Adaptability to participants' needs, such as the literacy issues of the Mennonite women, indicates that photovoice is a good method to use with rural populations who have limited English literacy and who might not have the ability or confidence to participate in other types of research. In addition, the method acted as a catharsis for some women, providing them with a beneficial opportunity to express troubling as well as inspiring experiences.

Several new methodological strategies were included in this photovoice study. Study participants were asked to introduce themselves in the camera orientation session. This information was not only inspiring but also acted as a source of health promotion knowledge about needs and strengths – who might need assistance and who could help. Audiotaping the camera orientation session, as well as the second focus group, was a new strategy that proved to be important since it ensured that all group interview data were captured. Asking participants to give their pictures titles was another new strategy; it effectively enabled participants to analyze and give meaning to their photographs, thereby facilitating accurate interpretation of data and empowerment of participants.

The use of three methods of analysis (Leipert and Smith 2008; Oliffe et al. 2008; Wang and Burris 1997) provided opportunities for deeper analysis by placing participants, photographs, narratives, and log books in context with each other. Not only were the participants able to analyze and provide detailed explanations of their photographs, but also the researchers were better able to situate participants in context with their pictures and vice versa. Using three methods of analysis supported rich mining of the extensive data and enhanced rigour and accuracy in the determination of findings.

Consent from vulnerable populations emerged as an issue in this study. Researchers must be particularly diligent in fully explaining, as much as possible, the nature of the research and its dissemination, especially to particularly vulnerable populations, such as those for whom English is a second language. Also, obtaining consent must be recognized as an ongoing process throughout the research rather than a one-time event. For example, even though the Mennonite participants provided written consent to publish pictures of themselves, their later comments revealed concerns about publication. We realized that the participants might not have accurately understood what this meant and that consent can be rescinded after pictures have been taken and discussed. Thus, dissemination of photovoice data needs to be done carefully and selectively in order to respect participants' understandings and preferences.

Regarding empowerment, the photographs helped participants in speaking more often and in more depth in the focus groups. The sharing of photos and discussions helped participants to realize the nature and importance of their experiences and perspectives, and this, too, was empowering. Thus, photovoice assists older rural women, who are often silenced and invisible, to feel confident, speak up, and experience empowerment.

Acknowledgments

We express appreciation to the rural women who participated in this study and to the Social Sciences and Humanities Research Council of Canada for funding our research.

References

Anderson, A. 2006. *Delivering Rural Health and Social Services: An Environmental Scan*, http://alzheimerontario.org/.
Caldwell, W., C. Brown, S. Thomson, and G. Auld. 2006. *The Urbanite's Guide to the Countryside*. Guelph: University of Guelph.
Canadian Institute for Health Information (CIHI). 2006. *How Healthy Are Rural Canadians? An Assessment of Their Health Status and Health Determinants*. Ottawa: CIHI.
Casey, J. 2009. "Rural Camera Work: Women and/in Photography." In *A New Heartland: Women, Modernity, and the Agrarian Ideal in America*, by J. Casey, 157-95. Oxford: Oxford University Press.
Clark, K., and B. Leipert. 2007. "Strengthening and Sustaining Social Supports for Rural Elders." *Online Journal of Rural Nursing and Health Care* 7, 1: 13-26.
Coward, R., L. Davis, C. Gold, H. Smiciklas-Wright, L. Thorndyke, and F. Vondracek, eds. 2006. *Rural Women's Health: Mental, Behavioral, and Physical Issues*. New York: Springer.
Dobbs, B., J. Swindle, N. Keating, J. Eales, and J. Keefe. 2004. *Caring Contexts of Rural Seniors: Phase 2 Technical Report*. Submitted to Veterans Affairs Canada, http://www.hecol.ualberta.ca/.
Forbes, D., and B. Janzen. 2004. "A Comparison of Rural and Urban Users and Non-Users of Home Care in Canada." *Canadian Journal of Rural Medicine* 9, 4: 227-35.
Health Canada. 2002. *Canada's Aging Population*. Ottawa: Minister of Public Works and Government Services Canada.
Hodge, G. 2008. *The Geography of Aging: Preparing Communities for the Surge in Seniors*. Montreal: McGill-Queen's University Press.
Karpan, R., and A. Karpan. 2002. *Western Canadian Farm Trivia Challenge*. Saskatoon: Parkland Publishing.

Keating, N., ed. 2008. *Rural Ageing: A Good Place to Grow Old?* Bristol: Policy Press.

Leipert, B. 2006a. "Rural Women's Health Issues in Canada: An Overview and Implications for Policy and Research." In *Canadian Woman Studies: An Introductory Reader,* 2nd ed., edited by A. Medovarski and B. Cranney, 552-64. Toronto: Inanna Publications and Education.

–. 2006b. "Rural and Remote Women Developing Resilience to Manage Vulnerability." In *Conceptual Basis for Rural Nursing,* edited by H. Lee and C. Winters, 79-95. New York: Springer.

Leipert, B., and J. George. 2008. "Determinants of Rural Women's Health: A Qualitative Study in Southwest Ontario." *Journal of Rural Health* 24, 2: 210-18.

Leipert, B., M. Kloseck, C. McWilliam, D. Forbes, A. Kothari, and A. Oudshoorn. 2007. "Fitting a Round Peg into a Square Hole: Exploring Issues, Challenges, and Strategies for Solutions in Rural Home Care Settings." *Online Journal of Rural Nursing and Health Care* 7, 2: 5-20, http://www.rno.org/.

Leipert, B., and J. Smith. 2008. "Using Photovoice to Explore Rural Older Women's Health Promotion Needs and Resources." In *Women's Health: Intersections of Policy, Research, and Practice,* edited by P. Armstrong and J. Deadman, 135-50. Toronto: Women's Press.

McCracken, M., K. Tsetso, B. Jean, K. Young, D. Huxter, G. Halseth, and M. Green. 2005. *Seniors in Rural and Remote Canada: Position Paper.* Ottawa: Canadian Rural Partnership Advisory Committee on Rural Issues.

McPherson, B., and A. Wister. 2008. *Aging as a Social Process: Canadian Perspectives.* Don Mills, ON: Oxford University Press.

Ministerial Advisory Council on Rural Health. 2002. *Rural Health in Rural Hands: Strategic Direction for Rural, Remote, Northern, and Aboriginal Communities.* Ottawa: Ministerial Advisory Council on Rural Health, http://www.phac-aspc.gc.ca/.

Ministry of Industry. 2006. *Women in Canada: A Gender-Based Statistical Report.* Ottawa: Statistics Canada.

Morgan, D., and R. Krueger. 1998. *The Focus Group Kit.* London: Sage.

Olesen, V. 2000. "Feminisms and Qualitative Research at and into the Millennium." In *Handbook of Qualitative Research,* 2nd ed., edited by N. Denzin and Y. Lincoln, 215-55. London: Sage.

Oliffe, J., J. Bottorff, M. Kelly, and M. Halpin. 2008. "Analyzing Participant Produced Photographs from an Ethnographic Study of Fatherhood and Smoking." *Research in Nursing and Health* 31, 5: 529-39, http://www.interscience.wiley.com/.

Parrett, C. 2006. "Evaluation of Nutrition Education and Exercise in a Health Promotion and Wellness Program for Older Adults." In *Rural Women's Health: Mental, Behavioral, and Physical Issues,* edited by R. Coward et al., 217-34. New York: Springer.

Patton, M. 2002. *Qualitative Research and Evaluation Methods.* 3rd ed. London: Sage.

Pringle, D. 2008. "The Future Is Aging: From Cell to Society." Paper presented at the Aging, Rehabilitation, and Geriatric Care and Faculty of Health Sciences Symposium, London, ON, February.

QSR International. 2006. *NVIVO 7.* Doncaster, Australia: QSR International PTY Ltd.

Romanow, R. 2002. *Building on Values: The Future of Health Care in Canada.* Saskatoon: Commission on the Future of Health Care in Canada.

Sarkella, J. 2005. *A Demographic and Socioeconomic Profile of Southwestern Ontario.* London, ON: Southwest Region Health Information Partnership.

Scharf, T., and B. Bartlam. 2008. "Ageing and Social Exclusion in Rural Communities." In *Rural Ageing: A Good Place to Grow Old?,* edited by N. Keating, 97-108. Bristol: Policy Press.

Statistics Canada. 1999. *A Portrait of Seniors in Canada*. Ottawa: Minister of Industry.
–. 2001. *Urban and Rural Population Counts for Provinces and Territories*. Ottawa: Minister of Industry.
Sutherns, R., M. McPhedran, and M. Haworth-Brockman. 2004. *Rural, Remote, and Northern Women's Health: Policy and Research Directions*. Winnipeg: Prairie Centre of Excellence for Women's Health.
Thorndyke, L. 2006. "A Research Agenda for the Future: Linking Mental, Behavioral, and Physical Health of Rural Women." In *Rural Women's Health: Mental, Behavioral, and Physical Issues,* edited by R. Coward et al., 253-74. New York: Springer.
Thurston, W., and L. Meadows. 2003. "Rurality and Health: Perspectives of Mid-Life Women." *Rural and Remote Health* 3, 3: 219, http://www.rrh.org.au/.
Turner, L., and I. Gutmanis. 2005. *Rural Health Matters: A Look at Farming in Southwest Ontario: Part 2*. London, ON: Southwest Region Health Information Partnership.
Wang, C. 1999. "Photovoice: A Participatory Action Research Strategy Applied to Women's Health." *Journal of Women's Health* 8: 185-92.
Wang, C., and M. Burris. 1997. "Photovoice: Concept, Methodology, and Use for Participatory Needs Assessment." *Health Education and Behavior* 24: 369-87.
Wang, C., M. Burris, and X. Ping. 1996. "Chinese Village Women as Visual Anthropologists: A Participatory Approach to Reaching Policy Makers." *Social Science and Medicine* 42: 1391-400.
Wang, C., W. Yi, Z. Tao, and K. Carovano. 1998. "Photovoice as a Participatory Health Promotion Strategy." *Health Promotion International* 13, 1: 75-86.
Ward-Griffin, C., and J. Ploeg. 1997. "A Feminist Approach to Health Promotion for Older Women." *Canadian Journal on Aging* 16, 2: 279-96.
Wenger, G., and N. Keating. 2008. "The Evolution of Networks of Rural Older Adults." In *Rural Ageing: A Good Place to Grow Old?*, edited by N. Keating, 33-42. Bristol: Policy Press.
Wirtz, E., H. Lee, and A. Running. 1998. "The Lived Experience of Hardiness in Rural Men and Women." In *Conceptual Basis for Rural Nursing,* edited by H. Lee, 257-74. New York: Springer.
World Health Agency (WHO). 2002. *Active Ageing: A Policy Framework*. Geneva: WHO.

Chapter 27   **The Future of Rural Health
Research: Concluding Thoughts**

J.C. Kulig and A.M. Williams

This first comprehensive volume about rural health issues in Canada illustrates both the vulnerability and the strength of rural people through examples of their health status and health issues; the health-care providers dedicated to caring for rural individuals, families, and communities; and the innovative programs and initiatives being developed and implemented in a variety of unique rural environments. This concluding chapter returns to the three sub-themes presented in the introductory chapter to suggest recommendations for future research and note examples of policy implications for the research findings presented in this volume. The chapter ends with a discussion on capacity building for the future of rural health research. As illustrated herein, a commitment to the needs of rural people must continue to be the basis of conducting collaborative, community-based research and delivering findings as key messages to decision makers responsible for policy development in rural Canada.

Lessons Learned: Recommendations for Future Research

In general, rural health research would benefit from a movement away from the emphasis on the "deficit model" so often used to describe rural health status. Thus, we hope that the studies presented in this volume, together with the current available baseline of studies on rural health status (Canadian Institute for Health Information [CIHI] 2004, 2006; Health Canada 2009; Mitura and Bollman 2003), become the platform for conducting studies that examine the variables within rural environments that positively impact the residents and build on their unique strengths, including shared life experiences, reciprocity, and extensive social networks (Phillips and McLeroy 2004). Which components of social support within rural communities, for example, have the most significance for reducing mental illness or for addressing socio-economic crises such as the impact of the pine beetle infestation on employees of forest industry-dependent towns?

Concomitant to this shift from the deficit model is the idea of ending the practice of comparing rural residents with their urban counterparts. Rural health needs to be examined on its own merits; the contextual backgrounds of the rural and urban environments make it difficult to assess health status with a simple comparison. And though the meaning of rurality is central to our concern as researchers, ongoing debates, some of them captious, about the definition of rural must not take precedence over the important work of engaging with rural individuals, families, and communities to determine their health issues. Our hope is that the established and flexible meaning of rural in health research be used productively to promote interdisciplinary and collaborative research.

We now return to the three sub-themes presented in the introductory chapter – *rural places matter to health, rural places have great diversity,* and *rural places are dynamic* – to offer our concluding thoughts and provide recommendations for policy and research.

The sub-theme rural places matter to health emphasized that there are health status differences among rural residents. What we can draw from the research findings is that there are less healthy behaviours (e.g., higher rates of smoking) and higher risks for specific health conditions (e.g., circulatory diseases) among rural populations. A number of the studies in this volume also make the point that rural residents access a different range of services across the country, from one rural community to another and in comparison with their urban counterparts. Regardless of which ones are used, services need to be developed according to the unique environment of the specific rural community to meet the current health needs of that population.

There are many topics yet to be explored within the realm of rural health. Health status differences across the range of rural communities and across our country's provinces and territories still need to be examined to develop and implement more appropriate, community-minded health-care delivery services. Choosing similar variables and health status indicators will help to provide comparisons in addition to establishing benchmarks to determine trends over time. This means that researchers across the country need equal access to datasets in their jurisdictions to conduct such studies. Comparing a range of rural communities enhances consistency in the way that we examine health. Future studies will also need to take better account of diverse groups, including Aboriginal peoples who live in both rural and remote settings; distinct religious groups, such as Anabaptists and Dutch Reformed groups who often hold agricultural occupations; and immigrants, such as the South Asians who are relocating to rural areas. Finally, viewing health status within a larger community context, one that recognizes the dynamic nature of rural communities, will lead to a more comprehensive understanding of the data being collected.

The challenges of recruiting and retaining health-care professionals within rural settings will always need to be addressed. The challenges begin in undergraduate programs across the full range of health-care disciplines, where content and clinical experience in rural and remote areas is often limited. It would therefore be beneficial to perform evaluations of the educational initiatives that have been implemented to prepare health-care professionals for rural and remote practice. Such evaluations would need to include the range of disciplines (e.g., medicine and nursing), provinces (e.g., British Columbia, Manitoba, New Brunswick, Ontario, and Saskatchewan), and basic and post-basic training programs (e.g., certificate rural programs). The Rural Health Training Institute discussed in this volume is an example of a professional training program designed specifically for rural health work. A careful evaluation of this program could assess its level of success and explore its potential to serve as a basic model to be implemented or adapted elsewhere.

We already know that education and technology can play an important role in increasing health service capacity and the uptake of new knowledge, including helping to ensure that rural and remote health-care professionals integrate research findings and evidence into their everyday practices while updating their skills. However, rural health-care providers are faced with significant barriers in accessing information and lack support in integrating new information into their practices. Again, evaluating an existing model, such as the Centre for Education and Research on Aging and Health, would be beneficial since doing so could help to determine its usefulness for capacity building of rural health-care professionals across different rural settings. We also need to identify the right combination of multiple factors (education, financial reimbursement, and other incentives) that helps to recruit and retain health-care professionals in rural locations.

There is limited knowledge about the appropriate health-care delivery models for the diversity of rural communities across Canada. It is by conducting scientifically sound evaluations of the community development initiatives used to create and implement health care in the rural environment that we can gain a better understanding of what is working and in which context. As Chapter 13 demonstrated through its discussion of initiatives dealing with mental health issues, community partnerships can be developed to tailor mental health services to the unique needs of rural communities. Such examples provided throughout that chapter can be used as a basis upon which to stimulate mental health program development in other rural areas and the subsequent evaluation of those programs.

The second sub-theme in this book, rural places have great diversity, emphasizes that not all rural communities are the same and that these differences are not currently well understood. Based upon the studies in this book, it is clear that Canadian rural researchers would benefit from conducting comparative studies with their counterparts in the international realm to generate much-needed information about rural health status, which can then be compared across nation-states. Furthermore, the development and delivery of innovative health services that work well in rural locales can be shared among researchers and decision makers to implement programs tailored to the specific rural context and then evaluated for their effectiveness. Certainly, sharing knowledge related to these evaluations will assist in the creation of rural health policies that will enhance the nation's ability to advocate for positive changes in other rural communities. One example of knowledge sharing that has proved successful in improving the health of a rural group is the Victorian Order of Nurses (VON) in Canada, which has purposefully developed relationships and programs that focus on Aboriginal and rural health needs of homecare clients across the country (VON Canada 2008, 2009).

Like many other industrialized countries, Canada has placed limited emphasis on understanding rural health issues from a regional or national level. Datasets are not always available, and when they are they do not allow for a comprehensive examination of rural health status; rural complexity has therefore not been examined for its impact on (ill) health (Rural Health Intelligence Program 2005). Mixed-method studies conducted within the context of the rural community will help researchers and decision makers to gain a more comprehensive understanding of rural complexity and rectify this current discrepancy. Interdisciplinary research teams conducting international studies on rural health issues are appropriate and can increase our understanding of, and attention to, common health issues across country borders.

What becomes obvious through the case studies herein is that focusing regional studies on specific conditions and health issues in rural areas will also enhance our understanding of the uniqueness of rural locations. One area of investigation that would forward much-needed information about regional differences in health practices, health-care delivery, and the presence (or absence) of specific conditions is an examination of physical and mental disabilities among rural residents. Another is studying environmental conditions (e.g., the use of herbicides) and drug use (e.g., the differences in drug use for depression among rural residents). Gender analysis of health conditions within rural areas is still needed to ensure that the breadth and depth are well understood for both women and men. Conducting comparative studies across regions of this country, as shown in Chapters 9 and 23, has the additional benefit of providing opportunities for policy makers within provincial and territorial health services to engage in conversations about health-care delivery in rural areas.

The final sub-theme, rural places are dynamic, focuses on the dynamism between the rural context and the experience of health and health-care delivery. The links between place and health became evident in the findings that discussed both negative and positive connections between place and health. In addition, supports for health-care professionals need to match the specific rural context, which can include access to telehealth systems or joining other health regions for continuing education sessions.

The possibilities for future research that highlights the dynamism of rural places are countless. Based upon the discussion in Chapter 10 on a web-based risk assessment system, we see the potential of technology in rural and remote areas for providing accessible health services, including care and continuing education for health-care professionals. The evaluation of technological innovations such as video-conferencing support for isolated clients and telehealth for educational opportunities can help us to understand the links to recruitment and retention of health-care professionals.

Further studies on social networks, neighbouring, and relationships within rural communities will also enhance our understanding of the acceptance, discomfort, or imposed stigma regarding specific conditions. One specific research question that warrants examination is the experience of dementia by diagnosed individuals and their family members. Conducting a study that generates information about community responses to individuals with dementia and needed caregiving and social support resources within the context of the changing demographics in rural locations would be beneficial. Additional studies that focus on the relocation of healthy (and often politically astute and vocal) retirees to rural areas and their perspectives on caregiving models for seniors who wish to age in place would also be warranted in regional areas of the country.

The ongoing demographic changes within rural communities also need to be examined continually to identify impacts on the *whole* community in terms of health status, health-care delivery, and sustainability of the social aspect of the community. Specific research questions to be addressed include the following. How will communities dependent on a single industry or tourism address the needs of aging seniors and young families? What is the impact of a crisis (e.g., wildfire) on rural health status and expectations of rural health-care systems?

The Future of Rural Health Research

Strategic planning for the continual development of rural health research in Canada would be beneficial only if there is available funding, skilled researchers, and political will to incorporate the findings into healthy rural policies. Some policy documents have called attention to fostering rural health research in Canada (see Ministerial Advisory Council on Rural Health 2002), but little progress has been made on the recommendations. Instead, rural health research is dependent on the personal connections that researchers make across this country (MacLeod et al. 2007) and on their willingness to navigate the field for research funding, research partnerships with communities, and appropriate research questions.

Other countries have focused attention on the development of rural training units (Humphreys and Nichols 1995), national organizations (e.g., the Australian Rural Health Education Network [ARHEN]) that provide rural research infrastructure (Wakerman and McLean 2005), universities that host centres of rural health (e.g., UHI Millennium Institute in Scotland [Centre for Rural Health 2005]), and the creation of issue networks with the aim of influencing policy regarding rural health (Hartley 2005). These international efforts can still be considered as possible models for Canadian rural health research, but investigators need to continue to put forward their own rural research agendas.

The virtual, interdisciplinary researcher will become more important to rural communities particularly as these communities' demographic and socio-economic profiles continue to change. Advances in technology provide rural researchers with the opportunity to live elsewhere but conduct their research in a variety of rural and remote settings in collaboration with local community members as research assistants and advisers. Learning the skills to conduct research in this way is likely best accomplished through mentoring relationships established between professors and their students.

Another aspect bearing consideration is securing funds for rural health research. Without a specific institute or personnel within Canadian Institutes of Health Research (CIHR) devoted to rural health research, it is easy to lose sight of the limited funding available from one of our largest national funding agencies (only 0.24 percent of its 2008 budget was committed to rural and northern research) (Kulig 2010). Rural health advocates need to work in tandem with funding bodies and other relevant agencies, such as corporations that are dependent on the natural resources of rural communities, to create interest in and commitment to funding rural health research. Assistance from organizations such as the Canadian Rural Health Research Society (CRHRS), which has devoted some of its time to advocating change, would also be helpful.

Indeed, the future of rural health research is largely dependent on the development of the next generation of researchers. Incentives, including mentorship programs and awards for enhancing the research capacity of new investigators and graduate students, are important in this regard. Few specific programs exist that help to prepare the next generation of rural health researchers. Exceptions include the Public Health and the Rural Agricultural Ecosystem (PHARE) Training Centre at the University of Saskatchewan with nationally based partners. PHARE provides funding for both graduate students and postdoctoral fellows and opportunities to work with rural health researchers at a host of participating universities.

There is one final word of caution to both seasoned and junior investigators when conducting rural health research. W.O. Mitchell's novel *Roses Are Difficult Here* illustrates the negative impacts of a researcher who arrives in a prairie town and studies its patterns and rhythms only through a limited lens. When the researcher, June, the protagonist of the novel, eventually leaves the town and publishes her perspective on the community, the residents are outraged by the inaccurate portrayal of their beloved community. Mitchell eloquently captures (both in front of and behind the scenes) the complex nature of the relationships within the fictionalized town of Shelby, Alberta, and in so doing reminds rural researchers of the importance of genuinely engaging with residents in the activities in which they partake to truly understand their unique context. This perhaps is the true beauty of conducting rural research – for many research topics that require interaction with rural residents, the researcher can enhance the depth and breadth of the study while truly understanding the unique and dynamic nature of the rural community.

Mitchell uses the difficulty of growing roses in this prairie town as an analogy of the strength and resilience of the people who inhabit the community. The analogy can also portray the challenges experienced by rural health researchers. These challenges include accessing research funding, appropriate databases, the political support of health services and government, and the social and political support of rural communities and residents. Learning about advocacy, the development of policy, how to engage with rural communities and their residents, and analyzing the findings within a unique rural environment are all necessary skills to move forward on rural health research questions that will expand our comprehension while helping to develop community-appropriate health-care services. Investing in and developing the next generation of rural health researchers and securing funding are essential. The future of rural places and their residents is dependent on such actions; all Canadians stand to benefit given the important role of rural places in our history, social makeup, and identity.

References

Canadian Institute for Health Information (CIHI). 2004. *Improving the Health of Canadians*. Ottawa: CIHI.

–. 2006. *How Healthy Are Rural Canadians?* Ottawa: CIHI, http://www.cihi.ca/.

Centre for Rural Health. 2005. *UHI Millennium Institute*. Inverness, Scotland: Centre for Rural Health, http://www.uhi.ac.uk/.

Hartley, D. 2005. "Rural Health Research: Building Capacity and Influencing Policy in the United States and Canada." *Canadian Journal of Nursing Research* 37, 1: 7-13.

Health Canada. 2009. *A Statistical Profile on the Health of First Nations in Canada: Self-Rated Health and Selected Conditions, 2002 to 2005.* Ottawa: Health Canada, http://www.hc-sc.gc.ca/.

Humphreys, J., and A. Nichols. 1995. "Education and Training: Role of Rural Training Units." *Australian Journal of Rural Health* 3: 80-86.

Kulig, J. 2010. "Rural Health Research in Canada: Assessing Our Progress." *Canadian Journal of Nursing Research* 42, 1: 7-11.

MacLeod, M.L.P., J.A. Dosman, J.C. Kulig, and J.M. Medves. 2007. "The Development of the Canadian Rural Health Research Society: Creating Capacity through Connection." *Rural and Remote Health* 7: 1-11, http://www.rrh.org.au/.

Ministerial Advisory Council on Rural Health. 2002. *Rural Health in Rural Hands: Strategic Direction for Rural, Remote, Northern, and Aboriginal Communities.* Ottawa: Ministerial Advisory Council on Rural Health, http://www.phac-aspc.gc.ca/.

Mitchell, W.O. 1990. *Roses Are Difficult Here.* Toronto: McClelland and Stewart.

Mitura, V., and R. Bollman. 2003. "The Health of Rural Canadians: A Rural-Urban Comparison of Health Indicators." *Rural and Small Town Canada Analysis Bulletin* 4, 6: 1-23. Catalogue No. 21-006-XIE2002006. Ottawa: Statistics Canada.

Phillips, C.D., and K.R. McLeroy. 2004. "Health in Rural America: Remembering the Importance of Place." *American Journal of Public Health* 94, 10: 1661-63.

Rural Health Intelligence Program. 2005. *Contemporary Rural Health Issues: Intelligence from Wales and beyond Cardiff.* Cardiff: Welsh Assembly Government.

VON Canada. 2008. *Health Starts at Home: VON Canada's Vision for Health and Home.* Ottawa: VON Canada, http://www.von.ca/.

Wakerman, J., and R. McLean. 2005. "ARHEN and FRAME Bring a New Era for RRN." *Rural and Remote Health* 5, 408: 1-2.

Contributors

Carol Amaratunga
Dean, Office of Applied Research, Justice Institute of British Columbia

Robert C. Annis
Former Director, Rural Development Institute, Brandon University

Alma I. Barranco-Mendoza
Chief Information Officer and Associate Faculty of Biotechnology, Computing Systems and Informatics, Trinity Western University, Langley, BC

Kenneth Beesley
Professor, Department of Rural Development, Brandon University

Leslie Bella
Honorary Research Professor, Memorial University

Cyndi Brannen
Research Associate, Centre for Research in Family Health, IWK Health Centre, Halifax

Meredith Burles
Research Assistant, Saskatchewan Population Health and Evaluation Research Unit (SPHERU), University of Saskatchewan

Wayne Corneil
Affiliate Scientist, Institute of Population Health University of Ottawa

Sarah Crowe
Affilliate, R. Samuel McLaughlin Centre for Population
Health Risk Assessment, University of Ottawa

Marie DesMeules
Director, Health Determinants and Global Initiatives Division,
Strategic Initiatives and Innovations Directorate, Public Health
Agency of Canada, Ottawa

Rhonda Donovan
PhD candidate, School of Geography and Earth Sciences,
McMaster University

Mary-Pat Dressler
Policy Analyst, Innovation Strategy, Health Determinants and Global
Initiatives Division, Strategic Initiatives and Innovations Directorate,
Public Health Agency of Canada, Ottawa

Karen Dyck
Associate Professor and Clinical Psychologist, Rural and Northern
Psychology Programme, Department of Clinical Health Psychology,
Faculty of Medicine, University of Manitoba

Jacquie Eales
Research Manager, Research on Aging, Policies and Practice,
Department of Human Ecology, University of Alberta

Julie Easley
PhD candidate, Department of Graduate Studies, Interdisciplinary
Program, University of New Brunswick

Dorothy Forbes
Associate Professor, Faculty of Nursing, University of Alberta

Julie George
Doctoral student, Department of Social Sciences, University
of Western Ontario

Laverne Gervais
Regional Coordinator, School of Health Sciences, University
of Northern British Columbia

Doris Gillis
Associate Professor, Department of Human Nutrition, St. Francis
Xavier University, Antigonish, NS

Pansy Goodman
Director, Academic Affairs, Lakeridge Health, Oshawa

Judy Read Guernsey
Director, RURAL Centre, Community Health and Epidemiology,
Faculty of Medicine, Dalhousie University, Halifax

Sonja Habjan
Research Affiliate, Centre for Education and Research on Aging
and Health, Lakehead University

Greg Halseth
Professor and Canada Research Chair, Geography Program,
University of Northern British Columbia

Colleen Hamilton
Project Coordinator, Saskatchewan Population Health and Evaluation
Research Unit (SPHERU), University of Regina

Neil Hanlon
Assistant Professor and Chair, Geography Program, University
of Northern British Columbia

Cindy Hardy
Associate Professor, Psychology Department, University of Northern
British Columbia

Roma Harris
Professor, Faculty of Information and Media Studies, University
of Western Ontario

Pamela Hawranik
Professor, Faculty of Health Sciences, and Dean, Faculty of Graduate
Studies, Athabasca University

Kristen Jacklin
Associate Professor, Human Sciences, Northern Ontario School
of Medicine

Bonnie Jeffery
Professor, Faculty of Social Work/Saskatchewan Population Health
and Evaluation Research Unit (SPHERU), University of Regina

Arminee Kazanjian
Professor, School of Population and Public Health, Faculty of
Medicine, University of British Columbia

Norah Keating
Professor and Co-Director, Research on Aging, Policies, and
Practice, Department of Human Ecology, University of Alberta

Mary Lou Kelley
Professor, School of Social Work and Northern Ontario School
of Medicine, Lakehead University

Kathy Kortes-Miller
Lecturer, Gerontology Program/Palliative Care Certificate,
Lakehead University

Judith Krajnak
Senior Evaluation and Research Consultant, Charis Management
Consulting, Inc., Edmonton

Daniel Krewski
Professor and Director, R. Samuel McLaughlin Centre for Population
Health Risk Assessment, University of Ottawa

Brigette Krieg
Assistant Professor, Faculty of Social Work, University of Regina

Judith C. Kulig
Professor, Faculty of Health Sciences, University of Lethbridge

Tamara Landry
PhD candidate, Faculty of Health Sciences, University of Western
Ontario

Josée Lavoie
Associate Professor, School of Health Science, University of Northern
British Columbia

Beverly Leipert
Associate Professor, School of Nursing, University of Western Ontario

Wei Luo
Senior Policy Analyst, Strategic Initiatives and Innovations
Directorate, Public Health Agency of Canada, Ottawa

Michael MacLean
Professor Emeritus, Faculty of Social Work, University of Regina

Doug Manuel
Senior Scientist, Ottawa Hospital Research Institute, Ottawa

Carol McWilliam
Professor, The Arthur Labatt School of Nursing, University of
Western Ontario

Alison Moss
Research Affiliate, Rural Development Institute, Brandon University

Lisa Murdock
Program and Policy Consultant, Aboriginal Initiatives, Healthy Child
Manitoba Office, Winnipeg

Christopher Mushquash
Assistant Professor, Department of Psychology, Lakehead University

Shevaun Nadin
Graduate student, Department of Psychology, Carleton University

Connie Nelson
Professor, School of Social Work, and Director of Food Security
Research Network, Lakehead University

Nuelle Novik
Assistant Professor, Faculty of Social Work, University of Regina

Aleck Ostry
Professor and Canada Research Chair, Faculty of Social Sciences,
University of Victoria; Senior Scholar, Michael Smith Foundation for
Health Research

Jungwee Park
Senior Analyst, Statistics Canada, Ottawa; Affiliated Investigator,
Centre for Rural and Northern Health Research, Lakehead
University

Deryck R. Persaud
Co-founder and Chief Scientist, Infogenetica Bioinformatics,
Coquitlam, BC, and Adjunct Professor of Biotechnology, Trinity
Western University, Langley, BC.

Linda Pisco
Education Planner/Team Leader, Centre for Education and Research
on Aging and Health, Lakehead University

J. Roger Pitblado
Professor Emeritus and Senior Research Fellow, Centre for Rural
and Northern Health Research, Laurentian University

Vera Pletsch
Retired, Women's Health Research Institute, Institute of Population
Health, University of Ottawa

Raymond W. Pong
Senior Research Fellow, Centre for Rural and Northern Health
Research, Laurentian University; Professor, Northern Ontario
School of Medicine

Tuija Puiras
Chief Executive Officer, North West Community Care Access
Centre, Thunder Bay

Frances E. Racher
Professor, School of Health Studies, Brandon University

Doug Ramsey
Associate Professor, Department of Rural Development, Brandon
University

Sheila Sears
Director, Public Health and Primary Health Care, Guysborough
Anitgonish Strait Health Authority, Antigonish, NS

Mark Skinner
Associate Professor, Department of Geography, Trent University

Wilma Sletmoen
Retired, formerly End-of-Life Care Coordinator, Northwest
Community Care Access Centre, Thunder Bay

H. Sullivan
Medical student, Faculty of Medicine, Dalhousie University

Tiffany Veinot
Assistant Professor, School of Information, University of Michigan,
Ann Arbor

Pamela Wakewich
Professor, Departments of Sociology & Women's Studies, Lakehead University

Feng Wang
Epidemiologist, Centre for Chronic Disease Prevention and Control, Public Health Agency of Canada, Ottawa

Wayne Warry
Professor, Department of Anthropology, McMaster University

Mamoru Watanabe
Professor Emeritus, Faculty of Medicine, University of Calgary

Allison M. Williams
Associate Professor, School of Geography and Earth Sciences, McMaster University

Stacey Wilson-Forsberg
Assistant Professor, Department of Human Rights and Human Diversity, Wilfrid Laurier University

Index

(t) indicates a table; (f) indicates a figure

herbs and medicinal plants, 349, 386
Herring, D.A., 399
high blood pressure, 2, 47(t), 180, 270, 322,
   356, 397-98. *See also* hypertension
HIV/AIDS, 3, 16, 222, 235, 299-315,
   314n1, 397, 411. *See also* palliative
   care
HMDB (Hospital Morbidity Database), 63,
   68, 72-73
Hoas, H., 284
hobbies, 490
holistic medicine, 349, 400, 414, 421, 443
homecare services: access to, 28, 61, 76,
   165-67, 171, 319, 413, 421, 484;
   aging population, 428; community-
   based, 131, 401; definition, 224;
   dementia, 449-51, 453; future research recommendations, 506; men,
   449-50; Métis population, 413, 415,
   421, 422; palliative care, 131-32, 222,
   224, 225, 233, 320, 324-26; resource
   communities, 470, 471(t); seniors,
   428; sustainability, 121, 131-32, 165,
   166; training models, 106, 113;
   women, 449-50. *See also* family
   caregivers
homeopathy, 349
Hosang, M., 151
hospice services, 222, 337, 347, 470, 471(t),
   477
Hospital Morbidity Database (HMDB), 63,
   68, 72-73
hospitalization rates, 60, 68-69, 69(t), 70-73
hospitals: Aboriginal population, 375, 379,
   391, 402; access, 207, 212, 324, 491-
   92; dementia patients, 454; health
   care expenditures, 61; *Hospital
   Report* radio program, 284; Indigenous healers, 349, 386; palliative/
   end-of-life care, 327, 345; resource/
   retirement communities, 468, 471(t),
   477; utilization patterns, 60, 68-69,
   69(t), 70, 72-75, 402
household income. *See* income level
HSAS (Health Services Access Survey), 63,
   64, 67(f)
Human Resources and Skills Development
   Canada, 260
Hux, J.E., 402
hypertension, 160, 184, 328, 397-98, 449.
   See also high blood pressure

immigrants: demographics, 25, 336; depression, 284-85, 290; future research
   recommendations, 504-5; literacy,
   264, 485; mental health, 282; mortality risks, 33, 34(t); social support
   networks, 284
in-migration, 198, 448, 464, 466, 468, 469.
   See also migration patterns
income level and health status, 33-38, 34(t),
   36(t), 38(t), 146, 266, 434(t)
Indian Act, 374, 377, 380, 391, 392, 403,
   405n1, 409, 410
Indian Health Policy, 380-81
Indian Health Transfer Policy, 381-85, 399,
   403-4
Indigenous knowledge, 377-78, 384
Indigenous Physician Association of Canada-
   Association of Faculties of Medicine
   of Canada (IPAC-AFMC), 374
Indigenous populations. *See* Aboriginal
   population; First Nations; Inuit
   population; North American Indian
   population
infants: Infant Mental Health Provision
   (Métis population), 251; mortality
   rates, 2, 3, 161, 375, 395
infectious diseases, 375, 377, 397, 399
Infogenetica Bioinformatics, 179, 192
information exchange. *See* networks/
   networking
information technology. *See* internet;
   technology innovation
Infoway (Canadian Health Infoway), 182
injury/poisoning: BSE-related impact, 356,
   364; mortality patterns, 13, 37, 49(t),
   50-53, 52(f), 53(f), 395; mortality
   risks, 32; urban-rural continuum,
   47(t), 48-50, 53, 56. *See also*
   accidents
instant towns, 15, 464, 465, 467-69, 477
Institute of Medicine (IOM), 261
Institutes of Aboriginal Peoples Health,
   378
insurance coverage, 176, 367
internal migration patterns, 83, 84, 87-88,
   95-97, 96(f), 97
internal migration rate, 88, 95-97, 96(f)
International Adult Literacy and Skills
   Survey (IALSS), 263, 277n1
International Adult Literacy Survey (IALS),
   277n1

Printed and bound in Canada by Friesens

Set in Syntax and Bembo by Artegraphica Design Co. Ltd.

Copy editor: Dallas Harrison

Indexer: Lillian Ashworth